Evaluation of Appraisal Techniques in Speech and Language Pathology

Editor

Frederic L. Darley   *Mayo Clinic*

Associate Editors

Warren H. Fay *University of Oregon Health Sciences Center*
Parley W. Newman *Brigham Young University*
Maryjane Rees *California State University at Sacramento*
Gerald M. Siegel *University of Minnesota*

Addison-Wesley Publishing Company

Reading, Massachusetts
Menlo Park, California
London · Amsterdam
Don Mills, Ontario · Sydney

This book is in the
ADDISON-WESLEY SERIES IN SPEECH PATHOLOGY AND AUDIOLOGY
Consulting Editors: Rita C. Naremore and Ira M. Ventry

Library of Congress Cataloging in Publication Data

Main entry under title:

Evaluation of appraisal techniques in speech and lang-
    uage pathology.

    1. Speech, Disorders of--Diagnosis. 2. Speech
disorders in children--Diagnosis. I. Darley, Frederic L.
RC423.E92   616.8'55'075   78-20918
ISBN 0-201-01276-6

ISBN 0-201-01276-6
ABCDEFGHIJ-AL-79

Preface

iii

The Domain of This Volume

This book is a compilation of critical reviews of 87 published tests designed for use primarily by professionals in the field of Speech and Language Pathology. The boundaries which delimit this field are not immediately evident. Communication skills are so fundamental to human enterprise that they reach into almost every aspect of personal endeavor—interpersonal contact, educational development, vocational progress. No single discipline can hope to prepare professionals in all aspects of the social, personal, educational, and emotional behavior that implicate communication in some way.

A volume addressed to speech–language pathologists must either by recourse to logic or to tradition attempt to delineate some loose boundaries. Not every member of the field will explore all the perimeters of these boundaries, and not all members of the profession will be contained by the boundaries drawn. Some professionals will find problems of stuttering, aphasia, or cleft palate so completely absorbing as to occupy them totally, but the work of others may take them into nontraditional areas such as child development, parental guidance, psychological counseling, and remediation of reading and writing.

This volume has been directed toward what has come to be the primary focus of our discipline: the development of vocal communication, dysfunctions that beset it, and those auditory skills that have been regarded as basic or prerequisite to speech and language function. Aural input and oral output are traditionally within the domain of Speech and Language Pathology. They constitute the behavior our members are most typically called upon to evaluate and treat. Our training programs most adequately prepare our students to deal with these areas. This view of the field will not fit all institutions and working environments and it may be quite out of touch with what the future holds, but it seems to us a fair representation of the primary responsibilities of our field at present.

This limitation of scope results in exclusion of consideration of tests that deal primarily with visual perceptual skills, motor skills, personality, cognitive functions, reading, and writing. Some users of this volume will quarrel with the limitation. Interesting and important though they are, the contribution of visual perceptual skills and motor skills to the acquisition of speech and language appears to be of less significance than is the contribution of auditory skills. The heavy involvement with language that has characterized the recent course of the profession has brought us into the arena of learning disabilities with increasing interest in reading and writing; but no major professional shift toward reading and writing has yet occurred, and our "language expertise" is clearly not directly related to school achievement in the three R's. It therefore seemed to the editors that it would be presumptuous to extend the boundaries to include test procedures used primarily by other than speech-language pathologists—by teachers, experts in special education, psychologists. Other volumes exist that provide fully adequate descriptions of these other measurement procedures. We refer particularly to the series of *Mental Measurement Yearbooks* edited by Oscar K. Buros (currently available is *The Seventh Mental Measurements Yearbook* (Gryphon Press, 1972)) and such specialized volumes as *Reading Tests and Reviews* (Gryphon Press, 1968) and *Personality Tests and Reviews* (Gryphon Press, 1970).

Our setting of the limits of this volume in the way described does not constitute a definitive statement as to what the shape of the profession will come to be. Clinical perspectives in Speech and Language Pathology are strongly influenced by developments in several basic disciplines that impinge on our field. Speech and Language Pathology reflects changing approaches, insights, and models in Psychology and Linguistics in its own concerns and remedial work. The course of our activities is as much influenced by neighboring disciplines as it is by our own, an inevitable result perhaps of its being something of a borrower from basic physical and social sciences. Furthermore, as an applied field, Speech and Language Pathology is vulnerable to the winds of change in social and political realms. As our society has developed new patterns of caring for the severely handicapped—for example, mainstreaming and the Right to Education laws—the demands on our profession have changed. Powerful forces shape the preoccupations of our field rather than inner pressures from the field itself. As a crossroads discipline we are sensitive to the influence of both social policy and intellectual controversy. The boundaries that describe us today will inevitably be altered by all of these influences. A whole new set of procedures may have to be included in some future revision of this book as a reflection of natural change of our interests, responsibilities, and skills.

Published Tests

With rare exception, the reviews contained in this volume pertain to tests which have been published, in English, in the United States, and considered to be commercially available. We have not reviewed tests that have gone off the market, however widely used they may have been in the past, nor have we reviewed tests that are in press or in process of revision with no version currently purchasable.

There are a great many appraisal procedures extant, described in research reports or presented in textbooks, that are no doubt as useful as the instruments herein reviewed. We do not, by neglecting to review them, denigrate these procedures. Their presentation here would have required lengthy descriptions and discussions that go beyond our defined purposes. The associate editors in their introductions to the several parts have in some cases indicated the relevance of procedures other than those prescribed by commercially available tests.

Our intention is certainly not to exalt the published tests as the sole or even the primary approach to the patient in a diagnostic and therapeutic setting. Tests constitute helpful first steps. They sharpen our observational skills. They provide leads for further exploration and intervention. Some test makers have done superior work in selecting and refining items, testing for reliability, occasionally determining validity, and preparing materials that are attractive and durable. But we recognize that we may be overimpressed by the simple fact that a test has been put into print. Tests are relatively easy to create and to sell. As Buros has said, "No matter how poor a test may be, if it is nicely packaged and if it promises to do all sorts of things which no test can do, the test will find many gullible buyers" (*Sixth Mental Measurements Yearbook,* p. xxiv). The more aware we become of the complexity of the human beings with whom we work, the more the tests we use lose credibility. We find that available tests are necessarily restrictive. For example, in the area of articulation, where our tests are probably most fully developed, published tests are unlikely to probe a particular phoneme in the depth the clinician might desire as an adjunct to therapy. So clinicians are presented here with an array of techniques, variable with regard to merit and usefulness—but not *all* the techniques available. They will want to maintain a liaison between the literature and the clinic and make translations of their own into clinical procedures. With a sufficient grasp of the areas being assessed, they can be creative and go beyond the limits of the formal tests here reviewed.

Nature of Reviews

The reviews presented here are critical reviews prepared by professionals in the field of Speech and Language Pathology who are independent of the test instruments they are reviewing and who are knowledgeable concerning the specific areas to which the tests apply. A single review of each test is presented in the belief that an independent, objective reviewer can share with us the important things we need to know about the values and limitations of a given test and in the conviction that to ask two or three similarly competent people to review the same test would be redundant and not sufficiently productive to warrant the effort or the space.

The tests here reviewed differ in the extent to which they are based upon some explicit theoretical system. Some tests are frankly atheoretical; they are pragmatic compilations of items or subtests which the authors have come to regard as important for the dimension being tested. Other tests are based on some more explicit theory or model of speech and language. It is generally more satisfying to have a theoretical basis for a test than not to have one, but to have one may lead to problems: the relationship between the test and the theory is often tenuous; the theory may not be a very good one to start with; sometimes the attempt to fit a test to a theory involves little more than adjusting the name of the test; theories develop, wane, and are supplanted by new theories, leaving as residuals tests that have found their way into print.

Reviewers who have prepared the evaluations in this volume differ in their sensitivity to theoretical issues and in the weight they place on underlying theory concerning individual tests. Obviously reviewers and readers, too, will not agree on the relative merits of the various theories that have held or currently hold sway in some aspect of our field. In some cases they attack a particular theoretical weakness. In other cases they attack a particular test weakness. In every case we have a confounding of test weakness with theoretical weakness, for if the theoretical base is weak so, too, is every instrument that purports to tap its properties regardless of the test's individual excellence.

The reviewers have no stake in the tests they are reviewing nor in any competing tests. They provide for the potential user of a test a documented opinion as to the merits and the demerits of the test in terms of its purpose and its achievement of its purpose, its adherence to requirements of proper psychometric techniques, its clinical usefulness, its practicality. Their insights and their frankness guide us in the adoption of these techniques for personal use. They also provide a kind of leadership toward the development of ever more appropriate, precise, reliable, valid, and clinically practical appraisal procedures as the field of Speech and Language Pathology develops.

Rochester, Minnesota   **Frederic L. Darley**
April 1979

Contents

Part IV

Part I
Appraisal of
Language Development

Introduction

The diversity of tests in this section reflects the variety of approaches one may take to the study of language development. As concepts and theories of language evolve, the tools available to clinicians change accordingly, bearing testimony to the fact that the clinical practice of speech–language pathology is intertwined with basic developments in theory and research. Some 30 to 40 years ago, when language was defined primarily in terms of count and tally procedures, diagnostic tests consisted mainly of phoneme and vocabulary counts, measures of the length and number of utterances, and various type-token ratios. The procedures that appear in the Johnson, Darley, and Spriestersbach (1963) *Diagnostic Methods in Speech Pathology* can be traced directly to the research methods then in use (McCarthy 1954). By contrast with current approaches to language assessment, those earlier methods were starkly empirical and atheoretical.

The language assessment methods of the last decade reveal the powerful influence of Chomsky's views of the nature of language. The tests constructed by Lee, Carrow, and Tyack and Gottsleben are outgrowths of the theory of transformational grammar and the new interest in developmental psycholinguistics. The tests focus on the sentence as the fundamental unit, rather than words or phonemes, and they attempt to probe the child's understanding and use of the grammatical rule systems.

In the years since Chomsky's major contributions to the theory of language, it has become apparent that there is more to language acquisition than is contained in a pure theory of syntax (Bloom and Lahey 1978). Children observe the world in context: agents operate on the environment and cause it to change; things appear and disappear. The child's earliest attempts at communication reveal an awareness of the events that occur in the child's perceptual and cognitive world. The child's early attempts at language, it is now argued, are best represented in terms of the semantic relations to be discovered in the world, rather than in purely syntactic constructions. Somehow, the semantic relations seem closer to the child's reality than do the categories of the strict grammarian. At least one test included in this section, the Environmental Language Inventory, is specifically concerned with assessing semantic relations, and we may expect to see other tests of this sort in the future. Even more recently, language theorists have drawn attention to the pragmatics of language, and Rees (1978) has already pointed out ways in which it may be advantageous for speech–language pathologists to exploit these new views of language.

The language tests constructed in any period inevitably reflect the prevailing concepts of that period. Tests that are out of touch with current theories or models seem empty of meaning. Indeed, even so prominent an earlier test as the Illinois Test of Psycholinguistic Abilities now seems to have scarcely any relationship to language. It may tap interesting and important behaviors, but they are not linguistic behaviors according to our current definitions (Kirk and Kirk 1978).

Not all tests were devised with a particular theory of language in mind, but every test maker must have some sort of construct or model to guide in the selection of those behaviors that will be sampled and those that will be omitted in the construction of the test. Every test, whether theory-based or not, is a map of sorts. Language is simply too vast and multifaceted a domain to be completely represented in any single test. A theory provides a set of guidelines as to how the map should be drawn. It directs the test developer to the areas that must be charted and gives the test user a basis for deciding how adequate and complete the coverage has been. The territory of language seems virtually inexhaustible, and while the map is clearly not the territory, a theory at least provides a basis for making a judgment about the probable accuracy and utility of the domain charted in any particular language assessment instrument. Of course, theories of language are not constant, and it is to be expected that approaches to testing will change as the territory is more fully explored. The assessment devices of any given period are likely to seem inadequate or misdirected in the next, and the alert clinician has little choice but to keep in touch with the literature in the field as well as with the specific tests available at any time.

The selection of assessment instruments included in this section is incomplete in several ways. Some tests were not available for review because they are still being developed or revised. This is the case with the Berry-Talbott Test, Comprehension of Grammar, which is out of print but is reportedly being revised. The Porch Index of Communicative Ability in Children was incomplete as we prepared this volume, but it has generated enough interest to warrant discussion of the test in its experimental form. There is also a body of tests that have been developed for bilinguals, particularly Spanish/English speakers. We have a sample of these in this section but it is by no means complete. Here too, tests were being published as this volume was prepared. In addition, there was the special problem of finding qualified reviewers who are competent in the language of testing as well as the languages being tested. There is a clear need, perhaps in a subsequent edition of this text, to include a comprehensive review of tests developed for bilinguals (and not only Spanish/English speakers).

This section is incomplete in still another way. The decision to evaluate only commercially available instruments has necessarily narrowed the field. There are many procedures reported in the language development literature that are potentially enormously useful to the clinician. Indeed, several of the published tests owe a direct debt to the research literature. The Grammatic Closure subtest of the ITPA is a direct outgrowth of the research reported by Berko (1958), and the Northwestern Syntax Screening Test is obviously related to the research protocol devised by Fraser, Bellugi, and Brown (1963). Similarly, though in a less direct way, the Carrow Elicited Language Inventory exploits the basic research on elicited imitation reported by Slobin and Welsh (1973), among others. The research literature on child language development is a rich reservoir of timely and useful ideas for language assessment, some of which may never be incorporated into a formal test framework. Any researcher who struggles with the attempt to sample and characterize some aspect of child language has a potential contribution to make to the speech–language pathologist. Commercially prepared tests are typically convenient and efficient ways to obtain preliminary information about a child's language status. However, by their very nature, such tests can seldom probe a given area of linguistic performance in great depth, and there may be some areas that are not addressed at all because they do not fit comfortably within the test format. Where this is the case, the speech–language pathologist should feel no hesitancy about devising additional and even novel means of studying the language characteristics in question. The available research literature can be a helpful source of ideas for such development. The system for grammatical analysis used by Brown (1973), the clever techniques for evaluating role taking and communication devised by Flavell and his colleagues (Flavell, Botkin, Fry, Wright, and Jarvis 1968), the methods of grammatical judgment reported by deVilliers and deVilliers (1972), and the wide array of tasks for studying pragmatics (Rees 1978)—all of these are in the literature and available to the clinician. A sprinkling of commercial tests, supported by knowledge of the literature and spiced by a resourceful clinician, are the basic ingredients for successful language assessment.

Gerald M. Siegel

References

Berko, J.   The child's learning of English morphology. *Word* **14**: 150–177, 1958.

Bloom, L. and M. Lahey   *Language Development and Language Disorders*. New York: Wiley, 1978.

Brown, R.   *A First Language, The Early Stages*. Cambridge, Mass.: Harvard University Press, 1973.

deVilliers, P. and deVilliers, J.   Early judgments of semantic and syntactic acceptability by children. *J. Psycholing. Res.* **1**: 299–310, 1972.

Flavell, J. H., P. T. Botkin, C. L. Fry, J. W. Wright, and P. E. Jarvis   *The Development of Role-Taking, and Communication Skills in Children*. New York: Wiley, 1968.

Fraser, C., U. Bellugi, and R. Brown   Control of grammar in imitation, comprehension, and production. *J. Verb. Learning Verb. Behav.* **2**: 121–135, 1963.

Johnson, W., F. L. Darley, and D. C. Spriestersbach   *Diagnostic Methods in Speech Pathology*. New York: Harper & Row, 1963.

Kirk, S. A. and W. D. Kirk   Uses and abuses of the ITPA. *J. Speech Hearing Dis.* **43**: 58–75, 1978.

McCarthy, D.   Language development in children. In L. Carmichael (ed.), *Manual of Child Psychology*. New York: Wiley, 1954.

Rees, N. S.   Pragmatics of language: applications to normal and disordered language development. In R. Schiefelbusch (ed.), *Bases of Language Intervention*. Baltimore: University Park Press, 1978.

Slobin, D. I. and C. A. Welsh   Elicited imitation as a research tool in developmental psycholinguistics. In C. A. Ferguson and D. I. Slobin (eds.), *Studies of Language Development*. New York: Holt, Rinehart and Winston, 1973.

ASSESSMENT OF CHILDREN'S LANGUAGE COMPREHENSION (ACLC)

Rochana Foster, Jane J. Giddan, and Joel Stark

Consulting Psychologists Press, 1969; 1973

Cost $13.50 for the kit, including stimulus plates, manual, pad of response sheets

Time Untimed test, should take 15–20 minutes for administration and scoring

Thomas M. Longhurst *Kansas State University*

Purpose The Assessment of Children's Language Comprehension was designed to enable the speech–language pathologist to determine how many word classes in different combinations of length and complexity a child is able to understand. The authors suggest that language-impaired children have very poor auditory memory. The ACLC determines the level at which the child is unable to process and remember lexical items in syntactic sequences and helps to isolate the nature of the items with which the child has difficulty. Items include words drawn from the semantic classes of agents, actions, relations, objects, and attributes. The authors call these "critical elements" and test items are made up of single critical elements (Part A) as well as combinations representing two (Part B), three (Part C), and four (Part D) critical element utterances.

Administration, scoring, and interpretation The ACLC consists of a series of 41 spiral-bound picture plates, a pad of single-page recording sheets, and a manual. The manual contains information concerning language development and impairment as well as guidelines for language training and clinical application of the ACLC. It also includes the usual information about test design, administration and scoring, and statistical properties of the test. An expendable group form booklet of 17 selected plates is also available for rapid screening purposes.

The first test plate contains five simple training items designed to acquaint the child with the task. The child is to look at each of the stimuli while the examiner reads the stimulus from the test form using a carrier phrase such as "show me" or "point to." The examiner does not indicate whether a response is correct or incorrect but provides general encouragement. If the child's responses are correct, the examiner goes on to the first test plate in Part A.

Part A tests single critical elements. It is made up of ten plates with five stimulus items per plate for a total of 50 items. The items were chosen because they were easily picturable, were commonly used, and contained no more than two syllables. At this level the child is required to identify 30 common count nouns (agents and objects), the present progressive form of ten verbs (actions), five prepositions (relations), and five modifiers (attributes). Part A is a vocabulary test and also pretests to be sure the child understands the single elements that are then combined in Parts B, C, and D. However, some of the foil items in Parts B, C, or D are not included in Part A and the test items change from shadow to line drawings and vice versa. It would be futile to continue with the test if a large number of the single elements are missed, but the authors do not give a cutoff for the allowable errors. An error on any item in Parts B, C, or D that contained a word that was missed on Part A would be difficult to interpret. The authors suggest that a child may be trained on error items in Part A before proceeding with the test, but this could be very time consuming. Correct performance on Part A assures that an error on Parts B, C, or D can be interpreted as something other than a vocabulary problem.

To respond correctly in Part B, the child must comprehend two critical elements by choosing one of four pictures on each of ten plates. Most of the possible syntactic combinations of agents, actions, attributes, and objects are included. Some examples of stimulus utterances are "horse standing," "broken cup," and "car and balloon." In addition to computing a percent correct for Part B, the examiner can determine whether the answer was correct, the first element was incorrect, the second element was incorrect, or both elements were incorrect. This procedure is particularly helpful in determining word order errors.

In Part C, a third critical element is added and relations now appear in the stimuli. In each of the ten test plates one element is varied in each of the four pictures. For each element in the stimulus utterance there is a foil on the plate. To choose correctly the child must comprehend all three elements. Some of the utterances include "ball under the table," " bird and dog eating," and "big broken fence." A percent correct is again computed and examination of the score sheet may reveal a pattern of errors in the first, second, or third element.

In Part D there are four critical elements and each of ten test plates contains five pictures. The child's choices include the correct answer and stimulus pictures with the first, second, third, and fourth element varying. The stimulus utterances express agent–action relations and include "happy little girl jumping," "dog eating and cat sitting," and "boy standing in the house." A percent correct is computed and an analysis of the child's error patterns is made.

Part A is scored by adding the number of correct responses. The other three parts yield a percent correct as well as an anecdotal description of the child's pattern of errors from the score sheet. In ACLC manuals printed subsequent to 1974 there are new normative data. The normative group consists of 311 nursery and elementary school children, 85 percent from the Tallahassee, Florida, area and the remainder from rural Vermont Head Start programs. These scores are divided into six-month age intervals from 3-0 to 6-5 with unequal numbers in each group ranging between 16 in the 3-0 to 3-5 group to 77 in the 5-0 to 5-5 group. The parents' socioeconomic and educational backgrounds are mixed with about 35 percent low level and the remainder low-middle to high-middle level. Thirty-eight percent of the children were black. The normative data should be considered tentative because of the limited number of scores at the age levels and because of the limited geographic sampling. The data suggest that most nonhandicapped children should have mastered the skills tested on the ACLC by the time they enter kindergarten. The level of difficulty increases from Part A through Part D for all age levels. No statistically significant sex or race differences are reported. Scores for 51 "neurologically or educationally handicapped" children between the ages of 4-0 and 6-11 are reported for the experimental edition, which was identical to the current version except for four items and some minor modifications on several of the plates. Even these children show improvement over age and Part D proves the most difficult. Scores for Parts A and B are only slightly depressed from the normal-age peers data with Part C and particularly Part D grossly depressed.

The ACLC Group Form was issued in 1973 to identify more quickly those children who may need follow-up testing. It consists of 17 plates from Parts B, C, and D of the ACLC in an expendable booklet. With the Group Form small groups of children can be screened. After simple instructions are given to the children, they mark the stimulus pictures with a crayon. After two trial items the children mark 12 additional stimulus items, four each from Parts B, C, and D of the ACLC. The examiner scores the children's responses on the cover sheet of the booklet. No normative data have been presented and there are apparently no data available comparing the ACLC with the Group Form. The authors suggest that if fewer than nine of the 12 items are marked correctly the ACLC should be administered. There is no information related to the selection of items from the ACLC.

Evaluation of test adequacy   The authors do not report any tests of examiner reliability nor are there any validity measures. Odd–even reliability coefficients were computed for the single element (Part A) items and for Parts B, C, and D combined to test whether the items were functioning consistently to measure the same skills. When the scores were corrected for attenuation, the computed correlation coefficients were .86 and .80 for odd and even respectively. These coefficients suggest there is sufficiently high internal consistency.

The rationale of the ACLC is logical but the test is not developed to anywhere near its full potential. Pictures are not ideal for testing language and the ACLC pictures are particularly poor. Most are black shadow pictures with little detail. There are also some line drawings, with some plates containing both types of pictures. Pictures representing the same object are not consistent throughout the test. Many utterances such as "happy lady sleeping" or "apple and shoe on the can" do not occur frequently in most children's environments.

Considerably more work needs to be done on test standardization. Better normative data with more extensive guidelines for interpretation of scores and error patterns would be helpful. Some standardization information on the Group Form is also necessary if it is to become a useful screening test for the ACLC.

Summary   As indicated, the main problems with the ACLC involve the preparation of the stimulus materials and the lack of supportive statistical data. There are features of the ACLC that justify its current popularity. It can be administrated easily and scored in 15-20 minutes. Part A helps to assure that the child understands the test vocabulary before the formal test items are presented. The ACLC is one of the few tests that probes auditory comprehension and memory for words in relatively simple syntactic constructions in a format of increasingly more difficult items. Our experience has shown that it is helpful in differentiating children who have problems in sustaining attention, processing verbal auditory stimuli, and pairing them to visual stimuli. Some clinicians and teachers have reported using the ACLC at periodic intervals to assess progress. Successive administrations require that the examiner begin retesting where the child began to fail at the previous administration and test upward until the child fails again. Bar graphs of percent correct for each of the parts at successive administrations present a good visual effect. Although it has not been used extensively, the Group Form may have some real strength in mass screening programs in kindergarten or preschools. Additional standardization would be useful if it is used for this purpose.

BANKSON LANGUAGE SCREENING TEST (BLST)

Nicholas W. Bankson

University Park Press, 1977

Cost Kit, $14.95. Extra test blanks and profile sheets, $5.00 per pad of 25

Manual bound with test materials, 13 pages; test blank and profile sheet bound with test materials, 5 pages

Time 25–30 minutes, administration and scoring

Roy A. Koenigsknecht *Northwestern University*

Purpose The Bankson Language Screening Test (BLST) is designed to be an efficient, broadly based screening device intended to provide preliminary information about expressive language abilities and selected auditory and visual skills in children. The need for and the nature of additional testing may be indicated by the profile of a youngster's performance on 17 subtests focused upon basic vocabulary and semantic knowledge, early acquired morphological and syntactic structures, and common visual/auditory tasks involving matching, association, discrimination, memory, and sequencing.

Administration, scoring, and interpretation Items are scored as either correct or incorrect, although the examiner is encouraged to note the nature of error responses. In the manual it is suggested that intelligent and perceptive individuals can be taught in a relatively short period to administer and score (though not to interpret) this individual test. This may be adequate with normally developing children but an understanding of child language problems, as well as experience in the handling of clinical children, is likely needed when testing children at risk for learning language. Stimulus materials for several of the items are confusing. For example, on Plate 7 the color of the block to be named purple is judged to be either black or gray by most adults. Norms are provided only for the expressive testing; however, instructions are provided for the use of several of the basic vocabulary and semantic knowledge subtests as receptive tasks, thus permitting the receptive testing of items missed expressively. No supporting evidence is provided for the guidelines contained in the manual specifying cutoff scores for those in need of further language assessment, those most certain to be enrolled for clinical language instruction, and those for whom a classroom enrichment approach directed to specific linguistic weaknesses may be appropriate.

Evaluation of test adequacy Normative data on the BLST were obtained on 133 four-year-olds, 174 five-year-olds, 165 six-year-olds, and 106 seven-year-olds from semirural counties adjacent to the Washington, D. C., metropolitan area. Eighty percent were white and 20 percent were from minority groups. The sample ranged from lower-middle to upper-middle socioeconomic levels. Means and standard deviations for raw scores by subtest are reported with subjects grouped in six-month age categories. Percentile ranks corresponding to raw scores are included only for the overall test score for the one-half year age groups. As acknowledged in the manual, the normative sample indicates that the instrument is sensitive to developmental differences at the lower age levels, but the scores plateau at the upper three or four one-half year age levels studied, thus indicating that the measure is most useful for children between four and six years of age.

No interitem or intersubtest correlations are reported; neither is the internal consistency within subtests reported. A general reference is made to a finding that 38 of the 153 items were most discriminating between age levels, although the age levels between which these items discriminated are not listed and no further item analyses are reported. Sketchy reports of favorable test–retest results and correlations with several widely used language tests are included for a sample of 70 children. Unfortunately, the ages and selection criteria of these subjects are not provided, thus limiting interpretation of these reports. Most important, no information is available concerning the use of the screening test with children demonstrating language problems.

A serious limitation of the BLST is that it does not assess the common, residual problems with language usage evidenced by children seen in speech and hearing clinics within the age range for which the test is standardized. That is, it does not tap language formulation skills; nor does it assess the relational, conditional, temporal, problem-solving, narrative, or descriptive aspects or uses of language. Early acquired grammatical features are sampled but more likely sources of difficulty such as modals, copulative verbs, reflexive pronouns, interrogatives, and forms of embedding and cojoining sentences are neglected. Useful information is missed also because of poor selection of stimulus items. For example, in sampling the use of past-tense inflections instead of having both verb stems end in consonants, it might have been more useful to have one item end in a vowel and one end in a consonant. Children are able frequently to provide a past-tense inflection in the former context but not in the latter. The contrast would yield a useful cue for language instruction.

Summary The BLST would appear to have greatest utility in the general screening of populations between the ages of four and six years. The test is not sensitive to developmental changes at higher age levels and does not yield extensive information about the language skills commonly impaired in children within the upper preschool and early elementary school years suspected or known to have language problems. Normative data for the test are incomplete.

CARROW ELICITED LANGUAGE INVENTORY (CELI)

Elizabeth Carrow

Teaching Resources Corporation, 1974

Cost $50 for the kit containing the manual, training guide, training tape, 25 scoring/analysis forms, and ten verb protocol forms

Time 20–30 minutes, administration; 45 minutes, scoring for sophisticated user

Laurence B. Leonard *Memphis State University*

Purpose The Carrow Elicited Language Inventory (CELI) is a diagnostic test aimed at measuring a child's productive use of grammar. This test provides a means of comparing a child's grammatical performance with peer performance and permits a determination of the specific grammatical structures that may be contributing to the child's inadequate test performance.

Administration, scoring, and interpretation The CELI consists of one phrase and 51 sentences which the child is asked to imitate. These stimuli range from two to ten words and from two to 11 morphemes in length. There are 47 sentences in the active voice, four sentences in the passive voice, 14 sentences involving negatives, 12 interrogative sentences, and two imperatives. The grammatical categories include articles, adjectives, nouns, pronouns, verbs, negatives, adverbs, prepositions, demonstratives, and conjunctions, as well as plurals and contractions. The verb category is most important and contains provisions for inflected and uninflected main verbs, copula forms, auxiliaries, modals, infinitives, and gerunds.

The CELI is administered by recording on audiotape the child's imitations of the test stimuli produced by the examiner. The child's responses are then transcribed onto a test form resembling a matrix where they can be classified according to the grammatical categories examined. The score derived represents the total number of errors made by the child. In addition, subscores can be derived representing the total number of errors made within each grammatical category. A verb protocol is provided that permits an even more detailed inspection of the child's difficulties in this area.

A manual accompanies the test and a training guide and training tape are included to facilitate accuracy in scoring.

Evaluation of test adequacy Content validity is not discussed at any length in the manual. Carrow comments only that pilot work on the test indicated that "the test yielded information about the grammatical functioning of children" (Manual p. 8). In fact, the CELI fares well in the area of content validity. There are grammatical features missing from the test, for example, sentences with embedded clauses and sentences whose deep and surface structure subjects differ; but a sufficient number of representative features are included. The CELI does not do quite as well in terms of the range with which each feature is examined. For example "and" is used in English not only in the combinatory sense (e.g., "Joel and Pedro entered the room") but also in the temporal (e.g., "Joel entered the room and Pedro handed him a sandwich") and causal senses (e.g., "Joel entered the room and Pedro panicked"). Only the combinatory sense of "and" is assessed in the CELI. Similarly, personal pronouns often play key syntactic roles in addition to "standing for" nouns. For instance, implied in the sentence "He knew that Gil was a dope" is the fact that "he" and "Gil" do not refer to the same individual, a condition not held in the sentence "Gil knew that he was a dope." Implied in the sentence "Dan jumped over Dave and then *he* jumped over the woman" is the fact that "Dave" did the jumping in the second instance, a condition not true if "he" was unstressed in the sentence. The grammatical features of the CELI were not examined with this kind of range.

Criterion-related validity is not dealt with in a direct manner in the CELI manual. Instead, Carrow relies on an indirect means of assessing criterion-related validity—an examination of the correlation between CELI performance and performance on Lee and Canter's (1971) Developmental Sentence Scoring (DSS), another measure of children's grammatical usage (and itself a tool whose predictive power has not been directly ascertained). Carrow reports an investigation by Cornelius that found a significant correlation between these two measures. Further details are lacking, a problem compounded by the fact that Carrow failed to include a reference section indicating where the Cornelius study and other studies cited can be located. In a recent study, Sinclair, Khan, and Saxman (1977) found that children's performance on the CELI and DSS did not closely correspond.

The construct involved in the CELI is never made explicit. Despite the fact that this is termed a "language" inventory, only certain aspects of syntax and morphology are assessed. While Carrow states that grammatical performance is examined, she also makes reference to the child's "grammatical system." Thus, it is not clear if the test is intended to examine verbal behavior or grammatical rules. Although the specifics of the construct serving as the focus of the test remain vague, Carrow found that the error scores on the CELI correlated negatively with age.

There is one difficulty with the age equivalencies of the test scores. From age 3-0 to 6-7 the expected test scores, based on the total number of errors, decrease, as one might expect. However, beginning at age 6-8, the expected scores begin to climb again in a highly consistent fashion through the highest age level, 7-11. Thus the expected score of a child age 7-11 is slightly poorer than that expected of a child age 5-3. However, for each 12-month span (e.g., 3-0 to 3-11, 4-0 to 4-11, etc.), Carrow provides separate percentiles and stanines. This provision ensures that a child will be compared only with other children of the same age. In addition, grouping in 12-month spans erases the reverse direction taken by the test scores beyond age 6-7.

The CELI test reports a very high correlation coefficient for test–retest reliability. Equally high coefficients are reported for interexaminer reliability of the transcription and scoring processes. No intraexaminer reliability is reported. Ordinarily, it is preferable to use item-to-item percentages of examiner agreement rather than correlation coefficients in order to provide a more accurate assessment of reliability. The high coefficients reported might suggest that the benefits of using percentages of agreement would not be worth the effort in this case. However, Carrow does not provide details regarding how the coefficients were obtained. Without these details the reported reliability is difficult to interpret. For example, one examiner might have transcribed an utterance as "Bill knew how to fix it" while another may have transcribed it as "Bill knew when to fix it." Both transcriptions contain the same number of words and the difference between them would be obscured in a correlation procedure.

In an effort to assess internal consistency, Carrow compared the subscores derived for each grammatical category with the total score. While this comparison may provide information regarding how each subscore contributes to a child's overall performance on the CELI, it does not constitute a measure of internal consistency. A more reasonable method would have been to perform a split-half reliability analysis of the items within each of the grammatical categories.

A major assumption behind the CELI is that an elicited imitation task can be used to gain a representative picture of a child's grammatical performance in an efficient and reliable manner. This assumption is based on earlier findings, such as those of Menyuk (1963) and Ervin (1964) that a child's imitations of adult sentences will closely resemble the manner in which the child would produce these sentences in spontaneous speech. This position was extended further by papers suggesting that imitation tasks should be used as a means of assessing a child's grammatical skills (Slobin and Welsh 1971). Yet, the use of imitation tasks is not without certain risks. A child's imitations may sometimes exceed spontaneous speech in grammatical complexity (Kuczaj and Maratsos 1975). There are also individual children who seem to display repetition deficits due to reduced auditory processing skills (Weiner 1972). For these children performance on imitation tasks may underestimate grammatical ability. These considerations suggest that the CELI should be supplemented with data from other tests or spontaneous speech.

The CELI, like other measures involving an imitation task, offers an advantage in the number of grammatical constructions that can be tapped using relatively few items. However, the scoring of the CELI is time consuming, particularly for those with little or no background in linguistics. Carrow states that 45 minutes is the average period of time required to administer, transcribe, and score the CELI. This seems more true for the experienced speech pathologist who is quite familiar with the CELI than for speech pathologists in general.

The classification scheme provided on the test form permits a visual inspection of any patterns that may exist in a child's grammatical performance. However, it has its drawbacks. Most notably, it may obscure other relevant variables operating on a child's grammatical usage. It has been well documented that a child's first use of a new grammatical feature occurs in sentence constructions that have been well established in the child's linguistic system (Slobin 1973). However, in certain cases the CELI's classification scheme misses this fact. For example, the test sentences "The big green ball is mine" and "The dog is under the house" are both classified as containing the copula unaccompanied by a modal or auxiliary. Yet, it seems likely that a child would acquire the copula in the second sentence prior to the former. The preposition "under" is acquired by the age of three years (Washington and Naremore 1976) while the use of two adjectives in their proper order does not appear in a child's speech until closer to five years (Ford and Olson 1975). Thus it is possible that the copula will be used by younger children only in the sentence "The dog is under the house." The CELI classification scheme, however, would permit only the conclusion that the child's copula usage was inconsistent, a conclusion that misses the systematicity of the child's use of this linguistic feature.

Some of the scoring conventions of the CELI fail to capture characteristics of child language. For example, a child's use of "cat" for "cats" is regarded as a substitution of the singular for the plural form. Such a decision is based on the fact that the singular in English is marked by the zero morpheme. Prior to the child's use of the plural form, plurality is unmarked. But this is not to say that the young child *intended* to produce a singular form where an adult would use the plural. Thus it would have been preferable to regard "cat" as showing the absence of the plural form rather than the substitution of the singular for the plural. A similar problem is seen in instances in which both substitutions and omissions occur. For example, in the CELI training guide a child's imitation "Where her dolls?" for the stimulus sentence "Where are the dolls?" is regarded as a substitution of "her" for "are" and an omission of "the." Familiarity with the fact that "her," like "the," is a noun phrase element (Jacobs and Rosenbaum 1968) and that the copula "are" is acquired later than these other elements and is more likely to be absent from a child's speech (deVilliers and deVilliers 1973) would have led to a different scoring decision—the substitution of "her" for "the" and the omission of "are."

Summary A firmer grounding in linguistics and developmental psycholinguistics would have improved the CELI. These difficulties, coupled with some of the test construction limitations noted above, suggest that the CELI should be used with some caution. However, considering the efficiency of the CELI, the variety of grammatical features examined in this test, and the fact that it tests such features in somewhat greater depth than most other assessment tools, the CELI should be regarded as one of the better tests available for assessing a child's grammatical usage.

References

Cornelius, S. A comparison of the Elicited Language Inventory with the Developmental Sentence Scoring procedure in assessing language disorders in children. Master's thesis, Austin: University of Texas, 1974.

deVilliers, J. and P. deVilliers A cross-sectional study of the acquisition of grammatical morphemes in child speech. *J. Psycholing. Res.* 2: 267–278, 1973.

Ervin, S. Imitation and structural change in children's language. In E. Lenneberg (ed.), *New Directions in the Study of Language.* Cambridge, Mass.: M.I.T. Press, 1964.

Ford, W. and D. Olson The elaboration of the noun phrase in children's description of objects. *J. exp. Child Psychol.* 19: 371–382, 1975.

Jacobs, R. and P. Rosenbaum *English Transformational Grammar.* Waltham, Mass.: Blaisdell, 1968.

Johnson, W., F. Darley, and D. Spriestersbach *Diagnostic Methods in Speech Pathology.* New York: Harper & Row, 1963.

Kuczaj, S. and M. Maratsos What children *can* say before they *will. Merrill-Palmer Quart.* 21: 89–112, 1975.

Lee, L. and S. Canter Developmental sentence scoring: a clinical procedure for estimating syntactic development in children's spontaneous speech. *J. Speech Hearing Dis.* 36: 315–340, 1971.

Menyuk, P. A preliminary evaluation of grammatical complexity in children. *J. Verb. Learn. Behav.* 2: 429–439, 1963.

Sinclair, S., L. Khan, and J. Saxman Do differing test conditions predict equivalent language ages? Paper presented at Boston University Conference on Language Development, Boston, 1977.

Slobin, D. Cognitive prerequisites for the development of grammar. In C. Ferguson and D. Slobin (eds.), *Studies of Child Language Development.* New York: Holt, Rinehart and Winston, 1973.

————— and C. Welsh Elicited imitation as a research tool in developmental psycholinguistics. In C. Lavatelli (ed.), *Language Training in Early Childhood Education.* Urbana, Ill.: University of Illinois Press, 1971.

Washington, D. and R. Naremore Children's use of spatial prepositions in two- and three-dimensional tasks. *Indiana University Working Papers* 1: 65–82, 1976.

Weiner, P. S. The perceptual level functioning of dysphasic children: follow-up study. *J. Speech Hearing Res.* 15: 423–438, 1972.

DEL RIO LANGUAGE SCREENING TEST, ENGLISH/SPANISH (DRLST)

Allen S. Toronto, D Leverman, Cornelia Hanna, Peggy Rosenzweig, and Antoneta Maldonado

National Educational Laboratory Publishers, Inc., 1975

Spanish and English versions are available

Cost $9.00

Examiner's manual with stimulus pictures, 125 pages

Time 12–15 minutes, administration; 5–10 minutes, scoring

Sara J. Barton *Illinois Institute for Developmental Disabilities*

Purpose The Del Rio Language Screening Test is designed to identify children with deviant language performance who are between the ages of three years and six years, 11 months. The test has separate norms for three groups of children: Anglo English-speaking, Mexican-American English-speaking, and Mexican-American Spanish-speaking children. Test items are consistent with the language and culture of the southwest United States. The DRLST can be administered in English or Spanish.

The authors state that the test can also be used to identify the Spanish-speaking child who has normal language development in the child's native language but has not yet learned English. The test is administered in English, and the score is compared with the norms for English-speaking Mexican-American children.

Administration, scoring, and interpretation The DRLST has a format of five subtests, each tapping a behavior important to the language learning process. The subtests cover (1) receptive, single-word noun and verb vocabulary; (2) repetition of sentences with length rather than complexity varied; (3) repetition of sentences that increase in grammatical complexity; (4) memory for increasing numbers of oral commands; and (5) story comprehension. Each subtest is constructed in both English and Spanish.

Specific directions for administration and scoring are presented in the manual. The test is easy to administer, with a clear and easy to use scoring form. Items are scored correct or incorrect, and the raw score is the number correct for each subtest. The test takes approximately 12 to 15 minutes to administer.

Separate norms are presented in the manual for each of the three groups of children. In order to interpret each subtest score, the examiner first determines into which group the child should be classified, then uses the appropriate set of norms. The normative data provide the following information for each subtest: age ranges in year intervals, percentile rankings, and distances one and two standard deviations below the mean. A score below the tenth percentile indicates the need for further diagnostic work, and a score two or more standard deviations below the mean indicates definite need for intervention.

Evaluation of test adequacy The DRLST was constructed by gathering items appropriate for each subtest that were typical of the language and culture of Del Rio, Texas. Items that discriminated by age were selected, following administration of possible items to 45 English-speaking and 45 Spanish-speaking children.

Standardization of the test was done on 384 normal children, 128 each of Anglo English-speaking, English-speaking Mexican-American, and Spanish-speaking Mexican-American children. The three cultural groups were balanced for age and male–female distribution. Each cultural group was divided into year-interval age groups. Thirty-two children were in each of the four age groups that ranged between three years and six years, 11 months. Statistical analysis indicated significant differences between language and age groups, with the variables of sex and individual tester being nonsignificant. The most discriminating subtests by age were receptive vocabulary and story comprehension.

Good reliability was established by a test–retest measure on 32 subjects from each cultural group. The correlation coefficients were significant at the .01 level of confidence for all subtests in each group. Internal validity was established by the ability to discriminate by age and by the reliability measures.

The Del Rio Test is a valuable addition to the limited number of screening and assessment tools available for use with Mexican-American children. Its ease of administration and scoring make it ideal for the screening purpose for which it was intended. It could be used by trained paraprofessionals and teachers. The DRLST will certainly be helpful in schools in which time is limited and the number of children to be seen is large.

Its uniqueness, and a limitation to its application, lies in its adherence to the cultural–language environment in which it was developed. The applicability of the test to other Spanish-speaking cultural groups, for example Cuban or Puerto Rican, remains to be demonstrated. It should not be used with Spanish-speaking children for whom it was not normed.

The format of the test with five independent subtests, each with separate norms, allows for flexibility of use. The receptive vocabulary and story comprehension subtests can be used as an even briefer screening procedure.

The DRLST samples a number of behaviors important to language performance in the areas of vocabulary recognition and ability to answer questions about short paragraphs. Memory for sequences of oral commands as well as the ability to repeat sentences is tested. Screening for syntax is accounted for by imitation of sentences that become increasingly more complex.

Summary   The DRLST was developed within the language and culture of the children whom it was designed to test. It goes beyond a translation of an English test. Because it was normed on three different language groups, it allows for deviancy to be defined by performance in the child's own language. The fact that it samples a variety of behaviors supporting language performance adds to the value of the test. Because each subtest is scored separately, and because the discriminative values of each subtest are available in the manual, the test has flexibility of usage. It is easy to administer and score. The DRLST is highly recommended as a screening test for language deviancy for the population on which it was normed. It should be used with caution, or not at all, with other cultural groups of Spanish-speaking children.

DEVELOPMENTAL SENTENCE ANALYSIS (DSA)

Laura L. Lee

Northwestern University Press, 1974

Cost Text, $13.50

Time Elicitation of the sample, up to an hour; scoring, indeterminate

Macalyne Fristoe *Purdue University*

Purpose Developmental Sentence Analysis (DSA) represents an attempt to apply the findings of psycholinguistic research to clinical needs in a form which will be useful in working with children with language problems. Lee (1974, p. xix) describes it more specifically as:

> A method for making a detailed, readily quantified and scored evaluation of a child's use of standard English grammatical rules from a tape-recorded sample of his spontaneous speech in conversation with an adult, in this case with his clinician. It provides a way of measuring a child's growth and progress throughout the period of clinical teaching. Because it is constructed upon developmental stages of language acquisition it allows a clinician to select appropriate teaching goals based upon an individual child's performance.

Administration, scoring, and interpretation Developmental Sentence Analysis, which is most often used clinically with children at the two-, three-, and four-year language age levels, employs two procedures: Developmental Sentence Types (DST) and Developmental Sentence Scoring (DSS). DST is based on 100 utterances and is used to see whether a child has the elements necessary for basic sentence development. DSS is based on 50 consecutive complete sentences and examines development of pronouns, verb tenses, negatives, questions, and conjunctions within the complete subject–verb sentence. DST is used when most of a child's utterances are "presentence" utterances. With DSS, the user can look at development of specific grammatical categories or, via the mean weighted-sum score, at sentence complexity, the "typical grammatical load contained in a child's responses." When at least 50 percent of a child's utterances are complete sentences, the DST is of less importance and can be omitted, except when a very thorough analysis is indicated.

According to Johnson and Tomblin (1975):

> The uniqueness of the DSS System is not that it can separate the child with deviant language from children with normal language, but that it has the potential of isolating specific areas in which the language user is having difficulty.

Unfortunately, however, there are no norms given for individual component scores.

The key to successful DSA lies in the elicitation and transcription of the language sample. When these have been accomplished, then classification of utterances can be carried out according to the rules (many rather arbitrary) that have been set out by Lee. The difference between the beginner and the seasoned clinician will lie mainly in the areas of sampling and transcribing. It is advisable for beginning clinicians to devote much time to scoring samples that have been elicited and transcribed previously by skillful clinicians. This is a criterion-referenced procedure, the criterion being use of adult language structures. The clinician must give the child every possible opportunity to use all the most advanced structures of which the child is capable. The scoring procedure was developed with this in mind.

Although the new weightings of the grammatical categories that appear in the 1974 version of the DSS seem to be an improvement over the previous weightings, it is still possible for a child to obtain a spuriously high score by such means as asking a variety of questions during the sample period or an unrepresentative low score by failing to produce forms within his or her repertoire. For this reason, the clinician must exercise judgment in interpreting the overall DSS score.

The chief practical disadvantage of DSA is the amount of time that is required to take a sample of adequate length, transcribe it, and then score it. One hour is the recommended time for obtaining an adequate language sample. If a child is so delayed in language development that she or he cannot produce 100 different utterances within the usual one-hour clinical session, then the DST is not an appropriate procedure and attention should be focused on vocabulary development to support production of combinations. The DSS sample, which consists of 50 complete subject + verb combinations, should be obtainable within a similar time period. Transcription of the sample takes varying lengths of time, depending on the child's intelligibility and the skill exhibited by the clinician in eliciting utterances. The time required for scoring the sample will depend on many factors, such as whether it is DST, DSS, or a combination that is appropriate, and how familiar the clinician is with the scoring conventions. This is not a procedure that yields immediate conclusions. One cannot obtain a sample, score it, and report the results to parents, all in the course of a morning's diagnostic session. DSS is far too complicated to be used satisfactorily as an initial diagnostic tool; rather, it is a means for tracing progress and for determining when to terminate therapy, according to Lee (1974).

Evaluation of test adequacy   The main value of the DSA procedures is that they provide a standard way of evaluating a child's expressive language skills with regard to syntactic development. One of the major shortcomings, acknowledged by Lee, is that it focuses more on surface structure than on underlying meaning. This has led to the criticism that it represents psycholinguistics as viewed in an earlier era and that it is difficult to identify an overall theoretical basis for choice of categories. Despite the shortcomings of requiring immense amounts of time and representing syntactic development somewhat superficially, it is still a useful tool from a clinical point of view. Tracking progress of a child in language development by repeating the DSA procedure at regular intervals gives a qualitative picture of progress or lack of progress, as well as an aid in making decisions concerning where intervention efforts should be concentrated next. However, because of the limited sample upon which the normative data were based, its use as a normative measurement device for determination of deviancy is of more limited value.

The normative group for the DSS consisted of 200 white children ages 2-0 to 6-11, with five males and five females in each three-month interval. They were from monolingual, standard General American-speaking, essentially middle income families residing mostly in the middle west (Illinois, Michigan, and Kansas) and in Maryland. (The number from each state was not reported, nor was a rural–urban breakdown given.) These children had "no unusual developmental or social histories," no suspected hearing-sensitivity problems, nor discernable behavioral problems, and could be

understood by the interviewing clinician. They also scored within one standard deviation of the mean on the Peabody Picture Vocabulary Test (qv) (Dunn 1965). Thus
this group was neither drawn at random nor representative of American children as a
whole in this age range. Reference to the norms can be made for children similar to
those on which the normative data were gathered, but some caution should be used in
applying these norms to other children. Lee cautions that "children from bilingual
homes or from communities where dialects differ significantly from standard English
should not be evaluated by this technique."

The lack of use of a standardized method of eliciting the language sample, particularly with regard to stimulus materials, has been of concern to many users. Koenigsknecht (1974) found that use of different stimulus materials does not appreciably
affect overall DSS score. It does, however, tend to change some individual grammatical
category scores to a significant degree.

Summary The need to determine whether or not a specific child is within normal
limits in syntax development, the need to measure change in a given child in order to
determine development and improvement over time, and the need to assess use of a
number of syntactic structures for clinical intervention planning have long been recognized. It was an attempt to meet these needs that led to the development of DSA. In
the hands of a well-trained and experienced user, DSA goes a long way toward meeting
the latter two needs. For children similar to the normative group, it can do much to
fill the first need, but this covers only a small portion of the children with whom such
a procedure is needed. If the user keeps in mind the limitations of DSA, then it can be
one of the most valuable tools available for measuring clinical progress in a child with
delayed language development.

References

Dunn, L. M. *Peabody Picture Vocabulary Test.* Circle Pines, Minnesota: American Guidance
Service, 1965.

Johnson, M. R. and J. B. Tomblin The reliability of Developmental Sentence Scoring as a function of sample size. *J. Speech Hearing Res.* **18**: 372–380, 1975.

Koenigsknecht, R. A. Statistical information on developmental sentence analysis. In L. L. Lee
(ed.), *Developmental Sentence Analysis.* Evanston, Ill.: Northwestern University Press, 1974.

Lee, L. L. *Developmental Sentence Analysis.* Evanston, Ill.: Northwestern University Press, 1974.

Scharf, D. J. Some relationships between measures of early language development. *J. Speech
Hearing Dis.* **37**: 64–74, 1972.

ENVIRONMENTAL LANGUAGE INVENTORY (ELI)

James D. MacDonald

Charles E. Merrill, 1978

Cost $7.95, spiral-bound, soft-cover manual

Time This is an untimed test which could take from 30 minutes to several sessions to administer. Scoring may take 30–60 minutes.

Shirley S. Doyle *University of Minnesota*

Purpose The Environmental Language Inventory is a diagnostic strategy for assessment and training of children with severe delay in expressive language. It is based on an analysis of the semantic–grammatical rules governing the early constructions of normally developing children. The rules describe the functional relations among word classes in emerging language and are based on the premise that words have semantic roles, not just grammatical categories. Distribution of these rules, utterance length, and intelligibility are assessed in three production modes: imitation, conversation, and free play.

The diagnostic model is the basis for the therapy model. Analysis of the assessment results determines which semantic–grammatical rules should be trained. The goal is to train spontaneous social use of these rules.

The ELI can also be used to measure language changes posttherapy and to investigate the early language development of normal children.

Administration, scoring, and interpretation The test is designed to evaluate a child's production of multiword phrases according to their semantic intent. Prior to administration, the examiner must be thoroughly familiar with the eight semantic–grammatical rules included in the assessment:

Rule	*Example*
1. Agent + action	block fall
2. Action + object	throw ball
3. Agent + object	daddy (wash) car
4. Modifier + head	
a) possession	my pants
b) recurrence	more pop
c) attribution	big ball
5. Negation + X	no cry
6. Agent or object + location	baby there
7. Action + location	push here
8. Introducer + X	hi baby

An assortment of nonlinguistic stimuli (toys, objects, and edibles) is necessary for administration of the ELI and it must be accumulated by the examiner. Specific items are designated to elicit each semantic–grammatical rule, but the items can be modified to meet the particular need and interests of each child.

A flexible administration format is recommended. The child may be seated at a table or playing on the floor. The test may be completely administered in one 30-minute session with a cooperative child, or divided into several sessions on separate days. The parent may or may not be present.

The examiner presents a total of 24 stimulus sets in order to test each rule three times. Each stimulus set consists of one nonlinguistic cue and two different linguistic cues. A nonlinguistic cue is defined as an environmental event that demonstrates the rules being tested. The linguistic cues are used to stimulate the rule in spontaneous conversation and in imitation. In each stimulus set two conversation tasks are separated by one imitation task. Responses to these three tasks are elicited by a linguistic cue. Prior to each task, the nonlinguistic cue (action or demonstration) is presented (Table 1).

When used as a clinical tool, the linguistic and nonlinguistic cues may be altered in order to obtain optimal language performance. However, all eight semantic-grammatical rules should be assessed in conversation, imitation, and play, and each linguistic cue should be preceded by presentation of the nonlinguistic cue in the conversation and imitation modes.

TABLE 1 Stimulus Set

Stimulus	Example	Child's response
1. Nonlinguistic cue	Examiner makes doll fall down.	Child watches action.
2. Linguistic cue 1	Examiner says, "Tell me what happened."	Conversation response 1.
3. Nonlinguistic cue	Examiner makes doll fall down.	Child watches action.
4. Imitation cue	Examiner says, "Say, 'baby fall down.'"	Imitation response.
5. Nonlinguistic cue	Examiner makes doll fall down.	Child watches action.
6. Linguistic cue 2	Examiner says, "Tell me what happened."	Conversation response 2.

A separate procedure is presented for language assessment in free play. It is suggested that 50 responses be obtained during a play session before or after administration of the ELI or during a play break. Materials from the ELI and toys from the child's home or school may be used. To facilitate analysis, contextual cues should be recorded and each response should be scored as imitation, conversation in response to a question from the examiner, or spontaneous.

An elaborate procedure for scoring ELI and free play responses is provided in the manual. The examiner can select those procedures which will yield useful diagnostic or experimental information for conversation, imitation, and play. The production measures that may be obtained include frequency, proportion, and rank order of each of the semantic-grammatical rules; mean length of utterance for total words and for intelligible words; proportion of intelligible words; frequency of unintelligible and multiple-word responses.

Performance on the diagnostic test indicates which semantic-grammatical rules and utterance lengths should comprise the initial objectives of a therapy program. Analysis of test scores indicates which rules are currently produced in the three different production modes.

Traditional normative data are not available for the ELI. However, the distribution of semantic-grammatical rules in free speech of normal and delayed speakers and distribution of normal and delayed language users' performance are described in the manual.

Evaluation of test adequacy The first edition of the Environmental Language Inventory procedure was introduced by MacDonald and Nichols in 1974. Reliability
and validity data using the 1974 ELI and the revised semantic–grammatical rules and
procedures from the current edition are discussed by the author in a series of studies
in Chapter 2 of the test manual. Test performance in imitation, conversation, and free
speech for several groups of normally developing children indicates that three semantic
concepts, agent, action, and object, dominated the responses.

In another study, production of the semantic–grammatical rules was analyzed by
comparing the ELI and a free-speech sample from five normally developing preschool
children and five mentally retarded children. For both populations the ELI procedure
elicited the same relative distribution of rules as occurred in free speech. In addition,
with some language delayed subjects the ELI procedures yielded a larger Mean Length
of Utterance (MLU) than the free-speech sample.

To examine reliability, the ELI was administered to a group of ten mentally retarded children whose MLU ranged from 1.0 to 4.0. Interexaminer reliability for utterance length and for semantic–grammatical rule content was 93 percent. Test–retest
results indicated that the ELI was relatively consistent for MLU scores over a one-week
interval, and the distributions of semantic–grammatical rules in all three modes were
similar.

The author cites several experimental language programs that effectively utilized
the ELI model to teach semantic complexity and expressive spontaneity. The clients
ranged from age two years to adulthood, and were characterized as hearing impaired,
autistic, vision impaired, and mentally retarded. In addition, the ELI has been used
in total communication programs, symbol systems, and other nonvocal language strategies. Details for application of the ELI model to these systems are provided in appendices in this reference.

In general, it is suggested that the ELI model would be effective for individuals
with good receptive skills but limited expressive skills that range from one to four
words in length.

The ELI model concurrently assesses (or trains) in imitation and conversation
modes, and simultaneously pairs linguistic and contextual cues. In addition, a second
conversation response is elicited immediately following the imitated response. Thus
rote imitation is avoided, and the examiner obtains immediate information about the
child's imitative skills. Since language programs that focus on vocal speech as the end
product rely heavily on imitation, relevant prognostic information is obtained.
Furthermore, generalization strategies are incorporated into the diagnostic and therapy
procedures.

The ELI model does have some inconsistencies. Each stimulus set assesses one
semantic–grammatical rule in three examples. In example 1, the imitation cue elicits a
two-word response; in example 2, the imitation cue elicits a three-word response; and in
example 3, the imitation cue elicits a four-word response. Sometimes the longer imitation cue elicits additional semantic content, and sometimes the increased length is
achieved by adding grammatical complexity. This is an inconsistency in the design of
the test, and the effects of the length or the grammatical or semantic complexity on
the child's ability to respond are unclear.

A second concern is that some of the imitative cues that the examiner provides are
"ungrammatical." Appropriate morphological markers, auxiliary forms, and articles
are omitted. The author discusses this issue in the revised edition of the ELI, but again,

the research to date does not adequately support either approach. The author suggests that the ultimate goal of this model is spontaneous social use of language, not correct grammatical use of articles, prepositions, auxiliaries, etc.

A third concern focuses on the procedures proposed for eliciting each semantic-grammatical rule. It is difficult to structure nonlinguistic cues that will elicit the desired semantic-grammatical rules in all of the stimulus sets. It is therefore possible that a child may know and use a particular semantic-grammatical rule, but the contrived cues may not elicit the desired response.

The use of the semantic-grammatical rules for analysis of spontaneous or free play language samples, in addition to the MLU data, appears to provide relevant information about a child's level of language development. If one accepts a semantic model, this approach then would be more informative than other free-speech analyses that focus primarily on grammatical content. In addition, the procedures for documenting intelligible versus unintelligible responses could have useful clinical function.

Summary Since this model focuses entirely on production, no information or suggestions were provided for adapting the procedures for individuals with limited receptive skills. However, for clinicians dealing with individuals with good receptive skills, functioning at a one- or two-word expressive level, the ELI model appears to be a viable assessment and therapy strategy. In order to administer the test and interpret the results, it is imperative that the examiner invest some time learning the semantic-grammatical categories discussed in the book. The investment of time is highly recommended.

Charles E. Merrill, 1978

Cost $7.95 for the spiral-bound, soft-cover manual

Time An untimed test that will take from 30 minutes to several sessions to administer; scoring, 10 minutes

ENVIRONMENTAL PRE-LANGUAGE BATTERY (EPB)

DeAnna Horstmeier and James D. MacDonald

Shirley S. Doyle *University of Minnesota*

Purpose The Environmental Pre-Language Battery is a diagnostic and training instrument designed for use with nonverbal or minimally verbal individuals who are functioning below or at the single-word level. The primary purpose of the test is prescriptive; placement in a language training program is indicated according to the results of the assessment and training techniques. A second suggested use is for language program evaluation by comparing pre- and posttherapy summary test scores.

Administration, scoring, and interpretation The EPB is divided into a nonverbal and a verbal section. Included in the nonverbal section are a brief history of early sound productions to be obtained from the parent; observation of preliminary skills, including eye control, sitting behavior, on-task behavior, and object permanence; observation of functional play with toys and objects; motor imitation; and assessment of receptive language, including identifying objects, understanding action verbs, identifying pictures, and responsiveness to instructions. This final task is optional and not included in the summary score.

The verbal section assesses sound imitation, noun imitation, noun production, action verb production, two-word phrase imitation, and two-word phrase production. In addition, other categories of words are reported by the parent but this information does not get included in the summary test score.

Prior to administration of this battery, the authors suggest that the Oliver: Parent Administered Communication Inventory (MacDonald 1978) be completed. This is a comprehensive written report to be completed by the child's parents or teacher. It provides initial information about the child's range of communication behaviors and interests in his or her home and school environment.

Information from the Oliver and examiner observations determine where to begin testing. An assortment of toys and pictures is necessary to administer the EPB and these must be accumulated by the examiner. Although specific objects and pictures are designated for each subtest of the EPB, other items may be substituted that better meet the needs or interests of the child. The battery can either be administered seated at the table in a formal setting or while playing informally on the floor. The parent may or may not be present.

Four test items are administered for each skill. The child who fails an item is immediately trained on that item. The EPB manual provides extensive, specific training suggestions appropriate for each skill for shaping the desired response. The techniques include physically manipulating the child through the item, modeling the response and pairing it with a verbal description, and verbal prompts. If the child responds correctly during the training procedures, the item is readministered. Total administration time for a cooperative client is approximately 30 minutes, but the battery may be administered in more than one session.

There are four items for each test level. Each item passed receives three points. An item that is passed following training receives one point. A test level is passed if a child receives 9-12 points, or 75 percent of the total possible score. A test level is considered emerging if the child receives 6-8 points or at least 50 percent of the total possible score. If a test level is not passed, the assessment continues until a second level is failed (ceiling).

Administration of the EPB does not result in a standard score or a developmental age score, but rather a behavioral description of a child's mastery of early prelanguage skills. Information obtained from the test items and the child's responses to particular techniques used during the training segments should determine appropriate placement in a language training program and help define specific goals.

For clinicians who feel compelled to assign a language age, the authors have included in the revised manual approximate age equivalents. These age equivalents are intended for information purposes only. They were obtained from previously published studies of normally developing children and include language skills usually learned from 12 to 30 months.

The manual states that those who have an interest in children and a willingness to familiarize themselves with the test procedures can administer the test. The authors urge examiners to be flexible and creative in adapting the task procedures to particular clients.

Evaluation of test adequacy   This is not a standardized test and normative data are not reported. No discussion of reliability or validity is presented. No justification is provided for including several of the skills tested other than the stated intent that the EPB was designed to be an assessment tool that would facilitate language programming and that only skills appropriate for an intervention program are included.

The authors report that the EPB has been used extensively with mentally retarded and language delayed individuals at the Nisonger Center for Mental Retardation and Developmental Delay in Columbus, Ohio, and that it has been successfully adapted for use with young or difficult-to-test children as well as children with visual, auditory, or physical impairment.

The preliminary EPB was published in 1975. The current edition (1978) includes several modifications in administration and scoring that improve its effectiveness. The manual provides explicit, even repetitive, directions for application and interpretation.

Because administration of this test involves the manipulation of objects, toys, and pictures, the examiner must be thoroughly familiar with the procedures in order simultaneously to interact with the patient, score the performance, and search for the next test item. When feasible, the presence of an assistant examiner may facilitate administration.

Furthermore, since the EPB utilizes appealing toys and objects, the examiner may occasionally need skill and finesse in encouraging some children to part with specific test objects in order to move on to the next phase of testing.

The EPB provides two sources of information that are relevant to behavioral diagnosis: (1) a careful evaluation of current behavioral status and (2) a measure of the rapidity of learning new skills. The goal is to derive not a diagnostic label but rather a behavioral description that will result in appropriate program planning. Useful information about teaching strategies is learned by incorporating teaching techniques into the actual assessment.

Summary   The EPB is unique in that it provides a creative, yet systematic procedure for evaluating a set of preliminary language skills that are often alluded to but not specifically evaluated. Thus it may be a valuable clinical tool for persons who are concerned about the language skills of very young or low functioning populations. It is specifically and highly recommended for clinicians who work in preschool settings with severely language-delayed children, or clinicians who work with clients for whom formal, standardized test procedures are inappropriate. It is particularly effective for children with nonadapting behaviors such as short attention span or hyperactivity. In addition, parents or teachers who participate in administering or observing the EPB battery may gain valuable information and insight about early language functioning and intervention strategies. A language program for parents, teacher, or speech clinicians, based on the EPB, is presented in *Ready, Set, Go—Talk to Me* (Horstmeier and MacDonald 1978).

References

Horstmeier, D. and J. D. MacDonald   *Ready, Set, Go—Talk to Me.* Columbus: Charles E. Merrill, 1978.

MacDonald, J. D.   *Oliver: Parent Administered Communication Inventory.* Columbus: Charles E. Merrill, 1978.

FULL-RANGE PICTURE VOCABULARY TEST (FRPV)

**Robert B. Ammons and
Helen S. Ammons**

Psychological Test Specialists, 1948

Two equivalent forms, A and B; C and D for research only

Cost $15.00

Manual, one page and 16 plates, $15.00; answer sheets, 1 page, pack of 25 for $2.50, pack of 100 for $8.00 (specify form)

Time 15 minutes, administration; less than 5 minutes, scoring

LuVern H. Kunze *Duke University Medical Center*

Purpose The authors have described the Full-Range Picture Vocabulary Test as an "... individual test of intelligence based on verbal comprehension with norms for CA two through adult level." They suggest its use as an estimate of verbal ability or a measure of auditory comprehension vocabulary.

Administration, scoring, and interpretation The test is administered individually. Test time is approximately 15 minutes. Four line drawings appear on each of 16 test cards. The testee is instructed to identify the picture that best represents each verbally presented word. Pointing or a yes–no response as the examiner points are acceptable responses. Correct and incorrect responses are recorded on a printed answer sheet.

Instructions to the examiner include appropriate methods for establishing basal and ceiling levels. The number of correct responses is used as a raw score. A table of norms on the back of the answer sheet converts raw scores to mental-age equivalents for children (two years through 16 years) and to percentiles for adults. Two comparable test forms (Forms A and B) are provided with the test materials. Two additional forms (Forms C and D) are available from the authors for use by reseachers interested in the study of superior adult levels. A scoring key is provided for each test form.

Evaluation of test adequacy Test construction was achieved by submitting 248 subjectively selected vocabulary items to 84 subjects. The subjects were two males and two females at each CA from two to 17 years and four adults at each of the following IQ levels: 99–109, 112–119, 121–129, 131–138, and 140–144 (Ammons and Huth 1949). Twenty-two items were eliminated as nondiscriminating. The remaining 226 items were listed in order of difficulty and were submitted to 589 white, American-born subjects ranging in age from two through 34 years (Ammons and Rachiele 1950). The sample was controlled for occupation, age–grade placement, and sex. From these results, 170 items were selected and divided to constitute forms A and B.

Three standardization studies (Ammons and Holmes 1949; Ammons, Arnold, and Herman 1950; Ammons, Larson, and Shearn 1950) provided the normative data published on the record sheets. The characteristics of these studies are summarized in Table 1.

Separate norms are also available for rural white schoolchildren (Ammons and Manahan 1950), black schoolchildren (Coppinger and Ammons 1952), and Spanish-American schoolchildren (Ammons and Aquero 1950). The characteristics of these studies are summarized in Table 2. Reference is made to norms for black adult males, but the study remains unpublished.

Intertest reliability comparing forms A and B ranged from .86 to .99 for the six standardization populations studied. (See Tables 1 and 2.) Reliability values in this same range are reported in studies of black adult males (Tucker unpublished) and children with reading disabilities (Smith and Fillmore 1954).

Estimates of validity were provided through correlation coefficients between FRPV scores and scores on selected criterion tests. (See Tables 1 and 2.) For all studies except the preschool study, other tests of vocabulary were employed as criteria. Correlation coefficients ranged from .82 to .88 for all populations except the white school-age group. For this group, correlation coefficients of .67 and .69 suggest somewhat more caution in the interpretation of test findings in the clinical setting.

The test has not been revised since its development in 1948. Because of the dynamic nature of language in general and vocabulary in particular, a revision would increase its clinical usefulness. This would also provide an opportunity to update the stimulus pictures.

This test is clinically useful as an estimate of an individual's receptive vocabulary, provided that the findings with white school-age children are interpreted with some caution. While the provision of norms for special populations (particularly the black and Spanish-American populations) is useful, caution must be exercised in interpreting results because of the small N at each age level in these studies.

No studies were found that correlated the FRPV with other measures of verbal comprehension or broader aspects of receptive language. Interpretation of test results as indicators of an individual's comprehension of linguistic rules seems unwarranted until such studies have been completed. There is no evidence to justify interpreting test results as indicators of expressive verbal abilities, since a clinical population will include many whose receptive and expressive capabilities will differ. Interpretation of test findings as indicators of intelligence with the language-impaired population also seems unwarranted since language impairment frequently appears as a specific learning disability that is independent of intelligence.

Summary For the purposes of the speech–language pathologist, the FRPV provides a reliable vehicle for estimating receptive vocabulary. Its use as an indicator of overall receptive language (including knowledge of semantic, syntactic, and morphologic rules) is unwarranted, particularly with language-defective individuals.

References

Ammons, R. B. and A. Aguero   The Full-Range Picture Vocabulary Test: VII. Results for a Spanish-American school-age population. *J. soc. Psychol.* 32: 3–10, 1950.

Ammons, R. B., P. R. Arnold, and R. S. Herrmann   The Full-Range Picture Vocabulary Test: IV. Results for a white school population. *J. clin. Psychol.* 6: 164–169, 1950.

Ammons, R. B. and J. C. Holmes   The Full-Range Picture Vocabulary Test: III. Results for a preschool-age population. *Child Develpm.* 20: 5–14, 1949.

Ammons, R. B. and R. W. Huth   The Full-Range Vocabulary Test: I. Preliminary scale. *J. Psychol.* 28: 51–64, 1949.

Ammons, R. B., W. L. Larson, and C. R. Shearn   The Full-Range Picture Vocabulary Test: V. Results for an adult population. *J. consult. Psychol.* 14: 150–155, 1950.

TABLE 1 Summary of Normative Studies. Data from These Studies Are Provided with the Test.

Group	Age	N and Sex	Ethnicity	Occupation	Between forms	Form A and criterion	Form B and criterion	Criterion test
Pre-school	2–5	15 M, each CA 15 F, each CA	White	Distributed	.93	.85	.83	Stanford–Binet (1937)
School	6–17	15 M, each CA 15 F, each CA	White	Distributed	.99	.67	.69	Stanford–Binet Vocabulary (1937)
Adults	18–35	60 M 60 F	White	Distributed	.96	.85	.86	WAIS Vocabulary

TABLE 2 Summary of Studies Providing Norms for Special Populations. Data from These Studies Are Not Provided with the Test.

Group	Age	N and Sex	Ethnicity	Occupation	Between forms	Form A and criterion	Form B and criterion	Criterion test
School	6–17	71 M and F	White	Distributed for rural population	.92	.88	.86	Stanford–Binet (1937)
School	6–13	5 M, each CA 5 F, each CA	Black	Distributed for Southern black population	.96	.81	.84	Stanford–Binet Vocabulary (1937)
School	7–16	4 M, each CA	Spanish-American	Distributed for Spanish-American population	.86	.85	.82	Stanford–Binet Vocabulary (1937)

Ammons, R. B. and N. Manahan   The Full-Range Picture Vocabulary Test: VI. Results for a rural population. *J. educ. Res.* **44**: 14–21, 1950.

Ammons, R. B. and L. D. Rachiele   The Full-Range Picture Vocabulary Test: II. Selection of items for final scales. *Educ. psychol. Measmt.* **10**: 307–319, 1950.

Coppinger, N. W. and R. B. Ammons   The Full-Range Picture Vocabulary Test: VIII. A normative study of Negro Children. *J. clin. Psychol.* **8**: 136–140, 1952.

Smith, L. M. and A. R. Fillmore   The Ammons FRPV Test and the WISC for remedial reading cases. *J. consult. Psychol.* **18**: 332, 1954.

Tucker, D. A.   A study of adult male Negroes with the Full-Range Picture Vocabulary Test. M. A. thesis, University of Louisville.

THE HOUSTON TEST FOR LANGUAGE DEVELOPMENT

Margaret Crabtree

The Houston Test Company: Part I, 1958; Part II, 1963

Cost Parts I and II, $27.00

Manual for Part I: 23 pages; manual for Part II: 34 pages; record form

Time 30 minutes, administration; 5–10 minutes, scoring

John T. Hatten *University of Minnesota, Duluth*

Purpose The Houston Test for Language Development was constructed to measure language development in children up to age six. It purports to provide the basis for the objective evaluation of language functioning.

Administration, scoring, and interpretation There are two parts to the test. Part I is for children up to age three years, and Part II extends the scale through the age of six. The test takes approximately 30 minutes to administer. Test items are presented for six-month age intervals up to 36 months and at year intervals to six years. Parents may assist the examiner in eliciting responses from infants one year of age or younger.

Both receptive and expressive language skills are included, involving such specific categories as melody, rhythm, accent, gestures, articulation, vocabulary, grammatical usage, construction, auditory judgment, syntactical complexity, sentence length, prepositions, counting, geometric designs, drawings, and others.

Each item is weighted relative to the total number of items at that age level. Scoring is accomplished by circling the correct responses on the provided record form, multiplying the number of correct items at each age level by the item value, and totaling the products. A basal age (age at which all items are passed), upper age (highest age at which any items are passed), and language age (total score in months) are obtained. "Test patterns" are determined by listing items under the age of the child's highest success to show areas of strength and weakness. Children are considered to have a language problem if they score two or more years below their chronological age.

Part I of this test was standardized on 113 white children from Houston, Texas. None were from bilingual homes, multiple births, or had "observable" mental retardation or physical defects. Part II was administered to 102 children from the age of two years, six months through six years, five months. All items were administered to all children.

The test manuals for the Houston Test provide specific information for test administration and the record forms allow direct and simple scoring. The test was first published in 1958 (Part I) and 1963 (Part II) and has not been revised to date. No particular training other than familiarization with the test appears to be required.

Evaluation of test adequacy Essentially no validity information is provided in the test manual for Part I although a rationale for item selection is provided. An interexaminer reliability correlation of .84 is reported although sample size and sampling procedures are not provided. The norms for Part II items were determined by three criteria: (1) a significant difference in the percentage passing the item from one age to another (presented as a measure of item validity); (2) over 50 percent of the age level passed the item; and (3) judgment. No reliability information is provided for Part II.

The Houston Test for Language Development may be used as a general measure of language development for children up to six years of age. Although the Houston Test is primarily designed to provide information about a child's language performance relative to other children of the same age, the inadequacy of the standardization data contraindicates its use. The test is too poorly standardized to be useful as a norm-referenced measure and too general to be used as a criterion-referenced test. The test is rather eclectic in its definition of language and relies on no specific theory of language. Although there is a heterogeneity of test items, no areas are tested with enough depth to provide adequate information regarding specific strengths and weaknesses.

The manual allows too much room for subjective judgment in scoring specific items, and many of the items for younger children are highly dependent on the cooperation of the child. Task demands appear to include many nonlanguage functions.

Summary   The Houston Test reflects an earlier era of language testing and is of limited use since more sophisticated measures of language functioning are now available. The test has not been revised since 1963 and reliability and validity data are inadequate. Standardization data are available on only a narrow segment of the population.

LANGUAGE FACILITY TEST

John T. Dailey

The Allington Corporation, 1977

Cost $15.00

Examiner's Manual: 43 pages; Spanish supplement, 12 pages; 12 picture plates accompany the manual

Time 10 minutes, administration and scoring

Harris Winitz *University of Missouri—Kansas City*

Purpose The Language Facility Test measures verbal responses to pictures on a continuous scale from mental ages two to 15. It was designed as a simple, short test that can be administered by teachers, aides, or others with little training in test administration. The test is said to be useful as an initial screening device. The author recommends its use in bilingual educational programs, foreign language programs, early education programs, programs for the deaf, programs for the physically handicapped, programs for the mentally retarded, and other programs for groups whose family language experiences have been atypical.

Administration, scoring, and interpretation The test consists of a set of 12 picture plates, grouped into sets of three pictures each. One set consists of photographs of preschool students and teachers in a school for children of migrant farm workers; a second set consists of rather stark drawings; the third set consists of scenes by old Spanish masters and is rich in shading and detail. Three extra plates are included for use as alternates. The author states that the different pictures give highly similar results and measure the same thing. The examiner presumably selects the set of plates judged to be most interesting to the child.

Subjects are prompted to tell a complete story about each of the three pictures in a set. Instructions are given as to how many prompts are to be used before a picture is withdrawn.

The test can be administered in Spanish, sign language, or other languages or dialects and scored by the same method. The examiner, of course, must be familiar with the language in which the test is administered.

The main scoring system involves assigning a rating from 0 to 9 according to the child's responses to each picture. Since each subject is administered only three pictures, test scores can range from 0–27. A detailed description for each scale value is provided in the manual. Also provided are numerous examples of responses. A supplemental manual provides comparable information in Spanish. Examples of the rating scale are:

0 No response, garbled speech, or only pointing at the picture.
5 A partial description consisting of two or more sentences with some description of movement or action as seen in the pictures.
9 A well-organized story with imagination and creativity. Need not be original. May use well-known fictional or historical characters.

Evaluation of test adequacy Examiner reliability was assessed on several occasions and Pearson product–moment correlations between .88 and .94 were obtained between examiners for homogeneous populations involving 100 children or more.

Test–retest correlations range between .46 (15-week interval) and .90 (12-week interval). Test–retest data for shorter intervals are not reported.

The least satisfying feature of the test involves the collection of the normative data. Over 4000 subjects between the ages of three and 20 years provided data. No description of these subjects is provided. Growth curves of several subsamples are illustrated, and a chart is provided in which raw scores for the entire sample are converted into percentiles. Growth curves are shown for groups of Head Start children, mentally retarded children in several summer programs, physically handicapped children, poor readers, and a group of children in a summer program for the deaf, as well as children enrolled in a middle-class private nursery school and first grade. These data are based on small samples and the characteristics of the children in the several subgroups are not described beyond the labels applied. The normative data for these special groups were obtained in 1966.

Validity is not explicitly discussed in the manual, but the performance of the various special populations differs from that of the normals and the test differentiates between disadvantaged children doing well in school and other disadvantaged children who are not doing well. This finding may be interpreted as indicative of a form of validity. In addition, the author reports correlations between scores on the Language Facility Test and several other instruments or ratings, such as SRA achievement ($r = .20$), Stanford–Binet ($r = .18$). These low correlations are presented but not discussed.

The samples of speech can also be scored to give a profile of frequency of common deviations from standard English. The author provides a preliminary diagnostic profile of common deviations and includes 24 error types that the examiner might look for, plus a brief example for each type. These include simple verb, wrong number; auxiliary verb, wrong number; *they* for *there* or *their,* etc. The error code is not standardized and is presented as only suggestive at its present stage of refinement.

Summary The rating scale which the author proposes is interesting. If the scale procedure were appropriately validated for representative populations, the test might prove to be useful since it can be administered and scored quickly.

LANGUAGE SAMPLING, ANALYSIS, AND TRAINING

**Dorothy Tyack and
Robert Gottsleben**

Consulting Psychologists Press, 1974

Cost Manual, $3.50; 25 sets of score sheets, $16.50. Specimen set consisting of manual and three copies of each of six score sheets, $5.00. The manual contains directions for obtaining the language sample, analyzing the language sample, designing remedial procedures based on the analysis, a series of appendices with specific instructions for counting words and categorizing constructions, and three sample analyses for practice

Time Will vary depending on experience of the examiner

Patricia A. Broen *University of Minnesota*

Purpose Language Sampling, Analysis, and Training is considered by the authors to be a handbook describing procedures for training children whose language delay is serious enough to warrant intervention. This test will not identify the child with delayed-language skill. Some other test should be used to separate the normal child from the delayed child. But once this determination has been made, Tyack and Gottsleben provide a way to identify those grammatical forms and constructions that the child has mastered, those that the child is beginning to master, and those that are absent from the child's speech. Guidelines are provided for choosing the grammatical forms and constructions to be taught, for designing teaching programs, and for testing the child's mastery when teaching is complete.

Administration, Scoring, and Interpretation The Language Sampling, Analysis, and Training procedure is applied to a 100-sentence sample of spontaneous speech obtained from a child in a more or less standard fashion. As with any other analysis of spontaneous speech, it can be only as good as the sample on which it is based. Tyack and Gottsleben provide some suggestions for obtaining the sample in a systematic and standard way but their suggestions do not seem to solve the problems inherent in such sampling. The use of 100 sentences rather than the more common 50-sentence sample is another attempt to make the sample more representative.

The sample of speech obtained from the child is transcribed on a special form that allows three lines for each sentence: one for any direct questions used to elicit the sentence, one for the sentence as spoken by the child, and one for a grammatical expansion of the child's sentence. Subsequent analyses are based on the transcription of the child's sentence and the grammatical expansion of that sentence. The child is assigned a "linguistic level," that is, a ratio of the mean number of words used in sentences to the mean number of morphemes used in sentences. This level sets the expectations for the child. The child is expected to use those structures that are used by other children at that linguistic level but not those structures that are used at higher linguistic levels. The levels described in the test range from 2.0 to 6.0. The procedure is most appropriate for children whose sentences fall within this range and would be used only in unique cases for children whose sentences were longer than six morphemes.

After the linguistic level has been determined, the child's speech is analyzed to identify those grammatical forms that are consistently correct, those that are sometimes correct, and those that are missing or consistently incorrect. The forms of interest include pronouns, prepositions, articles, conjunctions, plurals, possessives, modals, and various verb tense markers. Each form has been assigned a linguistic level that corresponds to the level at which most normal children use this form correctly. In this way, the child's performance can be compared to that of other children of the same linguistic level rather than to that of other children of the same age. The specification of level for various forms is based on previous research (Morehead and Ingram 1973).

The child's speech is also analyzed to determine which of a set of noun phrase, verb phrase, and noun and verb phrase constructions are used by the child. Linguistic levels are provided for the simpler constructions. In practice, the more complex constructions are difficult for the teacher or clinician to identify from the information in the manual and their description adds little to the treatment of the child.

This procedure is not standardized. The normative data used to assign grammatical forms and grammatical constructions to linguistic levels come from a study of 15 normal and 15 language-deviant children who ranged across the five linguistic levels.

Evaluation of test adequacy The information obtained from this analysis is to be used to design a remedial procedure to teach the child those forms and those constructions that are appropriate to his or her current linguistic level and current pattern of performance. Guidelines provide directions for the development of specific tests to explore the child's ability to understand and produce syntactic forms that are of particular interest or forms that may not have occurred in the speech sample.

This test is particularly useful for the description of a child's basic syntactic forms and simple syntactic constructions. It describes the child's use of just those structures whose misuse can make speech sound strange or immature.

Summary The manual provides detailed information for the transcription and analysis of the spontaneous speech sample but the user is assumed to have some experience or training in teaching language-delayed children. The ultimate validity of this procedure lies in the representativeness of the sample speech. If the sample represents the child's usual speech pattern, the analysis should describe his or her use of the forms and the constructions that are considered and this is all that the procedure claims to do. If the sample is biased in some way, the analysis will be similarly biased.

Reference

Morehead, D. M. and D. Ingram The development of base syntax in normal and linguistically deviant children. *J. Speech Hearing Res.* **16**: 330–352, 1973.

MICHIGAN PICTURE LANGUAGE INVENTORY (MPLI)

William Wolski and Louis Lerea

University of Michigan, Department of Communication Disorders, 1962

Cost $6.00
Twenty-five page mimeographed manuscript containing test description, instructions, and reliability and validity data. Thirty-five vocabulary test plates (mimeographed line drawings) and 50 language structure test plates (mimeographed line drawings)

Time One hour or longer, administration and scoring

Kenneth F. Ruder *University of Kansas*

Purpose The Michigan Picture Language Inventory was developed by Lerea (1958) and revised by Wolski (1962). The test is designed to measure two major components of language development in children: vocabulary and grammatical structures. Each of these components is tested in both verbal expression and verbal comprehension modes. The test is further designed to be developmental in nature, with normative data provided for children aged four, five, and six.

Administration, scoring, and interpretation The test is administered in two parts: a vocabulary subtest and a language structure subtest. Each subtest is further evaluated both receptively and expressively. Thirty-five vocabulary items selected from the Buckingham and Dolch word count for children comprise the content of the vocabulary subtest. The language structure subtest consists of 50 stimulus plates used to test 69 exemplars of various language structures: single and plural nouns (20 exemplars), personal pronouns (7), possessives (4), adjectives (12), demonstratives (4), articles (4), adverbs (4), prepositions (6), and verbs (8).

Administration of the vocabulary subtest begins with picture naming. Each of the 35 test items is pictured on a test plate along with two foil items. The examiner places the three-picture test plate in front of the child, points to the test item, and asks the child, "What is this a picture of?" Each correct response has a point value of one, yielding a total possible score of 35 for expressive vocabulary.

Receptive vocabulary testing follows the expressive testing. Credit is given for receptive vocabulary for all items that were correct on the expressive vocabulary test. Hence only items failed on the expressive test are further tested in the receptive mode. A standard comprehension format is used for the receptive testing wherein the child is presented with the three-picture test plate and is asked to show the examiner the item requested.

Each of the nine structures assessed in the language structure subtest is tested separately following a three-step sequence. First, the stimulus cards are described to alert the child to the context of the responses he or she will be required to give in that section. Next, the structure is tested in the expressive mode by asking the child to name the key item representing that structure. A modeling/grammatical closure type procedure is used to elicit the verbal response from the child. For example, given a set of pictures depicting a dog *in* a box and *under* a box, the examiner points to the first picture and provides a structural model by saying, "Here the dog is *in* the box." This is immediately followed by pointing to the second picture and saying, "And here the dog is _____." The child is to complete the statement by providing the appropriate verbal response, *under* the box.

The third part of the language structure subtest is the receptive test of the particular structure. As in the vocabulary testing, only items failed on the expressive portion of the test are further assessed in the receptive mode. Credit for receptive knowledge of the particular structure is given for all items correctly named in the expressive testing. The language structure subtest is scored the same as the vocabulary subtest. The receptive and expressive scores on each of the two subtests are compared to normative data provided in the appendix of the test in order to evaluate a particular subject's performance.

Evaluation of test adequacy Normative data on the MPLI were obtained from 180 children, 30 boys and 30 girls in each of the three age groups (4, 5, and 6 years). The authors also present data on reliability and validity. A claim is made for content validity on the basis of the manner of selection and the source of the test items. The fact that the older groups of children in the normative study did better than the younger children in both the vocabulary and language structure tests is taken as further indication of the validity of the test instrument. The authors followed acceptable procedures for standardizing their test; however, the normative subjects were all Caucasian singletons without siblings from the Flint, Michigan, area. One could question the logic of extending the findings from this rather select group to the diversities encountered within a language disordered population.

The content of the vocabulary subtest lacks representativeness, A preschool child could conceivably do quite poorly on this subtest and yet possess adequate vocabulary for communicative competence. It is not clear why this limited sample of 35 items was chosen over any other list of 35. The items are all nouns. Equally bothersome is the fact that the vocabulary items tested are not utilized in subsequent language structure testing.

In the language structure subtest, the list of structures tested is by no means exhaustive and no rationale for the selection is given. Considering the frequency with which children encounter problems with word-order syntax and the copula and auxiliary (is VERBing) structures, it is disconcerting to find such structures omitted from a language test.

The linguistic model upon which the test is based (Fries 1952) represents a superficial view of language structure that does not reflect the impact of transformational grammar (Chomsky 1965), case grammar (Fillmore 1968), generative semantics (Fillmore and Langendoen 1971), or the more recent emphasis on the pragmatic (Bates 1976) or functional (Premack 1970) bases of language. The consensus of current linguistic and psycholinguistic thought is that reliance on only surface structure features of grammar, such as is done in the MPLI, will yield an incomplete and unsatisfactory description of language behavior.

From a clinician's standpoint, a language test can serve three functions: (1) it identifies those who have language problems, (2) it identifies the nature and extent of the problem, and (3) it provides the clinician with adequate data to plan and structure training. The MPLI does not purport to meet the last two functions. Few language tests do, even though it is widely agreed that providing information upon which training can be based should be a primary goal of language testing.

The MPLI was designed to identify children with language problems, and it cites the validity and reliability data of the normative study as evidence of achieving this goal. However, even this claim deserves some scrutiny. As a part of the process of reviewing this test, three experienced language clinicians were asked to administer the test to five children with language problems and five children who were acquiring language normally. All were participants in a preschool language training program and familiar with the clinicians and test format. The clinicians individually familiarized themselves with the MPLI prior to administering it to the subjects. Comparison of test results from the three clinicians yielded agreement on identification on only one of the five language-impaired children. Two normal subjects were misidentified as having language problems by the three clinicians on the basis of the test results. For the other seven subjects, little agreement between the three clinicians was noted, either on total score or on specific structures or vocabulary items found to be deficient.

The data from this informal comparison are limited, but they highlight the questionable test–retest reliability of the MPLI and cast further doubt on the applicability of the test for identifying language disorders, particularly in borderline cases. All three clinicians agreed that they would not use the test again for clinical purposes. They found the directions and scoring procedures to be confusing and sometimes misleading. They also judged the stimulus pictures to be of poor overall quality. In some instances, particularly comprehension testing of demonstrative pronouns, a position preference could result in an inflated score since three of four correct responses occurred in the same position.

The three clinicians were likewise disturbed by the instructions to credit in comprehension all responses correct in production. As a follow-up to the test, the clinicians each assessed a subject for comprehension of items previously correct in production. All three subjects made errors in comprehension of items previously scored as correct on the basis of productive responses. In one case, the change in comprehension score was sufficient to change the child's diagnostic classification from "no problem" to "language impaired." The reason for this mismatch of production and comprehension is not clear. Psycholinguistic data of recent vintage indicate that children produce some linguistic contrasts they do not seem to comprehend. In addition, the problems of the comprehension test format, picture quality, and test reliability may have all contributed to the observed asymmetry of performance.

Summary   The MPLI is of limited clinical utility. It is a long test to administer and is of little clinical or linguistic relevance since sentential and/or communicative abilities are never directly assessed. The test may have adequately represented earlier views and data regarding language structure. The MPLI has not kept pace with recent advancements in the field of language and does not reflect current views of language and language intervention specialists. Though the MPLI may be of some historical significance, it cannot and should not be considered seriously as a functional clinical tool at this time.

References

Bates, E. *Language and Context: The Acquisition of Pragmatics.* New York: Academic Press, 1976.

Buckingham, D. R. and E. W. Dolch   *A Combined Word List.* Lexington, Mass.: Ginn, 1936.

Chomsky, N.   *Aspects of the Theory of Syntax.* Cambridge, Mass.: MIT Press, 1965.

Fillmore, C.   The case for case. In E. Bach and R. Harms (eds.), *Universals in Linguistic Theory.* New York: Holt, Rinehart and Winston, 1968.

Fries, C. C.   *The Structure of English.* New York: Harcourt Brace, 1952.

Lerea, L.   Assessing language development. *J. Speech Hearing Res.* 1: 75–85, 1958.

Premack, D.   A functional analysis of language. *J. Exper. Anal. Behav.* 14: 107–125, 1970.

Wolski, W.   Language development of normal children, four, five, and six years of age as measured by the Michigan Picture Language Inventory. Doctoral Dissertation, The University of Michigan, Ann Arbor, 1962.

NORTHWESTERN SYNTAX SCREENING TEST (NSST)

Laura L. Lee

Northwestern University Press, 1969, 1971

Cost $10.00

Spiral-bound manual composed of 14 pages of administration and scoring instructions and guidelines for use, 42 pages of test plates; record form, 1 page

Time Approximately 15 minutes, administration; 3 minutes, scoring

Carol Lynn Waryas *University of Mississippi*

Purpose The Northwestern Syntax Screening Test was designed to serve the dual purposes of being a screening instrument for use with large numbers of children and a means of providing a quick estimate of a child's syntactic development as prelude to a more comprehensive evaluation. The goal of the test is to identify those children between three and eight years of age who are sufficiently deviant in syntactic development to warrant further examination.

Administration, scoring, and interpretation The NSST is the outgrowth of a series of research studies conducted utilizing the procedures described by Fraser, Bellugi, and Brown (1963). The test consists of a receptive and an expressive component, each 20 items in length, that test the same linguistic structures (but with different contrasting sentence pairs) in both components. The linguistic structures which are assessed include personal pronouns, possessives, wh–question words, demonstratives, verb tenses, plural inflections, negation, yes–no questions, and contrasting word order in active and passive sentences and double-object constructions. No specific training is required to administer the test or interpret its results.

Test stimuli consist of ten four-choice plates for the receptive component and ten two-choice plates for the expressive component. All plates are black-and-white line drawings. The plates are in a spiral-bound booklet, which also includes administration and scoring instructions. Demonstration items for use in familiarizing the child with each task are included.

The receptive task is administered first. The child is shown the appropriate plate of four pictures and the examiner says the titles of two of the pictures (the tested contrast), without indicating to the child which picture goes with which title, and then repeats one for the child to point to. Scoring procedures involve only entering a "1" on the score sheet for each picture correctly identified.

In the expressive task, the examiner shows the child the appropriate test plate with two choices and says both picture titles, again without indicating which picture corresponds with which title. Then, the examiner points to one of the pictures and asks the child to name it. Expressive responses are scored as incorrect if the child makes any change in the examiner's spoken sentence that involves the contrast being tested, regardless of whether the resulting sentence is grammatically and semantically correct, and if there are any grammatical errors in the sentence, even if the tested contrast is correct. Items are scored correct if there are changes made that do not involve the test contrast and the sentence is grammatical, or if no changes are made. A single data sheet is used for both portions of the test.

The scores on each component of the test, once totaled, can be compared with the norms presented for each six-month interval from 3-0 to 7-11. These norms are based on the results obtained from 344 normal children and are reported in terms of the 10th, 25th, 50th, 75th, and 90th percentile as well as means and standard deviations for each group. Receptive and expressive norms are reported separately, in both tabular and graphic form. The author has also provided suggestions for interpretation of results. It is suggested that those children who score more than two standard deviations below the mean on either or both portions of the test probably are in need of language therapy. Scores between the 10th percentile and the second standard deviation are considered low normal. Guidelines for interpreting scores as well as illustrative test results obtained from 18 language-delayed children are also presented.

The test is short. Therefore it is suggested that the test be administered in its entirety for maximum accuracy. For use in screening large numbers of children, it is suggested that the test items may be administered until the child's accumulated score places him or her at or above the 10th percentile for his or her age. Thus the entire test would have to be administered only to those children who perform poorly on it. Administration of the entire test takes approximately 15 minutes. Half of this time may be saved if the alternate administration procedure is used.

Evaluation of test adequacy Ratusnik and Koenigsknecht (1975) conducted a study designed to evaluate the internal consistency of the two components of the NSST and the discrimination power of its individual items. The test was administered to 20 mentally retarded children and 20 children with severe expressive language delay. The results showed the Hoyt's reliability coefficients for the two groups of subjects on the expressive component to be .81 and .78, respectively, and on the receptive component to be .55 and .67, respectively. In addition, the test was administered to 20 normal children and the individual test items were analyzed to determine which ones served to discriminate between groups. Twenty-nine of the 40 receptive items and 39 of the 40 expressive items differentiated between the groups. Temporal reliability of the test as assessed by the retest method has not been reported.

Arndt (1977) suggested that the norms for this test are not readily generalizable to the general population since the standardization was performed on a group of subjects who were relatively homogeneous in terms of socioeconomic level and geographic location. In addition, the sample size in three of the five groups is too small to yield stable or representative estimates. Larson and Summers (1976) administered the NSST to 216 children in Northern Texas, some from lower socioeconomic backgrounds. The means were substantially below those reported for the population on which the norms were based, supporting the lack of generalizability.

Prutting, Gallagher, and Mulac (1975) provided an indirect indication of the validity of the test. The 12 children who served as subjects had all been diagnosed as language delayed on the basis of other standardized language testing procedures, and all scored below the 10th percentile of the test norms. However, Larson and Summers (1976) did not find significant differences in the means obtained for subjects in the age groups 5-6, 6-0, and 6-6. In addition, test norms are virtually identical in the 7-0 and 7-11 range. These facts cast some doubt on the developmental function that the test is stated to assess.

Prutting, Gallagher, and Mulac (1975) compared the results obtained on the expressive portion of the NSST from 12 language delayed children to results obtained from analyses of their spontaneous speech. Thirty percent of the syntactic structures that were incorrectly produced on the NSST were correctly produced in the spontaneous sample. Also, performance Forms A and B of the test (one or the other item in each pair) differed greatly. These results suggest that the NSST cannot profitably be extended beyond its originally designed use as a screening tool.

Byrne (1977) stated that the NSST does not meet the necessary criteria for being an objective measure of communication deficiency. Moreover, she suggested that task requirements may have confounded results at different ages. That is, the gap apparent in the normative data between receptive and expressive scores for the youngest subjects might have resulted from the greater memory requirements of the production task. She also pointed out that the production task is more a form of delayed imitation than of spontaneous language generation skills.

In a cogent reply to Arndt (1977) and Byrne (1977), Lee reiterated the following points regarding the NSST concerning issues which she said have arisen because the test has been put to uses for which it was never intended:

1   The NSST is a screening instrument only. It does not yield a language age, it cannot be used as the sole basis for classifying a child as language delayed, and it does not tap the full range of a child's syntactic abilities, let alone such factors as vocabulary, semantic intent, or mean length of utterance. What it does do is quickly screen out those who most probably need help.

2   Norms are doubtful beyond the 6-0 to 6-11 level.

3   Children from other socioeconomic levels and geographical areas may differ in their performance. Lee advised that clinicians should establish their own local norms.

4   The test does not predict the consistency of grammatical usage in spontaneous speech. If a child performs correctly on an item on the test, this does not mean that the child necessarily "knows" that grammatical rule.

5   It is useful only for standard English. Lee doubted that it would be possible to translate the test so as to render it applicable to speakers of black dialect.

6   The statistical support for the test is meager. Lee stated, in regard to this point, that by today's standards the NSST would not be considered a test at all, but rather an initial screening instrument or diagnostic indicator.

7   It has a place in a clinical evaluation procedure since it can be quickly administered and, according to clinical reports, tends to overselect rather than underselect children for further evaluation.

Summary   The NSST is a relatively inexpensive test which is easy to administer and score. It quickly yields a very rough estimate of some of a child's syntactic abilities in the receptive and expressive domains. The test's shortcomings, which Lee freely acknowledges, have resulted more from overextension of the test from the purposes for which it was originally designed and from the changing state of the art in the field of language assessment, rather than deficiencies in its original design. As a screening device to determine the need for further evaluation, the NSST has these advantages: (1) it is quick and easy to administer and score; (2) it involves forms of both reception and expression processes; (3) it covers a range, although admittedly somewhat restricted, of linguistic structures; and (4) it tends to produce false positives in terms of suspected language disorders rather than missing children who are later found to need help. Based on these factors, it can be recommended for use by clinicians, bearing in mind the caveats expressed by Lee (1977). It is strongly recommended that clinicians who use or comtemplate using the NSST read Lee's (1977) article.

References

Arndt, W. B. A psychometric evaluation of the Northwestern Syntax Screening Test. *J. Speech Hearing Dis.* **42**: 316–319, 1977.

Byrne, M. C. A clinician looks at the Northwestern Syntax Screening Test. *J. Speech Hearing Dis.* **42**: 320–322, 1977.

Fraser, C., U. Bellugi, and R. Brown Control of grammar in imitation, comprehension, and production. *J. Verb. Learn. Verb. Behav.* **2**: 121–135, 1963.

Larson, G. W. and P. A. Summers Response patterns of pre-school-age children to the Northwestern Syntax Screening Test. *J. Speech Hearing Dis.* **41**: 486–497, 1976.

Lee, L. L. Reply to Arndt and Byrne. *J. Speech Hearing Dis.* **42**: 323–327, 1977.

Prutting, C. A., T. M. Gallagher, and A. Mulac The expressive portion of the NSST compared to a spontaneous language sample. *J. Speech Hearing Dis.* **40**: 40–48, 1975.

Ratusnik, D. L. and R. A. Koenigsknecht Internal consistency of the Northwestern Syntax Screening Test. *J. Speech Hearing Dis.* **40**: 59–68, 1975.

THE ORAL LANGUAGE SENTENCE IMITATION SCREENING TEST (OLSIST) AND THE ORAL LANGUAGE SENTENCE IMITATION DIAGNOSTIC INVENTORY (OLSIDI)

Linda Zachman, Rosemary Huisingh, Carol Jorgensen, and Mark Barrett

LinguiSystems, Inc., 1976, 1977

Cost OLSIST, packets of 50 test forms for each of Stages III, IV, V, $3.00; packets of 50 score sheets for each of Stages III, IV, V, $3.00; Instruction Manual, $2.00; OLSIDI, Complete Test (one packet of each test structure, one packet of profiles, two instruction manuals), $79.00

Time OLSIST, 10 minutes administration; 10 minutes scoring
OLSIDI, 5 minutes per subtest, administration; 30 minutes or more, scoring, depending on number of subtests administered

Janis M. Costello *University of California, Santa Barbara*

Purpose The authors state the Oral Language Sentence Imitation Screening Test is designed to assess "whether a child's expressive language skills are within normal limits" and to provide information to inform the clinician whether further testing is necessary. The test is more accurately described as an indicator of a child's syntactical performance rather than the child's expressive language as a whole. While it cannot pinpoint whether a child's syntactical performance is within normal levels, since there are currently no norms, it gives the clinician a relatively rapid way to discover whether a child has difficulty in this area.

The purpose of the Oral Language Sentence Imitation Diagnostic Inventory, the test which is to be used following the OLSIST, is to provide a kind of "deep test" of the particular language structures screened by the OLSIST so that a clinician may select remediation targets. The OLSIDI is supposed to "yield information similar to language sampling" but to do so more extensively and more rapidly.

Administration, scoring, and interpretation Both tests are sentence imitation tests based upon the theory of language development described by Brown (1973). The screening test, the OLSIST, has three levels, Stage III, Stage IV, and Stage V versions, which are meant to correspond to Brown's theoretical developmental stages. Morpheme length is systematically varied throughout the sentences within each level of the test and is also controlled across these three levels.

Each of the three levels of the OLSIST contains 20 sentences and includes 24 consonant phonemes in controlled proportions. The Stage V version, designed to be administered to first grade and kindergarten children, tests 23 different morphological and grammatical language structures in sentences that range in length from six to 13 morphemes.* Generally each structure is tested several times throughout the 20 sentences. The Stage IV OLSIST, designed to be administered to preschool children (no specific ages given) and to children who fail the Stage V OLSIST, tests 22 morphological and grammatical language structures in sentences ranging in length from five to 11

---

*A list of the morphological and syntactic structures tested by the OLSIST and OLSIDI can be found in the appendix following this review.

morphemes. The structures tested are the same as those tested in the Stage V version (with some exceptions), and these structures are tested in generally the same proportions as found in the Stage V version, most being tested more than once. Different sentence forms and lexicon are used, although the same structures are tested. The primary difference between these two levels of the test is the morpheme length of the sentences to be imitated, thus allowing the examiner to determine whether sentence length was a determining factor in failure. The Stage III OLSIST, designed to be administered to young preschoolers (not below age three) and to children who fail the Stage IV test, includes 18 of the structures tested in the other versions of the test and has sentences ranging in length from four to nine morphemes.

The OLSIDI, the diagnostic test designed to be administered following the screening test described above, is composed of 27 individual sentence-imitation tests, each composed of ten sentences which test a particular morphological or grammatical structure. Five sentences in each test are eight morphemes in length and five are nine morphemes in length. All of the 270 sentences in the 27 subtests are different. Each structure is tested ten times in a particular subtest and then several times more in sentences occurring in other subtests. The 27 language structures tested are those which are screened in the OLSIST. The OLSIDI is designed so that when certain target grammatical structures have been identified by the OLSIST or by other means, the clinician may select whichever subtests are appropriate for further testing of specific morphological and grammatical structures which the child appears to have in error. Thus if administration of the OLSIST or some other test or observation of the child's spontaneous language production indicated that the child incorrectly produced, for example, third person regular forms of the verb, Subtest Nine would be administered requiring the child to imitate ten sentences that include this verb form. Subtests are given selectively, and it is not necessary to administer the entire battery.

The instructions for administration of both tests are the same and are simple. The child is told, "Today we are going to play 'Follow the Leader!' I want you to say exactly what I say. OK! Let's try it!" This is followed by examples of three sentences for the child to imitate, one at a time, until he or she clearly understands the task. Then the test begins with the examiner presenting the first test sentence for the child to imitate.

For scoring purposes the examiner marks on the protocol of test sentences the child's exact response. Certain words in each sentence are numbered, the numbered items corresponding to particular test structures (there may be more than one test structure in a given sentence). Any word changes, omissions, or additions occurring on these numbered items are scored as an incorrect response for that particular structure. On separate score summary sheets the examiner can rather easily summarize the child's responses to all instances of each of the tested structures. For each structure tested a percentage of correctness score is calculated, as well as a mean length of imitative utterance score.

The suggested guidelines for interpretation of the OLSIST results indicate that a child would pass the test if he or she showed few test errors and if these errors were randomly distributed across tested structures. Failure would be indicated by the presence of "numerous test errors" occurring throughout the test or consistently within particular structures. Further, it is stated that the examiner should watch for a child who consistently reduces the length or complexity of the response.

Regarding interpretation of the results of the OLSIDI, the authors state that any score "below 80 percent correct would demonstrate that a child was not demonstrating consistent knowledge and/or use of that specific test structure."

Evaluation of test adequacy   In general, it seems that these tests may offer some real value to the clinician working with children who display errors of syntax, a common component of the language-deficient child's disorder. The screening test is simple to administer, although there are no data to demonstrate whether it is truly sensitive in picking out children with real problems of syntax while ignoring children with normal syntactical performance. The diagnostic "deep" test, which clearly emanates from the screening test, provides a relatively rapid and systematic procedure for obtaining increased amounts of information regarding a child's production of specific structures. In this sense, the OLSIST and OLSIDI will be helpful to the clinician, especially to the clinician who is familiar enough with normal language development that his or her clinical judgment will be accurate in interpreting the results of these measures. There are, however, several important drawbacks to the design of these measures which must be pointed out.

Imitation as a Reflection of Spontaneous Production   One important issue is the question of the validity of a sentence imitation task as a correlate of a child's spontaneous language production. Certainly sentence imitation tests are popular (Lee 1971; Gray and Ryan 1973; Carrow 1974) because of the speed with which they can be administered, the variety of response forms which they can evoke, and the simplicity with which they can be analyzed and scored. However, intuitively there seem to be some critical differences between the behavior required of a child in imitating a sentence and in producing it spontaneously in a natural speaking situation. The absence of the meaningful semantic component of the sentence, that is, the child's intention to communicate a particular message, as well as the absence of the child's actual formulation of the sentence structure are two of the major differences in these two kinds of responses. Some research has indicated that children's responses on imitated sentences are comparable to their spontaneous language usage of the same structures (Brown and Fraser 1963; Lackner 1968; and Smith 1970). However, other researchers have argued against this finding (Menyuk 1963; Slobin and Welsh 1971). Perhaps the most recent refutation of this position is found in the work of Prutting, Gallagher, and Mulac (1975) who administered the expressive portion of the *Northwestern Syntax Screen Test* (qv) (Lee 1971) and compared the results with data obtained from spontaneous language samples from the same children. They found an average of 30 percent of the children correctly producing in their spontaneous speech grammatical distinctions that were in error on their NSST performances. Prutting et al. joined other researchers in stating that imitation tasks underestimate children's language performance.

The authors of the OLSIST and OLSIDI report a study conducted to address this particular issue. Twenty-three subjects, some of whom had either passed, failed, or performed at the borderline level of the screening test, were administered both the diagnostic "deep" test (OLSIDI) and a language sample. The methods of obtaining the language sample, the number of utterances emitted by the subjects, and the method of analyzing and scoring the language sample were not reported. The statistical analysis of the results of this comparison indicated that subjects who either passed or failed the

OLSIDI also passed or failed, respectively, the language sampling procedure. Although it is not clear how it was determined that a subject had failed the language sampling procedure, the fact that the authors demonstrated statistically that these two measures were not independent seems to be an irrelevant finding. Since the data were not analyzed structure by structure, one still cannot know whether the responses produced by the child on *particular* structures on the OLSIST or OLSIDI would be comparable with the child's spontaneous usage of those structures.

Test Construction Based on a Theoretical Rationale   A second issue of importance is the theoretical basis upon which these tests are based. Although the authors state that the test items are based upon the language development theories of Brown (1973), they test 23 morphological and grammatical structures while Brown has described the development of only 14 morphemes in the language of children through Stage V. It is unclear where the remaining structures tested come from. Whether the inclusion of these structures (indicated by the absence of asterisks on the morphemes listed in the appendix) is based on adult intuition, frequency of occurrence in the language of young children, or some other rationale should be clearly stated. Some of these structures, such as personal pronouns, Brown has stated cannot be pinpointed developmentally since they do not occur in obligatory contexts. Further, it is not clear from any data known to this reviewer that all of the 23 structures probed by these two tests should be present in the language produced by preschool, kindergarten, and first grade children. If all of these structures are not to be found regularly in the speech of normal language users of this age, how is the examiner to know which structures can be allowed to be in error?

Another theoretical issue which influences the design of these tests is related to the Mean Length of Utterance (MLU) variable that is so carefully controlled in these tests. It appears that the authors may be mixing the concepts of length and complexity by inferring that a child's omission of some of the sentence components necessarily reduces the complexity of the child's response. Brown has said that complexity and MLU are unrelated past the MLU of four morphemes. In the 290 sentences of the OLSIST and OLSIDI there are only three sentences of this length; all the rest are longer. Where variations in auditory memory span are concerned, however, systematic manipulation and control of MLU are probably relevant. However, the authors provide no data specifying the MLU which can be retained and repeated by normal subjects in the specified age range of three through seven years.

As is apparent from the above comments, little information regarding test construction is given in the two-page manual accompanying each test. Further, although the sentences included are generally interesting, no description of the vocabulary level of the tests' lexicon is given.

Clinical Judgment as a Replacement for Standardization and Normative Data   Another major issue is the importance of the examiner's clinical judgment in assessing the meaning of the tests' findings. Since no normative data have been collected by the authors, the examiner must rely on clinical judgment and the subjective guidelines provided by the authors for interpreting the test results. This is certainly a serious weakness of the tests but one which can be eliminated in the future if the authors or others were to undertake a rigorous normative study. It is the feeling of this reviewer that these tests would be worth the effort.

If the test were to be standardized, more information would have to be given in the manual regarding details of administration. An instruction is provided which the examiner reads to the child and then three imitative training trials are presented before the test begins. There are no guidelines as to whether stimulus sentences may be repeated, how to score a child's lack of response, or what to do regarding reinforcement. Edlund (1972) and Ayllon and Kelly (1972) have shown that positive reinforcement of correct responses increases a child's number of correct responses on standardized tests, thus inflating the final score. However, noncontingent presention of positive reinforcers is often appropriate and necessary to keep a child's attention to the task and evoke best attempts at performing. The instructions give no information to the examiner regarding the use or omission of stress in the modeled stimulus sentences. Several studies (Blasdell and Jensen 1970; Freedle, Keeney, and Smith 1970; Risley and Reynolds 1970; and Slobin and Welsh 1971) have shown children's imitations of certain portions of a stimulus sentence to be influenced by the emphasis given that portion of the stimulus sentence by the examiner.

Summary It is the impression of this reviewer that these two tests, a screening and diagnostic version of sentence imitation tests designed to sample the syntactic level of a child's language production, may be extremely useful to clinicians in terms of helping to select targets for treatment. These tests should also serve well as pre- and posttreatment measures to reflect changes in a child's language performance. Because of the problems discussed above it is suggested that these tests be used with caution and be supplemented by at least selective language sampling. Further development of these tests may alleviate many of the problems herein described.

Appendix: Structures tested in the OLSIST and OLSIDI

* present progressive	* contractible copula
* prepositions in	* contractible auxiliary
* prepositions on	pronouns
* plural (noun)	negatives—not, n't
* past irregular	wh-questions
* possessive	interrogative reversals
* uncontractible copula	modals
* articles	do insertions
* past regular	embedded sentences
* third person regular	infinitives
* third person irregular	coordinations or conjunctions
* uncontractible auxiliary	future tense

References

Ayllon, T. and K. Kelly Effects of reinforcement on standardized test performance. *J. Appl. Behav. Anal.* 5: 477–484, 1972.

* Morphemes described by Brown (1975). In Brown's listing, the prepositions in and on are counted as separate grammatical morphemes. In the OLSIST and OLSIDI, the two prepositions are combined and tallied as a single morpheme.

Blasdell, R. and P. Jensen   Stress and word position as determinants of imitation in first-language learners. *J. Speech Hear. Res.* 13: 193–202, 1970.

Brown, R.   *A First Language: The Early Stages.* Cambridge: Harvard University Press, 1973.

Brown, R. and C. Fraser   The acquisition of syntax. In C. N. Cofer and B. S. Musgrave (eds.), *Verbal Behavior and Learning: Problems and Processes.* New York: McGraw-Hill, 1973.

Carrow, E.   A test using elicited imitations in assessing grammatical structure in children. *J. Speech Hearing Dis.* 39: 437–444, 1974.

Edlund, C. V.   The effect on the behavior of children, as reflected in the IQ scores, when reinforced after each correct response. *J. Appl. Behav. Anal.* 5: 317–319, 1972.

Freedle, R. O., T. J. Keeney, and N. D. Smith   Effects of mean depth and grammaticality on children's imitations of sentences. *J. verb. Learn. verb. Behav.* 9: 149–154, 1970.

Gray, B. and B. Ryan   *A Language Program for the Nonlanguage Child.* Champaign, Ill.: Research Press, 1973.

Lackner, J. R.   A developmental study of language behavior in retarded children. *Neuropsychologia* 6: 301–320, 1968.

Lee, L. L.   *The Northwestern Syntax Screening Test.* Evanston, Ill.: Northwestern University Press, 1971.

Menyuk, P.   A preliminary evaluation of grammatical capacity in children. *J. verb. Learn. verb. Behav.* 2: 429–439, 1963.

Prutting, C. A., T. M. Gallagher, and A. Mulac   The expressive portion of the NSST compared to a spontaneous language sample. *J. Speech Hearing Dis.* 40: 40–48, 1975.

Risley, T. R. and N. J. Reynolds   Emphasis as a prompt for verbal imitation. *J. Appl. Behav. Anal.* 3: 185–190, 1970.

Slobin, D. I. and C. Welsh   Elicited imitations as a research tool in developmental psycholinguistics. In C. S. Lavatelli (ed.), *Language Training in Early Childhood Education.* Urbana: University of Illinois Press, 1971.

Smith, C. S.   An experimental approach to children's linguistic competence. In J. R. Hayes (ed.), *Cognition and the Development of Language.* New York: Wiley, 1970.

PEABODY PICTURE VOCABULARY TEST (PPVT)

Lloyd M. Dunn

American Guidance Service, 1965

Two equivalent forms, A and B

Cost $14.00, regular edition; $19.50, special plastic edition
Manual, 51 pages, $2.25; series of plates, regular edition, $9.40; series of plates, special plastic edition, $14.60; individual test records, 4 pages, pack of 50 for $3.65 (specify form); individual test records, pack of 50 with 25 of Form A and 25 of Form B for $3.65

Time 10–15 minutes, administration; 5–10 minutes, scoring

Paul S. Weiner *University of Chicago*

Purpose The Peabody Picture Vocabulary Test is intended, according to the manual, ". . . to provide an estimate of a subjects's *verbal intelligence* through measuring his hearing vocabulary" (Dunn 1965, p. 25).

Administration, scoring, and interpretation An individual, untimed test, the PPVT requires about 10 to 15 minutes to administer. It consists of a book of 150 test plates and three example plates, each containing four pictures numbered to allow for ready identification. The same set of plates is used for each of the two forms (A and B) of the test. The examiner administers the test by exposing a plate and pronouncing a word represented by one of the pictures. The subject points to or indicates in some fashion, the picture that has been named. The manual provides suggestions about the point on the word list at which testing might best begin for various age levels. The subject must respond to enough words to establish a basal and a ceiling.

The test blank lists the words to be read to the subject and the numbers of the correct choices. It provides spaces to mark the numbers of the pictures chosen and separate spaces to mark incorrect responses. This allows the examiner to determine the basal and ceiling readily. Space is also provided to note identifying information and other data that might be useful or necessary in interpreting the results.

The raw score is simply the sum of correct responses. Tables in the manual permit the conversion of the raw score into a mental age (age equivalent), intelligence quotient (standard score equivalent), or percentile equivalent. A classification table for intelligence quotients is also given (very slow learners, average learners, and so forth).

Evaluation of test adequacy In constructing the PPVT, the author of the test started with a search of the 1953 edition of *Webster's New Collegiate Dictionary* for words that could be depicted by means of line drawings. A total of 3885 words were found, and drawings were prepared for approximately half of these. On the basis of a tryout with 360 subjects, ages two through 18 years, 200 pretest plates were prepared from these drawings, each depicting four words. Pretesting with 750 subjects permitted the selection of the best 300 words and the final construction of the 150 plates used in the published test. These were arranged in order of difficulty based on empirical findings.

The final test was standardized on a sample of 4012 white children who lived in or near Nashville, Tennessee. They ranged in age from two years, six months through 18 years. The selection of the children was made according to different methods at various age levels. The preschool children were chosen on the basis of their residence in an area served by schools whose pupils had IQ scores on the Kuhlmann-Finch Intelligence Test which formed a composite normal probability curve. At the primary level scores on the Metropolitan Readiness Test were used for first and second grade children, while those on the Kuhlmann-Finch Intelligence Test were used in the third grade. Random samples were selected until a normal distribution of scores was approximated. Samples at the higher levels apparently included all the children in four elementary, two junior high, and two senior high schools. The Kuhlmann-Finch IQ's of the pupils in these schools approximated a composite normal probability curve. Except at the levels of two years, six months and three years, each age sample contained at least 100 children. All subjects were tested within a period of three months.

Since its publication, the PPVT has been popular both for clinical use and for investigation. In a search of entries in the *Psychological Abstracts* for the period 1967 through 1976, the reviewer found 121 published studies using the test. In a personal communication the author of the test noted that a 1974 computer bibliographical search turned up 258 abstracts on validity and reliability. Reviews of the PPVT are available in the Buros' *Sixth Mental Measurements Yearbook* (1965) and in Sattler's *Assessment of Children's Intelligence* (1974).

No attempt was made to cover all the literature on reliability and validity for this review. However, the studies covered and the material in available summarizations provide sufficient consistency to lend a considerable degree of confidence to the conclusions drawn. Reliability studies have generally been concerned with the equivalence of the alternate forms of the test. The manual lists reliability coefficients for the standardization group ranging from .67 for subjects at six years of age to .84 at 16 and 17 years. The median of .77 for this group is exactly that found by Sattler (1974) in 14 subsequent studies. The range in these studies was considerable, extending from .37 to .97. Test-retest studies reveal comparable temporal stability, the median coefficient being .73 (range, .28 to .97).

A number of aspects of the validity of the PPVT have either been discussed in the manual or formally evaluated in relevant research. Dunn presents the claim that content validity ". . . was built into the test when a complete search was made of *Webster's New Collegiate Dictionary* . . . for all words whose meanings could be depicted by a picture" (Dunn 1965, p. 32). He also claims support for construct validity in the repeated finding that vocabulary test results are the best single predictor of overall intellectual functioning and of school success.

Most formal validity studies have been concerned with concurrent validity. The most frequently used test for such comparisons has been the Stanford-Binet Intelligence Scale (S-B). The findings have varied greatly, with the median correlation coefficient between IQ results approximating .70. The results with the Wechsler Intelligence Scale for Children (WISC) have been comparable. As might be expected, the relationship has been closer with verbal IQ and lower with performance IQ. Interestingly, results on the recent revision of the WISC (WISC-R, 1974) and the restandardization of the S-B (1973) appear to show a closer relationship to the PPVT results than did those based on the earlier norms (personal communication from the author).

Equal in importance to the correlation coefficients are comparisons of intelligence levels found on the tests. The results have tended to vary according to the nature of the groups studied. Investigations of retarded subjects have usually resulted in PPVT IQ's higher than those found on the S-B or the WISC. In contrast, disadvantaged children have been found to have PPVT IQ's lower than those found on the S-B.

Some attempts have been made to relate performance on the PPVT to performance on other language tests. Unfortunately, the studies have been too few and the populations studied too varied to provide an adequate basis for evaluation.

Several studies have involved children with delayed language development. In one of these (Spellacy and Black 1972) children diagnosed as having "a primary language impairment" on neurological examination had significantly lower IQ scores on the PPVT than on a nonverbal intelligence test, the Arthur Adaptation of the Leiter International Performance Scale. The authors suggest that the difference between the results on the two tests might provide a useful estimate of the degree of language impairment.

There are many positive aspects to the PPVT. The pictures are clearly drawn and attractive. The administration of the test is brief and simple, requiring no special knowledge or extensive training on the part of the examiner. Scoring is objective and easily accomplished. The test blank is a model of simplicity and completeness, and the manual is well organized, simply written, and comprehensive. Test construction and standardization were carefully done. In addition the test is readily adaptable to the needs of various special groups of children who have limited ability to frame verbal or even motor responses. Finally, a wealth of information about the test is available in the research literature. It seems clearly to be the best of the currently available picture vocabulary tests. The pictures in the PPVT are far simpler and clearer than those in the Full-Range Picture Vocabulary Test (qv) or the Quick Test. Also the standardization seems to be much better than on either of these tests.

Inevitably there are also criticisms that can be made of the test. The IQ tables are unnecessarily limited. Through four years eight months (4-8 years), six-month age classifications are used (e.g., 3-3 to 3-8 years). Following one nine-month interval (4-9 to 5-5 years), 12-month intervals are used. The result is unacceptable leaps in IQ values. At the extreme, a child who is 5-5 years and achieves a raw score of 46 receives an IQ of 92; if the child is 5-6 years, the same raw score earns an IQ of 81. Further, the standardization group, however large and carefully selected, is a narrowly delineated one. It is clearly representative of only one ethnic group in one southern city in the United States. Supplementary studies are needed to determine how widely applicable the norms are.

While reliability seems to be acceptable both in relation to alternate form and temporal stability (though perhaps more for group studies than for individual diagnosis), validity is a far more complicated issue. The essential question is whether the PPVT is valid for the uses to which it is being put. When it is interpreted as a measure of the comprehension of receptive vocabulary, no major problems arise. If the standardization norms are appropriate for the group with which the test is being used, interpretation is essentially straightforward. The use of the test as a measure of general language adequacy (as suggested by Spellacy and Black) is more hazardous. The insufficient amount of research on the relationship of the PPVT to other language measures and the mixed results obtained make this an uncertain procedure.

The use of the PPVT as a measure of verbal intelligence is the greatest departure from the obvious content of the test. The correlational results with the S–B and the WISC, as already noted, have been variable but generally quite acceptable and indicate considerable overlap between the PPVT and these other tests in what they measure. However, scores on the tests are not interchangeable. For one, the correlations also indicate considerable independence of function in the various tests. Further, it has been found that the PPVT either overestimates or underestimates IQ scores on the major intelligence tests for several crucial groups, the retarded and the disadvantaged.

One frequent use of the test is as a screening instrument to select children who need a fuller evaluation. Another frequent use is to help decide whether a child might profit from a remedial or therapeutic program. In each of these instances it is not the specific IQ that is of interest but rather the classification of the child's level of functioning. What is of concern is the accuracy of classification judgments ("hit-rate") or the extent to which judgments made on the basis of the PPVT are borne out by succeeding events. Unfortunately little work of this sort has been done. In the one relevant study known to the reviewer (Shaw, Matthew and Kløve 1966), the classifications made on the basis of the PPVT did not accord well with those made from performance on the WISC. Additional studies of this type are much needed.

Summary   Because of its many positive features, the PPVT has been and remains a popular test. From the present survey of findings, it must be agreed that the PPVT cannot be used for all the purposes for which it has been suggested without considerable caution. It clearly may be used as a test of auditory receptive vocabulary with only the uncertainty occasioned by the restricted standardization sample. Its use as a test of general language adequacy is a much less certain matter. Much the same must be said about its employment as a measure of verbal intelligence. The PPVT is a "valid" test in the sense that it has considerable overlap in what it measures with the generally accepted individual intelligence tests. However, there is a lack of information on the use of the PPVT in making the kind of judgments that are most frequently needed in clinical situations. Nonetheless, with well considered use, the PPVT can measure up to its potential as a helpful, but not necessarily primary, clinical diagnostic instrument.

References

Buros, O. K.   (ed.), *The Sixth Mental Measurements Yearbook*. Highland Park, N. J.: Gryphon Press, 1965.

Dunn, L. M.   *Expanded Manual for the Peabody Picture Vocabulary Test*. Circle Pines, Minn.: American Guidance Service, 1965.

Sattler, J. M.   *Assessment of Children's Intelligence*. Philadelphia: W. B. Saunders, 1974.

Shaw, D. J., C. G. Matthews, and H. Kløve   The equivalence of WISC and PPVT IQ's. *Am. J. ment. Defic.* 70: 601–604, 1966.

Spellacy, F. and F. W. Black   Intelligence assessment of language-impaired children by means of two nonverbal tests. *J. clin. Psychol.* 28: 357–358, 1972.

PICTURE ARTICULATION AND LANGUAGE SCREENING TEST (PALST)

William C. Rodgers

Word Making Productions, 1976

Cost $18.00, includes picture booklet and 24 record forms

Record forms, 1 page; picture booklet, 13 pictures

Time 2-3 minutes, administration and scoring

Doris P. Bradley *Institute of Logopedics, Wichita, Kansas*

Purpose To screen pupils in classroom settings for language and articulation errors.

Administration, scoring, and interpretation This test is quick to give, is easy to manipulate, and has colorful pictures. Administration of the first six items is accomplished by pointing to a specific action depicted in a picture and asking a question to elicit from a child a complete phrase. The next six pictures are designed to elicit naming and thus single-word responses for later developing articulation skills. The last three pictures are designed to elicit the phonemes, /s/, /ʃ/, and /tʃ/ in isolation. Articulation errors are scored for initial and final positions and written in the seven columns of the score sheet. Language responses are recorded with a plus sign for complete phrase, a check mark for incomplete phrase or single word, and a minus sign for no response. Each plus is worth two points, each check is worth one point.

If a child achieves eight points on language responses on the first six pictures (twelve possible points), it is considered a passing score. Criterion is not stated for passing the articulation section of the test.

Evaluation of test adequacy Test construction is considered adequate in terms of selection of items, durability of materials, clarity of pictures, and instructions for administration. Test construction is considered inadequate in terms of the sampling obtained for language skills, criterion of pass/fail in articulation, and design of the score sheet which does not follow the presentation order of the items in the test booklet.

Strengths of the test are brevity of administration, convenience of recording results for seven children on the same score sheet, and durable and attractive stimulus material. Weaknesses of the test are the lack of a pass/fail score in articulation, inconvenience of score sheet design, selection of only the most frequent error sounds for testing, and severe limitation of language sample.

Summary This test may find its best application in age levels three through five years. Its simplicity makes its usefulness in school ages questionable. No data are offered in terms of the predictive value of the test or its reliability in identifying children with communication problems. The test guidelines do not indicate the age levels the authors believe appropriate.

PORCH INDEX OF COMMUNICATIVE ABILITY IN CHILDREN (PICAC)

Bruce E. Porch

Consulting Psychologists Press, 1975

Time   One hour

Norma S. Rees *Graduate School, City University of New York*

Purpose   The purpose of the Porch Index of Communicative Ability in Children, as stated in Volume 2 of the test manual, is to measure the child's communicative ability in a sensitive and reliable fashion. The results of the test may be used: (1) to determine the level of the child's communicative functioning; (2) as baseline data against which to measure changes over time or the effects of remediation; and (3) to provide "differential diagnostic, prognostic, and therapeutic information." The last listed is described by the author as the "ultimate purpose" yet to be fully realized as research using this instrument continues.

Administration, scoring, and interpretation   At the time of this review the PICAC was available only in a preliminary, and therefore incomplete, research edition. For that reason this review can be regarded only as tentative, raising some issues that may well be resolved in the final clinical edition. The research edition includes sufficient detail to permit an examiner to administer the test and score the responses, but interpretation of the scores is not possible because normative data are not given. Similarly, standardization studies and reliability data have yet to be published. In personal communication, the author indicates that Volume 1 of the manual, in preparation, will also deal with the test's clinical applicability and contain material useful for diagnostic, predictive, and remedial decision making.

The test consists of two batteries, Basic and Advanced. The Basic Battery, for preschool children, consists of 15 subtests; the Advanced Battery, for children from 6 to 12 years, consists of 20 subtests. Actually, 13 of the subtests appear in both batteries, with some variations in administration, so that the total number of different subtests in both batteries is only 22. All but one of the 22 subtests revolve around the same set of ten common objects arranged before the subject: comb, crayon, fork, key, pencil, penny, ring, scissors, spoon, and toothbrush.

The subtests are classified by "modality": verbal, gestural, reading, auditory, visual, and graphic. These modality groupings refer to the type of response required of the subject. In the five verbal subtests the child is required to give spoken responses ranging from single words ("Tell me the name of each of these") to sentences ("Tell me what you do with each of these"). The gestural subtest requires the child to pantomime ("Show me what you do with each of these"). Three subtests of reading require the child to read single words, words printed backwards, or sentences, in order to respond by placing cards correctly. The three auditory subtests require the child to follow directions spoken by the examiner. Two visual subtests require the child to match pictured objects with actual objects or to match duplicate objects with each other. The eight graphic subtests require the child to draw; to copy words, geometric shapes, or pictures; to write from dictation; or to write responses ("Write the names of each of these" and "Write what you do with each of these").

The test is administered individually. One hour is regarded as the usual total time for testing, but the child may be given as much time as needed. The test objects are placed before the child in predetermined order. The examiner administers each subtest in a standard order, instructing the child to respond according to the requirements of each subtest and recording the responses on a score sheet.

Because the PICAC is specifically designed to maximize an examiner's ability to derive quantified data about a child's communicative behavior, the procedures for administering the subtests and especially for scoring the responses are presented in great detail. The manual states that about 40 hours of training and practice are required for clinicians to achieve tester reliability, a concept central to the PICAC.

The principles and procedures for scoring are particularly elaborate. The author states that the scoring system is the "most important and the most difficult aspect of administering the PICAC." The system itself is described as multidimensional and binary. Briefly, subjects' responses are scored on five dimensions: accuracy, responsiveness, completeness, promptness, and efficiency. Using these dimensions as questions about the "rightness" of each response, the examiner selects one of 16 categories that best fits the response, recording the category as the score for that response. The higher the category on the 16-point scale, the better the response in terms of the five dimensions of "rightness." The scoring system can also be described as binary in that the examiner distinguishes between possible and impossible categories by answering questions like "Was the response accurate?" A yes answer, in this case, eliminates all categories below 8. By a series of successive questions producing such binary choices, additional categories are eliminated until only one category remains to be entered as the score for that response. Throughout the test manual, extensive examples of responses to each subtest and scoring guidelines are given to aid the clinician in learning how to use the scoring system.

From the subtest scores, mean scores for individual modalities as well as overall means may be derived.

Evaluation of test adequacy   In the introductory comments in the manual the purpose is given as measurement of the child's communication ability. Chapter III in Volume 2 of the manual includes a model of communication upon which, presumably, the test is based. The model is basically that of Osgood (1963), expanded to account for three types of input (visual, auditory, and tactile) and three types of output (graphic, verbal, and gestural). These input–output categories are the source of the "modalities" of the various subtests. No explanation is offered in Volume 2 for the overall structure of the test in terms of the specific subtests and their relation to the underlying model. It is possible that more information about this issue will be available in the final version of the test manual.

Whether the underlying model of communication is adequate to the test's purpose is a different kind of question. The author states his conclusion that this test may not assess language ability according to psycholinguistic considerations, and while it is certainly true that most recent tests of children's language have centered on aspects of syntactic structure and are thus very different from the content of the PICAC, it is also true that Osgood's model was the basis for the widely used Illinois Test of Psycholinguistic Abilities (qv) (1968). Current approaches to the study of language in communication have deviated both from the Osgood model and the syntactic emphasis. In any case, the Osgood-type model does not appear to provide an adequate framework for the study or the measurement of communication ability.

An examination of the subtests in terms of the PICAC's stated purpose also raises many questions. Reasons for so heavy an emphasis on visual and writing skills are not offered. Some of the subtests do not appear to tap any skill that may be considered communicative: among these are the tasks requiring subjects to copy geometric shapes, read words printed backwards, and imitate spoken nouns. Whether it is really necessary or even possible to measure perception as a separate "communicative" ability is also worth asking. On the other hand, in the case of a complex subtest like the one requiring the child to demonstrate the function of each test object via gesture, the manual states that this task requires the ability to "integrate a visual or tactile association with past experience and then to conceptualize, formulate, and express an idea gesturally." Regrettably, it would be difficult to know just which of these skills is weak when the child's performance on this task is poor. Some of the simpler subtests, moreover, appear to have more diagnostic than descriptive value: an example is the subtest requiring the child to match pictures with objects. Measuring a child's communication ability in terms of a given model of communication may not be the central purpose or ultimate usefulness of this test. Many of these and other questions about the subtests may be resolved when the theoretical background and task selection principles are more fully explicated in the final test version. What is needed is a more complete account of the principles underlying the decisions about what kinds of verbal (and related) behaviors are sampled, for what reasons, and to what ends.

The major contribution of the PICAC, insofar as it can be determined from the research edition, lies in the careful design of procedures for administering and scoring. No other test of child language offers the opportunity to assess so wide a range of behaviors in so systematic and refined a fashion, and with such meticulous attention to tester reliability. A minor point concerns the concept of a 16-point scale applied to easy tasks as well as difficult ones: for easy tasks the intervals between points on the scale are smaller than for difficult tasks, and the points on the scale therefore have different absolute values for each of the subtests. This potential problem can be overcome by developing normative data for each subtest on each battery separately, but as already noted the norms are not included in the research edition.

Summary The value of the PICAC for assessment as well as for diagnostic, prognostic, and remedial decisions has yet to be demonstrated. Until the final edition is available and clinical research utilizing this test is reported, no reasonable conclusions can be reached. In the research edition, the PICAC emerges as a combination of procedural strengths and theoretical weakness. Some of the latter may disappear in the final edition.

References

Kirk, S. A., J. J. McCarthy, and W. D. Kirk *The Illinois Test of Psycholinguistic Abilities* (Revised ed.). Urbana: University of Illinois Press, 1968.

Osgood, C. E. On understanding and creating sentences. *American Psychologist* **18**: 735–751, 1963.

PRESCHOOL LANGUAGE SCALE (PLS)

Irla Lee Zimmerman,
Violette G. Steiner, and
Roberta L. Evatt

Charles E. Merrill Publishing Company, 1969

Cost $5.00

Manual, 85 pages; Picture book, 34 pages; Scoring booklet, 16 pages

Time Dependent on establishment of basal age

Charlotte G. Wells *University of Missouri—Columbia*

Purpose The Preschool Language Scale was devised by a child psychologist, a child development specialist, and speech–language pathologist. The authors report that the scale can be used "with children of all ages who are presumed to be functioning at a preschool or primary language level." The scale was designed to isolate areas of strengths and deficiencies in two aspects of language—auditory comprehension and verbal ability. Hence it is really two scales, providing "language ages" for auditory comprehension (AC) and for verbal ability (VA) or a single "language age" for the combination of the two aspects.

Administration, scoring, and interpretation In each of the two parts of the scale, four items are used to assess a child's performance at each of ten age levels, from 1.5 years to 4.5 years at six-month intervals and at 5, 6, and 7 years. The examiner begins by administering the four items, for AC or for VA, for an age level slightly below the child's estimated ability. If the child misses an item, the examiner goes back to find the age level at which the child succeeds in passing all four items. This age level becomes the "basal age."

Testing continues from the "basal age" to the point at which the child misses all four items at an age level. If the child passes any item at an age level, the next group of items must be administered. Each of the child's responses is recorded in full in the scoring booklet to permit the examiner to review the scoring process and study the styles of the responses. Some items appear at more than one age level, but an item passed or failed the first time it is presented is shown as passed or failed at all subsequent levels on which the item appears.

The following are examples of items that are used in the scale: at the earliest age level (1.5 years), the child is required to follow two instructions given verbally (AC) or to name one picture (VA). At the 3.5-year level, the child is given such tasks as pointing to the wheels on a pictured car or giving his or her full name. At the 5-year level, the child is asked to show the examiner eight different body parts (AC) or to name six animals in one minute (VA). One item in the assessment of auditory comprehension at the 7-year level asks the child to touch the right thumb with the right little finger, and one item in the evaluation of verbal ability at the level requires the child to give his or her home address.

Each item is scored by determining, from directions in an accompanying manual, whether or not the response is acceptable. For each item at each age level, a value in months is assigned, one and one-half months of credit being given for each correct response at the first eight age levels, three months of credit being given for each correct response at age levels 6 and 7.

The total score for each of the two scales can be computed by adding credits for the basal age and those for items above the basal that were correct. Auditory comprehension age and verbal ability age can then be obtained. Each of these can be converted to a quotient (AC/CA × 100 or VA/CA × 100, where AC is the auditory comprehension age, VA is the verbal ability age, and CA is the chronological age). A total "language age" can be computed by summing AC and VA and dividing by 2, and a "language quotient" can be derived by using the formula LA/CA × 100, where LA is the "language age" and CA is the chronological age. The manual does not discuss interpretation of the various scores that can be obtained.

The two parts of the Preschool Language Scale are differentiated in terms of administration and scoring, appearing in parallel columns on the pages of the scoring booklet. The manual contains descriptions of the kinds of responses that can be considered correct and also provides a rationale for each of the items. References following the descriptions of the items in the manual indicate the sources from which the auditory and verbal language tasks were drawn.

Evaluation of test adequacy   No information on reliability or validity appeared in the manual available to the reviewer; but the authors state that "this scale is not a test, but an evaluation instrument, still in experimental form, to be used to detect language strengths and weaknesses." Explanations in the manual make administration of the items a relatively easy task, and no unusual amount of specialized training is required for the speech-language pathologist who wishes to use the Preschool Language Scale.

Although the scale cannot be considered a standardized test at this time, it can be useful for obtaining a variety of information about two aspects of a child's language if the child is functioning linguistically at or below the 7-year level, regardless of chronological age. The evaluation of verbal ability includes some items on the 5-, 6-, and 7-year levels that permit assessment of phonological skills but, in general, the scale focuses on auditory comprehension and verbal ability without regard to articulation.

Certain problems are inherent in any procedure for evaluating the performance of young children, and the authors recognize these in their instructions. They add that an interpreter might be used with children who do not understand nor speak English if the interpreter is trained to avoid giving clues or saying more than is stipulated in the standard directions.

The test provides the purchaser with a manual, a spiral-bound set of pictures to be used as stimuli, and one scoring booklet. Additional scoring booklets will be needed, one being used for each child evaluated. The manual contains complete directions for administering and scoring the items. The pictures are clear, in color, and on good paper stock; but the picture book takes only a limited amount of wear before losing its plastic spiral binding. The scoring booklets are of appropriate size for insertion in standard folders; and, like the manual, they contain directions for the administration and scoring of each item. The purchaser is expected to obtain the following additional materials: 12 one-inch blocks in the primary colors, one small piece of coarse sandpaper, a set of coins (penny, nickel, dime, quarter, and half-dollar), and a watch or clock with a second hand. None of these additional materials is costly, and none is difficult to obtain.

Summary   Certain characteristics of the scale differentiate it from such other instruments as the Houston Test for Language Development, the Northwestern Syntax Screening Test, the Denver Developmental Screening Test, the Communicative Evaluation Chart, the Receptive-Expressive Emergent Language Scale, and the Verbal Language Development Scale (qv). The Preschool Language Scale looks at two aspects of language, the auditory and the verbal. It covers a range from 18 months to seven years in terms of "language ages," and it can provide more information than can be obtained from "screening" tests. The limitation of the number of items to four at each age level shortens administration time. The scale obtains all of its information from direct observation of a child's performance rather than from reports by informants. In general, for its stated purpose, the Preschool Language Scale is a useful instrument.

RECEPTIVE-EXPRESSIVE EMERGENT LANGUAGE SCALE (REEL Scale)

Kenneth R. Bzoch and
Richard League

The Tree of Life Press, 1971

Cost Handbook and 25 recording forms, $17.50

Time 20 minutes, administration and scoring

James D. MacDonald *Ohio State University*

Purpose According to the authors, the motivation behind the Receptive-Expressive Emergent Language Scale was "the need for an effective means of identifying very young children who may have specific handicaps requiring habilitative and educational intervention." Beginning with the startle response (0-1 month), the test extends to a 36-month level. Six items (three expressive, three receptive) are listed for each one-month interval through the first year. The second year items span two-month intervals; the third year, three-month intervals.

Administration, scoring, and interpretation The REEL Scale is administered principally through a parent or informant interview. The instructions allow considerable license in probing for information on each item. The manual recommends but does not require direct observation of the child in order to confirm questionable parent responses. Individual items are scored as "plus," "minus," or "emergent." Adequate scoring requires clear communication between the interviewer and informant since the interviewer must reliably explain each item behavior in objective terms. Three scores are available: Receptive Language Age, Expressive Language Age, and Combined Age. A total language quotient is derived from an equation that weights the receptive and expressive items equally. The weighting makes the tenuous assumption that receptive and expressive skills are parallel at all levels of early development.

Evaluation of test adequacy The test items "were obtained, in part, through a search of the developmental literature. However, every item found in research reports or existing scales was reconfirmed through laboratory tests over several years" (Handbook, p. 19). The handbook does not state how the items were selected for each age range in the scale. Two of three correct reports qualify a child for an age level score; no report is made of the item–age match. Further, no information on the normative population is provided except the statement (p. 19) that

> the infants studied in the "normative item development" phase of the REEL project were selected to represent the probable norm of environmentally language-advantaged Caucasian infants. [No numbers, ages, or demographic information are provided. Support for the test's validity is limited to unpublished] pilot studies that reveal the REEL scores correlate positively with intelligence and social maturity scores.

Test–retest reliability was determined on 28 normal infants from linguistically stimulating environments tested by graduate students untrained in the REEL Scale. Test–retest agreement within plus or minus one age interval ranged from 90 to 100 percent. Limited description of procedures make interpretation of such reliability difficult. No clinical or diagnostic validity of the REEL Scale is reported in the manual.

In this reviewer's judgment, age scores are not warranted from a test that samples only three behaviors at each age range. No data are presented on the variability of the item behaviors, but one would expect great variability at early developmental stages. While the test is useful in identifying a sequence of behaviors in a child's repertoire, the procedures for item selection, the subjective administration techniques, and the limited validation efforts prevent any carefully reasoned reliance on the age score interpretations.

The manual specifies eight theoretical principles to follow in interpreting test results. These principles come from observational studies of normal infants and from the authors' interpretations of data from early developmental studies. No direct research support is offered for the principles. Certain of the principles, in fact, are highly questionable. For example, the one (p. 32) stating that receptive language development is "more dependent upon genetic factors and the integrity of the nervous system" could have serious implications should clinicians follow the authors' interpretive suggestions. Another principle states that patterns of discrepancy among receptive language, expressive language, and chronological age have significant diagnostic meaning. The authors do not document this principle but simply state that such discrepancies indicate specific disorders such as retardation, autism, and deafness. Little in the theoretical or empirical development of the test seems to warrant use of the age scores.

The REEL Scale provides a sequence of 66 behavioral items each for expressive and receptive language performance for the purported age periods of birth to 36 months. While the scale appears to have serious limitations in item selection, theoretical support, and validation, it is clinically useful as a report of a range of early vocal, symbolic, and communicative behaviors. Clinicians with sound developmental training should be able to use the scale as a screening device for clients needing further assessment.

The REEL Scale should not be viewed as a diagnostic tool. The items and age determinations have such minimal empirical and theoretical support as to render it virtually useless in diagnosing particular disorders or prescribing language program direction. One clinical use may be in a rough differentiation between receptive and expressive language performance. The gap between what a child knows and what the child communicates may be tapped by the REEL Scale in a way that can direct a clinician to further diagnostic probing. Another potential use of the REEL Scale may be as an interview format for establishing a common ground between parents and professionals concerning a child's language development.

Summary The REEL Scale allows informants to report on a range of behaviors involved in expressive and receptive language development. While it makes the important distinction between reception and expression, it presents a rather random sample of behaviors not clearly related to any theories of development or empirical support. The test does not clearly distinguish among speech, language, and communication behaviors; such a failure makes systematic diagnostic follow-up difficult. Heavy emphasis on vocal speech aspects may limit its use with populations (e.g., cerebral palsy, Down's syndrome) whose speech production skills may be physiologically limited. As an initial screening instrument, the REEL Scale is easy to administer and yields potentially useful points for later diagnostic testing. The validity of the age scores is highly questionable; a strong recommendation must be made that they not be used.

THE RILEY ARTICULATION AND LANGUAGE TEST (RALT)

Glyndon D. Riley

Western Psychological Services, 1971

Cost $8.50

Examiner's manual, 5 pages; test booklet, 4 pages

Time 2–3 minutes to administer and score

Thomas J. O'Toole *Montgomery County (Maryland) Public Schools*

Purpose The Riley Articulation and Language Test (RALT) is designed to accomplish the following:

1 Use but 2–3 minutes of administration time. (This time was revised from 1–2 minutes in the original edition because an estimate of language proficiency and an estimate of intelligibility are now obtained.)

2 Provide an estimate of language proficiency.

3 Provide an estimate of intelligibility.

4 Provide an objective articulation loss score that can be an index of speech loss and speech function. Such an objective score can serve to determine the possibility of spontaneous remissions.

5 Provide a standardized language loss score and language function score.

The RALT has been standardized on children in kindergarten, Head Start, first grade, and second grade. It provides normative data for boys and girls coming from homes of low and middle socioeconomic status.

Administration, scoring, and interpretation The examiner must have sufficient knowledge of articulation disorders to recognize quickly differences between substitutions, distortions, and omissions, and be able to decide when a sound has been produced correctly after stimulation. A knowledge of phonetics is essential if substitutions are to be noted accurately.

The examiner begins by obtaining a language sample, Subtest A: Language Proficiency and Intelligibility, by asking the child to tell a familiar children's story, such as "The Three Bears" or by showing pictures in a children's book and having the child tell a story about them. Such a procedure allows the examiner to obtain a Language Proficiency Estimate and Intelligibility Estimate, neither of which is normed. The Language Proficiency Estimate is made by deciding whether the child's language is normal, somewhat abnormal, or severely abnormal with regard to: (1) willingness to talk, (2) length of phrases, (3) complexity of phrases (use of plurals, pronouns, prepositions, verb forms, etc.), and (4) ability to follow directions. If unable to determine the child's ability to follow directions, the examiner can ask the child to perform a simple and a complex task appropriate for the child's age. The examiner rates each area on a three-point scale: 0 = Normal, 1 = Somewhat abnormal, and 2 = Severely abnormal. A total score of two or more points indicates that further language assessment should be undertaken. The Intelligibility Estimate is determined by marking on a five-point scale: Complete Intelligibility = 100 percent; Intelligible except for a word now and then = 76 to 99 percent; about Half Intelligible = 25 to 75 percent; Unintelligible except for a word now and then = 1 to 24 percent; Completely unintelligible = 0 percent.

Next, the examiner moves to Subtest B: Articulation Function by saying each of eight words and having the child repeat each one aloud. If the child makes an incorrect response, it is noted in the "incorrect" column. Columns are included for substitutions, omissions, and distortions. Each sound error is given a predetermined weighted number or loss score. The degree of stimulability of each sound is given a weighted score. Errors are scored only for the sounds underlined in the test words. The author cites as an example: "mov" for "smooth" would be scored as "v" for "th" and be a substitution error; the "s" omission would be ignored in the scoring. If errors are made, the examiner tests the child for stimulability by saying the word and having the child "say the word just like I do." The child has two tries on each word. If the child fails to say the sound correctly, the number in the "Not Stimulable" column in the Protocol Booklet is circled to indicate that additional points are to be substituted for this sound, thus increasing the loss score. The Articulation Function is determined by adding the loss score for each word and then adding the total and subtracting from 100.

Next the examiner goes to Subtest C: Language Function and says the first of six sentences and directs the child to "listen carefully and say it after me." The examiner is reminded to reassure the child as the child approaches his or her limits. Each sentence also has a weighted score. The sentences have the following numbers of syllables: (1) four, (2) six, (3) eight, (4) ten, (5) twelve, and (6) fourteen. All but the first sentence are personalized by use of the pronoun "I," deal with topics of interest to children, and contain simple words. The last sentence is more complex as it contains four multisyllabic words, including the comparative "better." If the child fails to repeat a sentence but makes some attempt that is not phonetically accurate, credit is not given for the first try but a second try is offered. To receive credit, syllables must have stress and intonation resembling the examiner's model. Failures are circled in the Protocol Booklet. The first and second sentences have the same first try weighted score and all others have different weighted scores. Failures on two consecutive items constitute the ceiling; testing is halted and all the remaining numbers are circled. If two consecutive items are passed on the *first* try, this constitutes the floor, and errors prior to this are not counted. For example, if a child scores correctly on the second and third sentences on the first try, after missing the first sentence, the first sentence error is not counted against the child. Language Function score is determined by adding all the circled numbers and subtracting the sum from 100.

The author suggests three possible classifications based on the RALT scores but notes that the limitations of such classifications must be considered. A high score on articulation and low scores on language often demonstrate central nervous system damage on further diagnosis. Low articulation and high language scores may have peripheral etiologies such as malocclusion or cleft palate. Low articulation and language scores may indicate mental retardation.

Evaluation of test adequacy The RALT, which was revised in 1971, is accompanied by a manual and a protocol booklet. The revision appears to have addressed some earlier shortcomings in that a language proficiency measure has been added and an intelligibility estimate is made utilizing a specified language sample. However, even though the first grade sample population has been expanded, standardization data are still interpolated from those of adjacent age subgroups. Age, geographic, and ethnic data of the standardization groups are still unspecified. The test has been expanded for use with a Head Start population. The sounds tested in the articulation functions section are appropriate. The validity of the clinical observations related to test interpretation is in need of investigation.

A review of the literature, including an ERIC search, failed to turn up more than one reference to the use of the test. The test is easy to administer and to score. The norms for language and articulation are given on the score sheets, adding to the rapidity of scoring. The research potential is apparent; however, in over ten years, little evidence of widespread use is found. The biggest weakness is that the test fails to give the amount of information that the speech–language pathologist working in the schools needs in this time of Individual Education Plans and parental permission. Other tests such as the McDonald Deep Test of Articulation (qv), the Goldman-Fristoe Test of Articulation (qv), and the Bankson Language Screening Test (qv), while taking a bit longer, give more of the kind of information needed.

Summary This test is easy to administer and easy to score. It would be of value in certain research studies. Its value in the public schools must be weighed with the matter of how much information one should obtain during the initial contact with the child referred for evaluation. Other tests take longer but give much more information. If screening of all children in a class or at a grade level is the goal, then this test has much to offer.

SCALES OF EARLY COMMUNICATION SKILLS FOR HEARING IMPAIRED CHILDREN	Central Institute for the Deaf, 1975
	Cost Manual with 1 scale, $7.50; 25 scales, $3.00 per package
	Examiner's manual, 42 pages; test blank, 4 pages
Jean S. Moog and Ann V. Geers	Time Depends on stage of child's development

Julia Davis *University of Iowa*

Purpose The authors describe the Scales of Early Communication Skills for Hearing Impaired Children as a test that provides a means of evaluating the "speech and language development" of young hearing impaired children between the ages of two and eight. It is designed for use by teachers or others who have extensive contact with the child being tested and who can evaluate the child's customary performance on the items included.

Administration, scoring, and interpretation This test is not "administered" in the true sense of the word. Descriptions of oral communication behavior are provided and the evaluator, based on experience with and knowledge of the child, rates each item as follows:

+ = child demonstrates the described skill in several instances

± = child has demonstrated the skill on occasion, but not often enough to warrant a rating of +

− = child has not demonstrated the skill, except accidentally

The test consists of four scales: Receptive Language Skills, Expressive Language Skills, Nonverbal Receptive Skills, and Nonverbal Expressive Skills. Each of the nonverbal scales, however, consists of only three items and involves the understanding and use of gross gestures. The ratings given on these scales are not used in computation of the raw scores.

Two levels of items exist for the receptive and expressive skills subtests: "A" level items describe the use of a skill within a structured situation; "B" level items represent the use of the skill in a spontaneous manner. Items are arranged developmentally so that a ± or a − rating must always be preceded by a + rating. A + rating cannot follow a ± or a − since the child must be able to demonstrate success on earlier items before later ones can be present, according to the authors. Although the manual does not say so specifically, each series (A or B) within a subtest (receptive or expressive) should be terminated as soon as a rating of ± or − is given. Three receptive and three expressive raw score subtests are generated as follows:

Receptive	*Expressive*
"A" scale (identification)	"A" scale (imitation)
"B" scale (comprehension)	"B" scale (spontaneous production)
Combined "A" and "B" scale	Combined "A" and "B" scale

Raw scores are used as entry points into tables of percentile ranks and standard scores for each of the categories listed above, for seven age groups (2-0 through 8-11)

at yearly intervals. These norms were established on 372 children enrolled in 14 oral programs for the hearing impaired. A mean hearing loss and standard deviation for each of the seven age groups are given. The mean hearing loss level is greater than 90 dB in all cases; ranges are not provided.

Evaluation of test adequacy   The test was published in 1975 and the available manual is the original one. Detailed instructions for using the scale are given. Each item under the receptive and expressive scales includes a rationale for inclusion of the item, criteria for rating the item, and examples of behavior that would earn a + rating.

Items were chosen on the basis of experience in teaching deaf children and no evidence of validity measurement is provided. The rationales given for each item appear to be an attempt to establish face validity, but the questions of content, criterion-related, or construct validity are not addressed. The assumption is implicit that "identification" (A items) and "comprehension" (B items) of spoken utterances constitute two separate, observable aspects of language reception while "imitation" (A items) and "spontaneous production" (B items) constitute two separate, observable aspects of language expression. The receptive categories are less clear-cut than the expressive, a fact that probably contributes to the somewhat lower reliability measures obtained for the receptive subtests. Each item contributes equally to the total score, leading to the assumption that each contributes equally to overall language development. Children receive as much credit for attending to the face of the examiner, for example, as they do for demonstrating comprehension of the meaning of stories.

Reliability estimates are based on ratings of the communication behavior of 31 deaf pupils between four and eight years of age. Raters were two teachers of the deaf at the Central Institute for the Deaf. Reliability coefficients are highest for Expressive A items (imitation), .91, and lowest for Receptive A items (identification), .76. No reliability measures are reported for different age groups, and children younger than four are not included in the reliability data provided.

The test is most useful for a limited population, i.e., severely to profoundly deaf children who are enrolled in special classes. Examiners must have extensive exposure to the child being tested and are most likely to be teachers of the deaf. Norms are appropriate for use only with children whose hearing losses average 90 dB or greater. Not only must the child's oral communication behavior be familiar to the examiner, but the child's speech must be intelligible as well. This requirement will eliminate many young deaf children from evaluation, at least on the expressive subtests.

Because reception of language is measured only by response to spoken utterances, it can be argued that the receptive subtests measure lipreading and/or audition rather than language. Similarly, the measure of expression of language is based on the child's speech alone. The authors seem to recognize this limitation in the title of the test by their use of the term "early communication skills" rather than "language." Unfortunately, once the title page is turned, the terminology used is "receptive and expressive language" and the normative data are so labeled. The test is not designed to measure use of language forms other than speech in deaf children and would be more appropriately titled Scales of Early *Oral* Communication Skills for *Deaf* Children. This is not to suggest that the test *should* measure other forms of language usage. The terminology employed, however, should recognize that there are other important communication skills used by many deaf children that can be measured and that contribute to overall language knowledge and use.

The strength of the test is that it provides a means of quantifying observation of language behavior by teachers for gross classification. The authors contend that deaf children move through the skills sampled in a predictable manner. Therefore, the teacher can determine the next step in language teaching by observing the point at which the child's performance breaks down. It is questionable, however, that a teacher who needed such guidance would be able to determine that the next step in language development for a child who used "phrases of 4 or more words in spontaneous speech" (Item E VII, B) would be to imitate or recall "practical sentences of 6 or more words," (Item E VIII, A).

Indeed, the greatest weakness of the test may be the authors' view of language development in the deaf. Imitation of words, phrases, and sentences appears to be considered a necessary step in the development of expressive language, a view that is not held by all educators of the deaf and that ignores the generative grammar and cognitive approaches to language teaching that are in widespread use at present. Greater emphasis is placed on the number of words in a string that the child understands and produces than the sentence structure and semantic relationships involved. In essence, the scales are designed to test that which has been taught or is being taught by a specific method.

Summary The test may be useful to oral educators of the deaf. It can provide a general evaluation of a deaf child's ability to identify and understand spoken words and sentences. Performance on the scales can be compared only with that of deaf children being trained in oral programs. Ratings are subjective in nature and based on long-term observation of the child being tested. Detailed instructions as to rating criteria are described in the manual and must be read carefully before ratings are assigned. Validity of test items as adequate measures of language development is questionable.

SEQUENCED INVENTORY OF COMMUNICATION DEVELOPMENT (SICD)

Dona Lea Hedrick,
Elizabeth M. Prather, and
Annette R. Tobin

University of Washington Press, 1975

Cost Kit, $95.50; separate manual, $8.50; packages of 50 response booklets, $7.50
Test Kit contains Examiner's Manual, 100 pages; Expressive Communication Age Scale Response Booklet (packages of 50); Receptive Communication Age Scale Response Booklet (packages of 50); *Photo Articulation Test* Stimulus Cards (large and small)[*]; Collection of stimulus items

Time For children under two, 30 minutes, administration; 10 minutes, scoring. For children over two, up to one hour, administration; 10 minutes, scoring

[*]Pendergast, K., S. Dickey, J. Selmar, and A. Soder, Photo Articulation Test. Danville, Ill.: Interstate Printers and Publishers, 1969.

James E. McLean *Bureau of Child Research, University of Kansas*

Purpose The Sequenced Inventory of Communication Development is designed to quantify the communicative development of normal and retarded children who are functioning between four months and four years of age.

Administration, scoring, and interpretation The SICD samples a wide range of behaviors that typify communicative interactions between young children and the entities in their environment. The instrument inventories both *expressive* and *receptive* responses using informant reports about children's behavior at home and evoked responses in the testing situation.

On the receptive side, the SICD samples motor responses to both environmental sounds and communicative speech. These responses are classified as reflecting awareness, discrimination, or understanding of incoming auditory stimuli. The earlier receptive behaviors sampled include such items as the observation of sound localization responses, differential child responses to a refrigerator being closed and a door to the house being closed, and responses to negative intonation in the examiner's voice. Later developing receptive behaviors which are sampled include responses to several types and levels of verbal directives, singular–plural contrasts, and even speech sound discriminations.

On the expressive side, the SICD samples developmental responses that include prelinguistic "talking" to people and things, use of upward inflection for presyntactic questions, and imitation of play routines such as block stacking. At the higher end of the expressive continuum, the SICD samples such things as picture naming responses, answers to "What if?" questions, and responses to such test questions as "What is this for?"

In addition to highly specific inventory items, the SICD directs the taking of a language sample and provides for scoring it along a full range of syntactic constructions. It also provides for an articulation inventory and its scoring along a developmental continuum.

All told, the SICD has 32 data points on the receptive scale and 67 points on the expressive scale, excluding the articulation sample. The authors make it clear that this inventory of responses was not generated to be representative of any one theory of language. Rather, the items and classes of behavior sampled are considered to have obvious face validity as developmental milestones along the continuum of communication development by young children.

The SICD provides norm-referenced scales for the test items based on its administration to 252 children ranging in age from four months to 48 months. The items on the test are scored yes/no and a comparison of the yes items with the norm-referenced scale provides the examiner with a score for both the expressive scale and the receptive scale. These scores are represented as the Expressive Communication Age (ECA) and the Receptive Communication Age (RCA) that can then be compared with either or both the child's chronological age (CA) or mental age (MA), derived from another instrument.

The articulation test is scored separately and is not subsumed in the ECA. The articulation norms included for this test were obtained on the 147 children of the 252 child sample who were 24 months or older.

Evaluation of test adequacy   The adequacy of a norm-referenced instrument rests almost totally with the adequacy of its norms as representative of the overall population to which it is referenced. The normalization sample of 252, while not exhaustive, appears to be reasonable in terms of its support for a first edition of an evaluation instrument. This aspect of the SICD will certainly be strengthened as the pool of data is increased and the norms revised accordingly.

The validity of this instrument poses some interesting questions. Since the authors' intent was purely toward sampling representative milestones along the developmental continuum of communication acquisition, it is most difficult to quarrel with the content of this test. In fact, the pragmatic philosophy that undergirds this particular instrument seems to make it consonant with more language theories than many other tests are. The SICD's sampling of play behaviors, for example, makes this test highly compatible with the more cognitive approaches to early child language. This test's concern with prelinguistic communication behavior makes it similarly more acceptable to those who view language and communication in these early stages as basically socially determined behaviors. The language sample included within the test should satisfy those who consider language primarily in terms of its morphological and syntactic structures. Thus by staying eclectic in its identification of milestones in communicative development, the SICD has managed to provide something for every theoretical persuasion.

Test validity and clinical utility are often considered to be mutually covarying. In the sense that a test which is of questionable validity has questionable clinical value, this mutuality is true. It is possible, however, that a highly valid test might not have much clinical utility. It seems that the SICD is a valid instrument and that it has real clinical utility. However, it also seems that its clinical usefulness is unique and must be carefully evaluated.

The SICD is not a highly specific *prescriptive* instrument in that its items cannot be routinely translated into specific clinical targets. On the other hand, this instrument can be most useful in the identification of broad areas in communication development that require intensive clinical prescriptive development. For example, if the SICD indicates that a child has very few prelinguistic communicative responses, the social and cognitive precursors of communication and language might be carefully applied to generate a clinical program. Similarly, if receptive responding is demonstrated to be low, the clinician is directed toward intensive analysis of auditory acuity or auditory processing problems that might be clinically attenuated. Some of the later test items relating to syntax and morphology might be directly translated into clinical targets.

All of this is simply to say that the SICD is intended to be a measure of general communicative development that is useful in and of itself and, in addition, because of its broad, pragmatic view of communication, it can be of considerable utility in directing the *broad* thrust of clinical programming. Thus, while the SICD is not the finally definitive instrument for clinical prescription in early language and communication training, it does seem to offer important data in that area, data that are unique in their base perspectives of early communicative development as a process of interaction between a young child and the environment. Although this instrument predated the most recent breakthroughs in language theory that concentrate on cognitive and social primacy in language development, it is surprisingly resonant with them, albeit in relatively gross fashion.

Summary The SICD seems to be a valuable instrument for quantifying a developmentally young child's relative place on the communication behavior continuum. Highly pragmatic in its selection of test items, this instrument would appear to test developmental milestones in areas of high validity if one views communication development as best measured in terms of its interactive function among children and their environmental audiences and initiators.

Clinicians who view language as more than a collection of syntactic and morphological structures should find this instrument most helpful in placing a child along developmental grids and for identifying the areas of communicative functions in which fine-grained analyses and clinical target development must be carried forth.

TEST FOR AUDITORY COMPREHENSION OF LANGUAGE (TACL), ENGLISH/SPANISH	Teaching Resources Corporation, 5th edition, 1973

SCREENING TEST FOR AUDITORY COMPREHENSION OF LANGUAGE (STACL), ENGLISH/SPANISH

Elizabeth Carrow

Cost $39.95 includes: test manual containing 32 pages and 101 test plates; 25 scoring/analysis forms, 4 pages each; $3.95 STACL test manual; $0.80 STACL test booklet

Time TACL, 20 minutes, administration; 10–15 minutes, scoring

Jon F. Miller *University of Wisconsin—Madison*

Purpose The purpose of the Test for Auditory Comprehension of Language is to allow the examiner to assign a developmental level to the child's auditory comprehension of vocabulary and linguistic structure and to provide diagnostic information leading to therapeutic intervention.

Administration, scoring, and interpretation The TACL consists of 101 plates of line drawings, three drawings to a plate, in a test book including instructions and separate scoring forms. The language categories measured by individual test items are grouped into four subscales, (1) Form Class and Function Words, (2) Morphological Constructions, (3) Grammatical Categories, and (4) Syntactic Structure. The three pictures on each plate represent the linguistic form being tested (e.g., "The girl is jumping") and the referents for the contrasting forms (e.g., "The girl has jumped" and "The girl will jump"). The test items are sequenced by grammatical levels and not by level of item difficulty. "Consequently, the entire test must be administered in order to utilize the normative data" (Test Manual, p.23).

According to the author (Test Manual, p. 7),

> Most of the lexical items used in the test are those learned early in the language development sequence. Inclusion of these items insures that the words used in testing linguistic structures will be tested first as separate items; failure on subsequent items indicates lack of knowledge of the grammatical form and not lack of knowledge of the lexical form used.

No scoring mechanism is provided, however, to distinguish lexical versus grammatical errors for individual subject responses.

The test is administered in a one-to-one setting. The examiner reads aloud the stimulus items and the child responds by pointing to the appropriate picture. Responses are recorded on a separate scoring form. The picture pointing format requires no verbal language of the child, only that he or she recognize and point to the picture best representing the verbal stimulus.

Individual responses are scored as correct or incorrect. The total raw score may be converted into an age score equivalent and percentile rank. The scoring form provides an analysis section for studying an individual's performance on specific classes of items (form class and function words; morphological constructions; grammatical categories and syntax). The scoring form also provides the age at which 75 and 90 percent of children pass each item.

A screening version of this test is also available entitled Screening Test for Auditory Comprehension of Language: English, Spanish (STACL) (1973). The screening procedure is organized in the same format as the TACL. Twenty-five items have been selected from the TACL to represent a wide range in difficulty. Test–retest reliability of .60 is reported on 100 children. The STACL is designed for group administration. Percentile ranks corresponding to raw scores are presented for the standardization group of 418 children. No information is given about the standardization population. It is suggested that children scoring at or below the 10th percentile on the STACL be given the TACL.

Evaluation of test adequacy   The standardization sample for the TACL consisted of 200 middle-class black, Anglo-American, and Mexican-American children, ages three through six. There were 50 children at each age level, 3, 4, 5, and 6 years. Neither the exact age intervals employed nor the distribution of subjects within age categories is described. No geographic information is explicitly provided for the standardization sample. The normative data presented are for the English version only.

The reliability data reported were obtained from the 1971 or earlier versions of the test. Test–retest reliability coefficients for total score of .93 and .94 are reported for the English and Spanish versions of the test, respectively. Test–retest intercorrelations reported for the four subscales are .92 for form class and function words, .77 for morphological constructions, .87 for grammatical categories, and .58 for syntactic structures. All of these measures are reported to be significantly different from zero. No reliability data are reported for the 1973 version of the test.

Construct and criterion-related validities are discussed briefly in the test manual. Test scores increase significantly with age and several studies report that the test distinguishes between normal and linguistically deviant children. (See Davis [1977] for a study of hard of hearing children; Weiner [1970] for a study of dysphasic children; Marquardt and Saxman [1972] for a study of children with articulation deficits; and Bartel, Bryen, and Keehn [1973] for a study of moderately retarded children.) The data reported relate to earlier versions of the test with the exception of Davis (1977).

No item selection criteria are provided except for the statement, "[Items] were selected and maintained if, by agreement of experts, they evaluated knowledge of specific grammatical structures." The rationale for the selection of specific grammatical structures to include in the test is not discussed at all. This omission represents a serious problem in determining the construct validity of this test for several reasons. First, presumably items were originally selected for their ability to reveal the developmental sequence of language comprehension. Given the general assumption that comprehension precedes production in development (Test Manual, p. 3), the facts necessary for item selection must have come from the developmental literature on language production available at the time. A discussion of developmental change in language production and the selection of items to reveal developmental change in comprehension is conspicuously absent. The result severely limits the relating of performance on this test to analyses of language production in individual children. The second problem related to construct validity is the limitation on item selection imposed by the testing format. A number of grammatical and syntactic constructions in English, such as personal pronouns and Wh-questions, cannot be accurately represented by pictures.

This test can be a helpful beginning step in the assessment process. The limitation of the items included in this and all other picture comprehension tests requires that they be considered as first step or screening procedures for general comprehension development. Children evidencing problems on this test must be further evaluated with multiple presentations of the linguistic construction(s) in question, varying the mode of presentation, context, meaning, and sentence length.

Interpretation of performance on individual items is questionable for several reasons including length of stimulus sentences, method of stimulus presentation, the order of stimulus items, and guessing rate.

Sentence length: Clinicians should be aware that the stimulus items included in this test vary in length. In general, the longer the stimulus item the later its mastery by 75 to 90 percent of the children in the standardization sample. The relationship between sentence length and grammatical complexity is unclear in comprehension. It i clinically important, however, to determine whether errors are related to grammatical complexity, as is assumed by the test, or to increasing processing demands introduced by the longer stimulus items. This is a particularly critical issue for children demonstrating problems in auditory memory skills.

Stimulus presentation: A procedural question is raised by the testing manual on page 10. Stimulus items are to be presented only once unless misstated. Since young children frequently fail to respond to the first presentation of a stimulus, this may result in scoring a "no response" as an error. There is some evidence to suggest that for young children, 1-8, to 2-8 years of age, the response characteristics on second stimulus presentations given "no response" to the first are almost the same (Chapman and Miller 1975). These data suggest that initial "no responses" should not be scored as errors and that to do so would result in underestimating the child's comprehension of language.

Order of item presentation: The stimulus items of the TACL are organized for presentation by type of linguistic construction. For example, all locatives are presented consecutively (Items 44–49). This raises the possibility of order effects. Clinicians should consider a second administration of the test with the stimulus items randomized for presentation.

Guessing rate: Individual grammatical contrasts are tested by only one item, on which the guessing rate is .33 (one of the three pictures is correct). As a result, we cannot conclude that passing an individual item is evidence for comprehension of that item.

The limited size of the standardization sample, particularly the failure to report the norms for boys and girls separately, limits the flexibility of the TACL. A recent study (Koenigsknecht and Friedman 1976) of productive syntax found girls significantly advanced over boys at five age levels, 2, 3, 4, 5, and 6 years. This study suggests that norms for boys and girls need to be reported separately. Due to the limited size and geographical distribution of the standardization sample, the failure to report norms for boys and girls separately, possible order effects, and single stimulus item presentation, it is suggested that local norms be gathered.

Summary   Given the nature of the comprehension process, all comprehension tests have limitations. The TACL remains the best commercially produced language comprehension test available to date. Its use is recommended within the limitations stated in this review.

References

Bartel, N. R., D. Bryen, and S. Keehn   Language comprehension in the moderately retarded child. *Exceptional Children* **39**: 375–382, 1973.

Chapman, R. S. and J. F. Miller   Word order in early two- and three-word utterances: does production precede comprehension? *J. Speech Hearing Res.* **18**: 355–371, 1975.

Davis, J. M.   Reliability of hearing-impaired children's responses to oral and total presentations of the Test of Auditory Comprehension of Language. *J. Speech Hearing Dis.* **42**: 520–527, 1977.

Koenigsknecht, R. A. and P. Friedman   Syntax development in boys and girls. *Child Development* **47**: 1109–1115, 1976.

Marquardt, T. P. and J. H. Saxman   Language comprehension and auditory discrimination in articulation deficient kindergarten children. *J. Speech Hearing Res.* **15**: 382–389, 1972.

Weiner, P. S.   The perceptual level functioning of dysphasic children: a follow-up study. *J. Speech Hearing Res.* **15**: 423–438, 1972.

TORONTO TESTS OF RECEPTIVE VOCABULARY: ENGLISH/SPANISH (TTRV)

Allen S. Toronto

Academic Tests, Inc., 1977

Cost Manual and stimulus plates, $24.95; pack of 30 score sheets, $3.50

Manual, 7 pages of text, 3 English practice plates, 40 English plates, 3 Spanish practice plates, 40 Spanish plates; score sheet, 1 page

Time 10 minutes, administration; 3 minutes, scoring

Thomas A. Linares *New Mexico State University*

Purpose The purpose of the Toronto Tests of Receptive Vocabulary is to "identify English- and Spanish-speaking children whose performance in identifying orally presented vocabulary words is significantly below that of their peers" (Manual, p. 1). The tests may be administered to (1) Anglo-American children, (2) English-speaking Mexican-American children, and (3) Spanish-speaking Mexican-American children, between the ages of four years and ten years.

Administration, scoring, and interpretation The test consists of an English section and a Spanish section, each composed of 40 plates of black and white line drawings. Subjects are required to identify one picture from among three on each plate. Because of the shortness of the test, no basal or ceiling is required. The stimulus words are ordered from easy to difficult.

Standardization of the test items was based on a sample of 1276 children from three different cities in Texas. Equal numbers of males and females were tested at each age level for each of the three groups. Norms for each group were independently obtained, no child belonging to more than one group. A subject's raw score is interpreted according to a percentile rank or as a standard deviation. Administration of either section takes approximately ten minutes.

Evaluation of test adequacy Test–retest reliability of administrations to approximately 50 children in each group yielded Pearson r's between .82 and .92. Validity of the test was .66 (Pearson r) for the entire group of 1276 children when it was compared with the Toronto Bicultural Test of Non-Verbal Reasoning. (The latter test was apparently standardized on the same children at the same time.)

The criterion for selection of the Spanish-speaking Mexican-American children was that they spoke "Spanish at home at least 75 percent of the time" (Manual, p. 3). This basis leaves much to be desired for several reasons. First, speaking Spanish 75 percent of the time at home doesn't mean that these children don't speak English at school, especially in the case of "balanced" bilingual childern who speak the language of their immediate environment. Secondly, no information is given about how much receptive/expressive language the Spanish-speaking children had in English. Third, no information is given as to how the "75 percent" was determined or by whom. Similar comments apply to the selection and determination of the "English"-speaking Mexican-American children. For all three groups, no information is given about their socioeconomic levels, years of living in the United States, or immediate geographical environments. This is important to know because many Mexican-American children (at least in the reviewer's hometown) are "migrant" children who do not represent the "typical" child in the community.

Toronto states that in order to give the TTRV, one should "determine whether the child is Anglo-American, English-speaking Mexican-American, or Spanish-speaking Mexican-American" (Manual, p. 3). However, he does not give guidelines for classifying children into these groups. Classifying a balanced bilingual child is difficult, since this child does not fit into any of the above three groups. After one has given several tests to determine whether a child can be included in one of the above groups, the administration of the TTRV would probably be redundant. Perhaps these children should be given both English and Spanish sections, but the testing of balanced bilingual children is not specifically addressed in the manual. Children who are close to being truly balanced do not necessarily function at an age-appropriate level but are likely to be "delayed" to some extent in both languages and, therefore, need to be evaluated just as much as the three groups suggested by Toronto.

As with any picture vocabulary test, some of the test items are less then satisfactory. The greatest problem lies in the selection of the words. Administration of the test to two children in the reviewer's city, as well as personal evaluation, revealed several differences in vocabulary (not necessarily more correct or incorrect). Regarding this matter Toronto warns,". . .the farther away one gets from matching the standardization sample (geographically or ethnically), the less confidence one can have in the score" (Manual, p. 3). Obviously differences in vocabulary will "penalize" children who are not familiar with the test items. Here again, it is the responsibility of the examiner not to misinterpret the results. A primary concern, therefore, is the possible inappropriate utilization of the TTRV throughout the United States. Many diagnosticians would be tempted to change a test word to the word used in their immediate area. However, substituting a word without standardizing the new word would invalidate the test.

A second problem with the test pictures is the "figure–ground" relationship. Because of the use of black and white line drawings, some of the pictures might be visually confusing to children (e.g., English plates 3, 14, 22, 35, 36; Spanish plates 16, 18, 21, and 33). Utilization of better pictures, perhaps with color, would be an improvement. In some instances, the test item is ambiguous or poorly represented. For example, the far right picture in English plate 8 might be interpreted as a "Father" (especially by Catholic children) instead of "judge." All three pictures in 13 could represent "removing" depending on the child's interpretation. "Erasing" in 19 could have been better illustrated. Plate 24 poorly represents "escaping." Similar observations may be made concerning some of the pictures in the Spanish section.

Although the TTRV was standardized on children between the ages of four and ten, little discrimination in performance exists among the ages eight, nine, and ten. Toronto discusses this limitation on page 5 of the manual.

Validity is often checked by correlating a new test with an already existing and similarly constructed test. Toronto validated the TTRV against his own Toronto Bicultural Test of Non-Verbal Reasoning. This procedure is questionable since the validity of the Bicultural Test has not yet been fully established.

Toronto did an exceptional job with the statistical and reliability analysis of the TTRV. Reliability values are quite acceptable.

It would have been helpful had guidelines or suggestions been given for follow-up procedures with children identified as having a vocabulary deficit. The test items are nouns and verbs, but no detailed error analysis procedure is included in the manual. Once the score is obtained, no further procedures are suggested other than that "the child should be evaluated further to determine whether he or she requires special education services" (Manual, p. 3).

Summary The TTRV is a well developed receptive vocabulary test. The major limitation is its extent of applicability to areas where a somewhat different vocabulary is used. Some of the test items could have been better represented, while other items need improvement with regard to figure–ground relationship. More information should have been given on selection and backgrounds of the children comprising the three groups. Possibilities of incorrect use of the test or misinterpretation of test results should have been emphasized more. Testing of balanced bilingual children should have been addressed. Guidelines regarding follow-up procedures would have been beneficial.

UTAH TEST OF LANGUAGE DEVELOPMENT

Merlin J. Mecham, J. Lorin Jex, and J. Dean Jones

Communication Research Associates, 1967

Cost Test kit with 23-page manual and 25 4-page score sheets, $20.00

Time Untimed, varies with child

Rita C. Naremore *Indiana University*

Purpose The Utah Test of Language Development was designed to provide "the clinician with an objective instrument for measurement of expressive and receptive language skills in both normal and handicapped children." According the the authors, "It not only provides a broad overall picture of expressive and receptive skills, but utilizes the developmental approach for appraisal of language readiness" (Manual, p. 1).

Administration, scoring, and interpretation The test is administered verbally by the examiner, who gives the child instructions, sometimes using a set of toys or pictures provided with the test, and sometimes using paper and crayons or pencils provided by the examiner. The test can be administered in less than one hour and may be completed in more than one sitting if necessary. The examiner scores the child's response to each item as + (correct) or − (incorrect) on a score sheet provided with the test. The examiner begins testing items approximately at the child's chronological age level (items are age-graded on the score sheet) and tests up from that point. If the child fails to achieve eight consecutive correct responses above CA level, the examiner moves downward from CA level until eight consecutive correct responses are achieved. The basal score is the highest consecutive correct response. Items are tested upward from the basal score until at least eight consecutive incorrect responses occur, at which time testing is discontinued.

The total raw score on the test is calculated by counting the total number of correct responses above the basal score and adding this number to the basal score. Raw scores can be converted to language age scores (ranging from nine months to 16 years) by referring to a conversion table provided in the manual. A language quotient may be obtained by dividing the child's language age by the chronological age. Standard scores and percentile equivalents are not available because of the small size of the normative sample.

Evaluation of test adequacy The standardization of this test is subject to question, primarily because of the small size and limited geographical distribution of the normative sample. The authors recognize this in the instruction manual (p. 6) when they state:

> It is the realization of the present authors that unrestricted use of the test as a diagnostic instrument is not feasible until a larger collection of normative data is available. It is with this idea in mind that the present test is being "launched" in its present form with the hopes that additional normative data will be forthcoming from users.

Reliability of the testing instrument, based on split-half correlations and correlation of scores in the direct-test edition with scores from the informant interview edition of the test, appears adequate. Validity of the instrument, however, remains questionable. The authors assume that, since all items on the Utah test were taken from other standardized tests, the Utah test has good face validity. This assumption would hold only if the items selected from other tests had been shown to measure language development. In many instances, this is a questionable assumption. A child's ability to mark on paper with a pencil without either tearing the paper or breaking the pencil point (Item 3) may be an index of social or motor development, but its ties with language development are not clear. The same could be said of Item 27, which requires the child to print simple words, or Item 41, which requires the child to give rhymes in response to instructions such as "Tell me the name of a color that rhymes with head." The authors checked the performance of children in their sample against the performance of children in the normative samples used in the "source tests" by correlating the age-equivalents of the items derived in their testing with the age-equivalents of the items as they appeared in the original sources (Manual, p. 5). These correlations, while high, still do not ensure that the items in question are measures of language development. Furthermore, the fact that a normal child's performance on such tasks may correlate with performance on tasks directly related to language development does not make such items useful indices of language development for children who have fine or gross motor problems or visual problems or hearing loss.

This, then, brings the clinical usefulness of the test into question. Of the 51 items on the test, 23 are items which demand fine motor skills, test memory for digits or word lists, require repetition of rote material (counting from 1 to 50, naming the days of the week), or appear to be testing something other than the child's knowledge of language (rhyming, spatial orientation of directions). For the remaining 28 items, there appears to be little attention given to a systematic presentation of various aspects of language to which the child might respond. These items include naming colors and body parts, labeling pictures, and following simple directions ("Give me the ball."). In conjunction with these tasks appear such tasks as that in Item 23:

Procedure: After getting up from the chair and moving *with* the child to the center of the room, say, *"Now I want you to do something for me. I want you to shut (open) the door; and then bring me the box which you see over there* (pointing in turn to the objects designated). *Do you understand? Be sure and get it right. First you put the pencil on the chair, then shut (open) the door, then bring me the box. Go ahead."*

Do not repeat the instructions again or give the child any further aid whatever, even by the direction of the gaze. If the child stops or hesitates, it is never permissible to ask what comes next.

Score: All three commissions must be executed and in the proper order for item to be scored plus.

Given such an item, with the scoring suggested, it is not clear what one would know about the language development of a child who failed the task. Could the child get two parts of the command but not three? The scoring procedure does not allow such analysis. Did the child simply stand and stare? The scoring sheet will not allow one to know.

Summary Given the nature of the items on this test and a scoring system that does not encourage attention to the exact nature of a child's response, the Utah test does not appear to be useful in clinical situations in which one wishes to know how a child uses language or what a child does in response to language. No attempts appear to have been made to present an ordered sequence of language forms which the child is expected to use or respond to. Rather, a range of behaviors which may correlate with language development is being tested. Due to the numerous items requiring visual discrimination and fine motor skills, this is not a test that should be used with any child suspected of being impaired in either of these areas of development.

This test might be useful as a preschool screening instrument, if the "language ages" can be taken with a grain of salt. Its usefulness even in this situation is impaired because one does not know what kind of difference between chronological age and language age would indicate language impairment or delay. Furthermore, since screening tests are available that more directly focus on language behavior than does the Utah test, the Utah test is not recommended.

VANE EVALUATION OF LANGUAGE SCALE (VANE-L)

Julia R. Vane

Clinical Psychology Publishing Co., Inc., 1975

Cost $15.00

Manual, 32 pages, $5.00; record sheets, 2 pages, pack of 50 for $3.50; test kit, $8.00

Time 10 minutes, administration; 5 minutes, scoring

Lauren M. Carlile *Sunlight, A Preschool for Children with Communication Disorders Oklahoma City, Oklahoma*

Purpose The Vane Evaluation of Language Scale is a screening device that measures language skills in children aged two-and-a-half to six years. It assesses receptive and expressive language as well as memory and handedness and may be used as a diagnostic, teaching, or research instrument.

Administration, scoring, and interpretation The test was designed to be administered by preschool and kindergarten teachers to assess the level of language development of individual children as well as the progress of children as a group. Testing time is about ten minutes. The Vane-L consists of a receptive language and an expressive language scale, and a test of auditory and visual memory. Test items were selected from a wide range of language constructs that were field tested during a four-year period in nursery schools, day-care centers, Head Start centers, kindergartens, and first grades. For example, field testing revealed that children responded more readily to "put your finger on" and "show me" than to "point to," so the first two commands are used almost exclusively throughout the test.

Test items have been carefully designed so that all the elements in the stimulus sentence are known to the child except the concept(s) to be tested. As an example, "Show me your elbows" is scored for knowledge of body part and understanding of plural form. Likewise, "Put two fingers beside your nose" is scored for the concepts "two" and "beside." Traditional items from language measures such as "What do you do when you get sleepy?" are not included because if a child fails to respond to such a question, it is unclear as to whether the child does not understand "what," "do," "when," "sleepy," or all of these.

The receptive language scale is given first and depends on nonverbal responses. Expressive language items require the child to repeat sentences of increasing length and complexity and to define vocabulary items. The teacher evaluates each child's speech in terms of "good," "fair," and "poor," and "initial" and "other" sound substitutions. Auditory and visual memory are assessed by asking the child to repeat a block tapping sequence and by observing whether the child watches, listens, or both. Scores on the three subtests are converted to percentile equivalents. Throughout the test the teacher records which hand the child chooses for pointing and picking up objects. Depending on the percentage of time the hand is used, the child is "consistently" right or left (100 percent), "predominantly" right or left (75 to 95 percent), or has not established dominance (below 75 percent).

Evaluation of test adequacy While the Vane-L is primarily an edumetric test, one that measures language gains in preschool children, normative data are provided for those who prefer to use it as a psychometric instrument. The standardization sample consisted of 740 children from New York, New Jersey, and Vermont. The sample conforms closely to the 1970 Unites States census data with respect to variables of age, sex, race (white or nonwhite) and occupation of parent. The urban–rural distribution is somewhat biased in favor of urban children.

The author draws no comparisons between the Vane-L and other language measures. Low correlations found between scores on the *Vane Kindergarten Test,* a measure of intellectual ability, and the Vane-L are presented as evidence that the two tests are not measuring the same phenomena.

The Vane-L has in its favor a self-contained, childproof test kit, carefully designed receptive language items, and short administration time. Its main weakness is teacher-administration of a language instrument. No mention is even made of the role of the speech–language pathologist in diagnosis and remediation of language disorders. Referral is not suggested if, for example, the teacher judges a child's speech to be poor in comparison with that of the child's classmates. The assumption underlying the test is that proper classroom teaching will enable language delayed children to reach competence in language usage. There is much research, however, to indicate that this is not the case. Since the Vane-L is given by the classroom teacher, only functional language is evaluated. No assessment is made of the child's production of phonemes or use of grammatical rules.

Summary Use of the Vane-L is recommended. It would be an even more useful instrument had it been designed with a speech–language pathologist in mind.

Reference

Vane, J. R. Vane evaluation of language scale (the Vane-L). *Archives of the Behavioral Sciences, Monograph No. 49,* 1–30, 1975.

VERBAL LANGUAGE DEVELOPMENT SCALE (VLDS)	American Guidance Service, 1971
Merlin J. Mecham	**Cost** Manual, 16 pages, $ .75; 25 3-page score sheets, $2.00
	Time 15 minutes, administration; 2 minutes, scoring

Bruce R. Hanson *Mankato State University*

Purpose The purpose of the Verbal Language Development Scale (VLDS) is to provide an indirect method of assessing the language of children who "cannot or will not respond to direct testing methods" (Manual, p. 2). Included in this category are normal preschoolers and children who have physical, emotional, or mental handicaps.

Administration, scoring, and interpretation The VLDS was designed initially to serve as an extension of the communication section of the Vineland Social Maturiy Scale (Doll 1947), and procedures for administering and scoring the VLDS are nearly identical to those used for the Vineland.

Like the Vineland, the VLDS uses the informant–interview method of testing. The examiner asks someone who is familiar with the child (preferably a parent or teacher) to indicate the extent to which the child has developed each of several age-appropriate communication skills. The examiner reads or paraphrases from memory the test manual's description of each skill in question. On the basis of the informant's response to the description of the item, the examiner scores the item as *passed, emerging,* or *failed.* Emerging items are given half as much credit as passed items toward the child's total score.

The test consists of 50 items arranged in ascending order of development from infancy through age 14. More items are tested at ages 0–1, 1–2, and 2–3 than at any of the older age levels. More than two-thirds of all items test speech skills. The remaining items test reading, writing, or listening abilities. Examples of test items include imitation of sounds, recognition of objects when named, use of plurals, printing simple words, reading words at the preprimer level, and telling a familiar story.

The test is untimed and requires no specialized training of the examiner. Administration time averages about 15 minutes.

The test manual contains a table for converting the child's total score to a language-age equivalent score. The age equivalent scores are based on normative data obtained by administering the VLDS to 237 white, normal-speaking children from central and mid-northern Utah. A stratified random method of sampling was used to maximize the likelihood that the subjects were representative of their regions in sex, socioeconomic status, and residence. Approximately 20 subjects were tested at each age level between 2 and 12 years. Ten or fewer subjects were tested at ages 1, 13, and 14.

Evaluation of test adequacy The manual reports data on test–retest and alternate forms reliability. Two studies of test–retest reliability were reported. One study involved children from the normative sample whereas the other study involved mentally retarded children. In both cases, correlation coefficients of .96 were obtained. Three studies of alternate form reliability were reported. In each, scores on the VLDS were compared against scores on an early form of the Utah Test of Language Development (qv) (Mecham, Jex, and Jones 1967). The Utah is basically a "direct-test" version of the VLDS. Correlation coefficients of .97, .72, and .81 were obtained on samples of normal children, educable retarded children, and institutionalized retarded children, respectively.

Most of the items in the VLDS were drawn from the Gesell Developmental Schedules, the Stanford–Binet, and the Vineland Social Maturity Scale. Other evidence offered in support of item or content validity is that the VLDS items yielded relatively small standard deviations in a study involving mentally retarded children. Construct validity is reported in terms of the ability of scores on the VLDS to (1) increase with increases in age, (2) correlate highly with Form L of the Stanford–Binet, and (3) correlate highly with judges' ratings of language development.

When used in conjunction with direct observation of the child's behavior, the VLDS may provide useful information about the development of communication skills in young normal children or in children whose handicaps make direct, formal testing impractical. The test also may be useful as a substitute for less standardized methods of conducting parental interviews. However, in using the VLDS the examiner needs to be aware of several potential problems.

A potentially serious problem with the VLDS is that the scoring may in some cases be inaccurate. Scoring error can be introduced by the examiner, the informant, or both. In this reviewer's experience as an examiner, it is particularly difficult to differentiate between "emerging" and "passed" items on the VLDS. The problem seems to stem from the fact that the manual gives several behaviors as examples of each tested skill. It is not clear from the scoring instructions whether the skill is to be scored as emerging or passed when the child consistently performs some but not all examples of the skill. It is impossible to know how seriously this problem affects the scoring process since no information on examiner reliability is presented in the manual.

The informant may contribute to scoring error in obvious ways. In some cases, the informant may simply not recall a skill that the child nonetheless has developed. In other cases the informant may intentionally or unintentionally exaggerate the child's abilities.

A second disadvantage of the VLDS is that the language age-equivalent scores may be misleading. These scores are derived solely from the means of the normative data and provide no information about variability around the mean. Without standard deviation or percentile information it is impossible to interpret the normality or deviance of a child's score. For example, it is not possible to know how low a score can be before it becomes a matter of clinical concern.

A third disadvantage of the VLDS is that it does not appear to measure "language" as language is presently viewed. Few items provide information about the child's use of specific syntactic and semantic language structures. The VLDS might best be viewed as a functional communication scale rather than a language scale.

Summary The VLDS is an informant-based method of assessing the language of children from infancy to 14 years. It is readily administered in a brief time. Though no special training is required of the examiner, there is a strong possibility of examiner and informant bias in the test. The scores are not very revealing and the test taps little that would be designated as "language" according to current interpretations. The VLDS appears to have little utility as a language assessment device.

References

Doll, E. A. *Vineland Social Maturity Scale.* Circle Pines, Minn.: American Guidance Service, 1965.

Mecham, J. M., J. L. Jex, and J. D. Jones *Utah Test of Language Development.* Salt Lake City, Utah: Communication Research Associates, 1967.

VOCABULARY COMPREHENSION SCALE

Tina E. Bangs

Teaching Resources Corporation, 1975

Cost $40.00 for kit containing objects, puppets, cardboard farm building, score sheet (4 pages), and manual (32 pages)

Time 45 minutes, administration and scoring

Christine Harris and Philip Levinson *Children's Hospital of Los Angeles*

Purpose The Vocabulary Comprehension Scale is designed to assess comprehension of pronouns and words of position (e.g., in, behind), size (e.g., big, thin), quantity (e.g., all, less), and quality (e.g., soft, different).

Administration, scoring, and interpretation The test uses toy objects rather than pictured representation. It requires from 20 to 45 minutes to administer. There are no standardized administration procedures. There are 61 items and scoring is pass/fail.

The test was standardized on 80 preschool children aged two to six. There were ten children in each six-month interval. A summary sheet is provided on the scoring form that lists the age level at which 80 percent of the standardization sample passed that item, allowing one to compare an individual child's performance to the sample population.

Items within each category (e.g., size, quantity, etc.) are scaled according to the percent of children passing the item in the standardization sample. This can provide a rough index of a developmental performance level. However, these interpretations must be made with caution. The standardization sample size is small, and no validity or reliability data are reported.

Evaluation of test adequacy The scale has some advantages. First, it provides a survey of vocabulary words (namely, pronouns and words of size, quantity, etc.) that are not well represented on pictorial vocabulary tests such as the Full-Range Picture Vocabulary Test (qv) or the Peabody Picture Vocabulary Test (qv). The use of real play objects rather than pictures also is advantageous in that these materials can be more meaningful to some groups of children who might not comprehend or be motivated by pictorial tests. The reviewers have found this to be true in the case of some mentally retarded children and some children who are passive or simply unwilling to point to pictures.

There are several limitations to the scale. First, the administration and scoring procedures are not standardized in any way. The instructions in the manual could be clearer and more specific. As it is, much is left to the judgment of the examiner, resulting in considerable variation in administration and consequent possibilities of biasing results. This problem is even more apparent on a test that requires that the child manipulate the objects in some way (an open format), as opposed to the traditional picture test that requires pointing to one of three or four choices. For example, one item requests that a child "Put the dog high on the ladder." Some children examined by this reviewer placed the dog between the roof and ladder where it can be positioned without falling. The dog was placed "high" but not exactly "on" the ladder. It appeared that this was a logical place for the children to place the dog because the dog would stay there and not fall. On previous items the child had learned to place the dog some-where and then let go of it. Was this their intention on this item? Did this take priority over an exact response to the direction?

Some problems come from the ambiguity of language itself. One child when asked to "Take the cars apart" (cars being presented side by side together), picked up a car and tried to take off a wheel. The correct response was to separate the cars. Obviously, there's more to the meaning of "apart" than the test elicits. A further limitation is that there is just one item testing each word form. It is highly probable that a child may have some understanding of a word in some semantic contexts not represented in the test and may respond with that meaning as opposed to the one tested. In addition, there is no way of knowing whether a particular item is emerging in a child's vocabulary.

The absence of more than one item for each word means that there is no internal reliability within the test itself. Some responses, particularly on the opposites like "thin-fat," have a high probability of being correct by chance. Credit is given for two of three correct responses, but this in no way eliminates the chance factor because the items are presented in exactly the same way allowing for perseverative responses.

Another limitation, at least for clinical populations, is the pass/fail scoring method. It does not allow for abstracting more qualitative aspects of performance such as re-sponse latency or number of repetitions given. Another potential problem is that the materials are so interesting that many children do not comply with the directions. They prefer to handle and play with the materials in their own way; this is particularly true for children under five. Of course, a skillful clinician can work with this situation and elicit the data, but then the assessment becomes the kind of informal testing through play that can be done in any case.

Summary   The instrument may be most applicable for nonclinical preschool popula-tions that are language delayed but are not exhibiting behavior that suggests a language learning disorder. It also may be useful in assessing vocabulary in some mentally re-tarded populations. However, it is not a diagnostic test nor is it conclusive in any way. It can only be one of several indicators used. Its results should be compared against the examiner's own informal observations, as well as other standardized measures.

Part II
Appraisal of Articulation

Introduction

Traditionally, speech clinicians have devoted the majority of their professional time to the remediation of functional disorders of articulation. In addition, persons with organic conditions such as dysarthria, cerebral palsy, cleft palate, and hearing loss also experience disordered articulation that requires assessment. It therefore seems defensible from a historical perspective to suggest that the primary assessment tool of speech pathology has been the test of articulation. It is perhaps the unique tool of speech pathology. Nearly every other test or technique used by speech–language pathologists is also part of the armamentarium of other professions. Examples come quickly to mind. Speech clinicians administer some types of hearing tests that are the contribution of audiology. They conduct examinations of the oral speech mechanism as do dentists and physicians. They administer various other kinds of tests borrowed from psychology and psycholinguistics. It is probably unnecessary to supply further commonalities. The point is that tests of articulation have played a central role in the development of the profession of speech–language pathology.

The seemingly simple task of listening to a person's speech and noting errors of speech-sound production readily opens the testing of articulation to a wide variety of approaches. Nevertheless, a concern that no speech sound be overlooked in an assessment probably motivated the creation of systematic procedures to elicit all speech sounds in an orderly fashion. A system designed to elicit each speech sound in the repertoire of a client also yielded an economy in test time. A systematic sequence of elicitation of words containing specific sounds probably takes less time than waiting for each sound to occur in spontaneous conversation. Ensuring that all speech sounds were tested in a brief span of time was perhaps the original reason for the development of tests of articulation. These were often constructed by individual clinicians. The construction of a test was time consuming. Pictures representing stimulus words for nonreaders needed to be drawn or cut and pasted. It was necessary to obtain durable, easily manipulable materials. The selection of appropriate stimulus words was required. One of the original reasons for the emergence of commercial tests was probably to save the practicing clinician from this chore.

To the earlier tests designed primarily to elicit target sounds in particular words, important improvements have been added. Among the early contributions to test development beyond simple error identification was the provision of normative data to assist a clinician in deciding whether a child's misarticulation signalled a problem or was merely a sample of normal, immature speech. Some attention has more recently been given to establishing the validity and reliability of tests. However, these matters still need more emphasis. Knowledge of the fact that speech sounds are produced differently in different contexts casts doubt upon the validity of minimal elicitations of target sounds in a few selected words. Also, the challenge of phonological analysis of the production of suprasegmental phonemes in addition to evaluation of production of segmental phonemes lends further awareness to the inadequacy and doubtful validity of the more traditional forms of testing.

Other purposes and contributions of tests of articulation have been defined and created. These include indexes of intelligibility, provision for identifying the influences of coarticulation, assessment of palatopharyngeal valving for speech, means to predict spontaneous mastery of articulation, estimates of language proficiency, simple analysis of errors by distinctive features, and attempts at phonological assessment as part of more comprehensive tests of language and communication. These test purposes and functions are elaborated and explained in the reviews that follow.

The increasing contributions that creative test makers have made to the profession provide reason for predicting the future appearance of more tests with more definitive purposes. Another premise upon which to base this prediction is the accumulating knowledge of phonological processes coming from research. As the complex processes of phonology become better understood, new tests will appear reflecting improved insights. The desire to obtain a more complete assessment of phonology in its entirety and not just its segments will probably bring about the development of more comprehensive tests of phonology. These will likely require new approaches to sampling oral language performance in different communicative contexts to provide suprasegmental information overlooked in today's tests. Current interest in analysis of distinctive features also provides cause to predict the appearance of more commercial tests in this area.

Present tests are an index of current professional status. As this rapidly changing profession undergoes its continuing metamorphosis, so will its tests. This chapter and this book capture this moment in time. The need for future revision is practically guaranteed but, for now, the published articulation tests of today are here reviewed.

Parley W. Newman

ARIZONA ARTICULATION PROFICIENCY SCALE (AAPS)

Janet Barker Fudala

Western Psychological Services, 1963, 1970, 1974

Cost $17.50 per set of cards, 25 record booklets, 25 survey test forms and manual

Time Approximately 20 minutes, administration

Frank J. Falck *University of Houston*

Purpose The purpose of the Arizona Articulation Proficiency Scale is to provide a rapid and precise determination of misarticulations and of total articulatory proficiency. The rationale upon which this particular test is based is that the more frequently a misarticulation occurs in speech, the greater is the articulatory problem. The AAPS provides a numerical scale of articulatory proficiency by weighting misarticulations according to the frequency with which a particular sound occurs in American speech. The test may be used to (1) serve as an aid in the identification of and selection of children for speech therapy, (2) assist in the determination of speech therapy progress, (3) help in the comparison of articulation therapy and techniques, (4) provide a frame of reference for discussing speech development and speech therapy with persons who are nonspecialists in the area of communication disorders, and (5) facilitate research studies.

Administration, scoring, and interpretation The AAPS consists of a set of cards containing line drawings of objects or common events, one to a page. These are shown to the child in sequence with instructions to "tell me what they are." The examiner records only the child's misarticulations.

Consonant errors are recorded in a printed protocol booklet in the appropriately indicated column. Substitutions are recorded, sound omissions are indicated by a dash (—), and distortions by an x.

Vowels are not tested separately but are evaluated as they appear with certain consonants. Vowel errors are recorded in a column provided in the protocol booklet for that purpose.

In addition to the basic naming of objects or events there are four questions asked the child during the test based on certain drawings or card colors. These questions are used to elicit the responses "green," "red," "yellow," "this" or "that," and "cold."

Spontaneous speech can be elicited through the use of two special drawings that stimulate conversation. In addition, a sentence test is included that can be administered by having the person read aloud. Consonant and vowel errors are recorded on another section of the protocol booklet. The sentences are comprised of words taken from vocabulary lists contained in several basic readers up to the third grade level.

Each tested consonant and vowel has an assigned value determined by the number of times it probably would occur in 100 consecutive speech sounds. These values are derived from studies done at Bell Laboratories. Each misarticulated sound receives its assigned value. The error values are added and recorded in the appropriate Total Consonant Score and Total Vowel Score boxes on the back of the protocol booklet. The two scores are added together and subtracted from 100 to provide the AAPS Total Score.

The AAPS Total Score is interpreted according to the following categories:

95–100	Sound errors are noticed occasionally in continuous speech
85–94.5	Speech is intelligible, although noticeably in error
70–84.5	Speech is intelligible with careful listening
60–69.5	Speech intelligibility is difficult
45–59.5	Speech is usually unintelligible
0–44.5	Speech is unintelligible

In addition to the frequency of use value assigned to each sound, there is also an age level assigned that represents in years the age by which 90 percent of the children tested in the normative activities had mastered the sound. Mastery level was chosen rather than an average developmental level to assist the speech-language pathologist in determining sounds that will not develop through maturation. It was hoped that this might be useful in reducing parental anxieties and possible inappropriate pressures to produce perfect articulation prior to developmental readiness.

Evaluation of test adequacy Standardization of the AAPS included attention to reliability and validity and appropriateness of test material. Age norms were determined from data obtained by 19 speech-language pathologists testing 702 children ranging in age from 3-0 to 11-11 years of age. Children tested were members of "average" Seattle Public Schools excluding children with gross deviations in hearing, mental ability, emotional stability, or neurological functioning. The test manual states that children in 16 preschools in the Seattle area were also tested. There is no report of racial or ethnic distribution in the samples employed.

A reliability coefficient of .96 (test-retest interval within one week) was reported based on the testing of 105 children by 19 public school speech-language pathologists. Assumption of validity is based on a reported correlation of .92 between AAPS scores and a judgment by ten speech-language pathologists of defectiveness on brief recorded samples of spontaneous speech of 45 children.

The AAPS has the potential of being a valuable addition to a speech-language pathologist's set of tools. It may be slightly more difficult to administer and record than some other articulation tests in common usage. However, it provides much more information and there are uses to which the information gathered can be applied not found in other approaches to articulation testing.

The AAPS would appear to be particularly of value in the comprehensive planning activities that are evolving in public schools under the mandate of PL 94-142. Exchange of relevant information among team members and parents or parent advocates can be facilitated using the AAPS total score and the concept of specific sound values and age mastery. Comparison of scores obtained over specified periods of time will be helpful in evaluation and accountability procedures. Included in the protocol booklet is a formula with work space for determining a percentage of speech improvement, and this may be found to be useful if used judiciously.

It is to be hoped that continued research will be done on and with the AAPS. Further information is needed relative to the intelligibility weighting of each sound based not only on frequency of use but also on its importance to the overall intelligibility of conversational speech. As is true with almost any test instrument, further normative data are needed. The age mastery data especially need further elaboration and diversification relative to the varied populations with which most speech-language pathologists work.

Summary   The AAPS is recommended as a tool that should be familiar and available to speech-language pathologists. The test author has made a valuable contribution to the field with an obvious attempt to provide for useful and practical application.

AUSTIN SPANISH
ARTICULATION TEST (ASAT)

Elizabeth Carrow

Teaching Resources Corporation, 1974

Cost $16.95
Examiner's manual and test stimuli, 130 pages;
test booklet, 4 pages

Time 25 minutes

Allen S. Toronto *Southwest Texas State University*

Purpose The Austin Spanish Articulation Test (ASAT) provides material for evaluating articulation of Spanish phonemes, including single consonants, vowels, diphthongs, and consonant clusters that occur in Spanish.

Administration The ASAT consists of 59 pictures with corresponding incomplete sentences, each intended to elicit a test word containing the target phoneme. The child concludes each sentence with the test word. The ASAT was field tested on 20 Mexican-American children between the ages of four and seven in Texas to assure that the illustrations were appropriate. No attempt is made to account for different Spanish dialects.

Evaluation of test adequacy The ASAT presents a good set of materials for its stated purpose. The pictures are clear and the sentences are well constructed. The words selected for elicitation are generally known in all Spanish dialects. The words *globo* and *andar*, however, have common alternate words in many dialects. Avoiding vocabulary variations for particular pictures is impossible for this type of test. Some adaptation would have to be made when using the test with children of different dialects.

The ASAT does not provide a means of assessing articulation in running speech, which is an essential aspect of adequate phonological evaluation. This would have to be done by informal observation of the child's speech. Some speech-language pathologists who use the test indicate that older children respond well to the sentence stimuli, but that children between the ages of four and five years do not. No provision is made to assess more than one phoneme per test item making the test fairly long to administer (25 minutes).

Summary The ASAT is an adequate test for elicitation of single words, but it suffers the same inadequacies of all articulation tests in Spanish, namely, variations in Spanish dialect exist mainly in the consonant system, making many allophonic differences of the same phoneme acceptable. This confuses speech-language pathologists not familiar with local dialects. Additionally, the success of any articulation test depends not so much on the adequacy of the materials as on the listening and phonetic skills of the speech-language pathologist.

A DEEP TEST OF ARTICULATION: PICTURE FORM, SENTENCE FORM, AND SCREENING DEEP TEST OF ARTICULATION

Eugene T. McDonald

A Deep Test of Articulation, Picture Form
Eugene T. McDonald, 1964
Cost $7.50

A Deep Test of Articulation, Sentence Form
Eugene T. McDonald, 1964
Cost $6.00

Screening Deep Test of Articulation
Eugene T. McDonald, 1968
Cost $8.50

Articulation Testing and Treatment: A Sensory-Motor Approach, 1964
Cost $8.00

Individual record sheet, screening (50 sheets per pad), $ .75; teacher report form, screening (50 sheets per pad), $ .50
All available from Stanwix House, Inc.

Empress Y. Zedler *Southwest Texas State University*

Purpose The purposes of the Deep Test of Articulation are (1) to permit evaluation of speech sounds as the audible end-products of a series of overlapping, ballistic movements; (2) to sample representatively the phonetic contexts in which the sound being observed might occur including those contexts in which the sound is one of an abutting pair; and (3) to provide a test long enough to permit observation of the degree of variability present in the speaker's production of the sound.

Administration, scoring, and interpretation The Picture Form Test is used with persons whose reading ability is below third grade level. It consists of two sets of picturecards mounted side by side so that either picture can be turned to expose the next. It is explained to the testee that the pictures can be turned to make "funny big words out of two little words," i.e., tubvase. One card is kept stationary while the adjacent cards are turned providing the opportunity to test one sound in several contexts.

For those whose reading level is at or above the third grade, the Sentence Deep Test is used. Thirty sentences are provided for testing each of 11 consonant sounds in various phonetic contexts.

The record sheet provides blanks for recording type of misarticulations and correct or incorrect articulations of the sounds tested. Scoring provides a percent of correct articulations for any sound tested. The progression continuum for any sound from Almost Never Correct to Almost Always Correct permits evaluation of therapy.

The Screening Deep Test purports to assess a speaker's ability to articulate nine commonly misarticulated consonants by eliciting ten productions of each consonant.

Evaluation of test adequacy Standardization validity and reliability of the test are explained in *Articulation Testing and Treatment: A Sensory-Motor Approach,* which should be read before using the test. The existence of overlapping movements of different muscle groups during connected speech, upon which McDonald bases his test, has become well documented in the research upon normal articulation processes or coarticulation (Daniloff 1973). Juxtaposing words and requiring the subject to speak them in an unbroken syllabic stream characteristic of normal utterance has a high degree of logical validity as a test procedure. With most tests of articulation, face validity appears to be so obvious that little, if any, effort is made to establish any form of empirical validity. However, McDonald does provide data showing substantial correlations between results of four different forms of a deep test. Such measures can be taken as evidence of empirical validity, not for his test specifically, but for deep testing in general. In addition, correlations such as these lend support to the assumption that deep testing is a reliable procedure.

The manual emphasizes the motor rather than the perceptual aspects of articulation. Results of the Deep Test, however, may be used as readily for investigating perceptual aspects of phonology. It is a lengthy and tedious testing procedure but worth the investment of time for a clinician interested in investigating phonetic surroundings of the various phonemes in connected speech. When a phonetic context is discovered in which a child can articulate an error sound correctly, such a "key word" can provide the basis for therapy. Successes on the Deep Test can be analyzed to reveal the distinctive features responsible for success.

Summary   The Deep Test of Articulation is the result of a thoughtful analysis of existing data concerning articulation processes. It is a creative test procedure that has several valuable applications including (1) discovery of a context in which a misarticulated sound is produced correctly to provide a therapeutic base, (2) a measure of articulation proficiency, and (3) an index of therapeutic progress.

Reference

Daniloff, R. G. Normal articulation processes. In F. D. Minifie, T. J. Nixon, and F. Williams (eds.), *Normal Aspects of Speech, Hearing, and Language.* Englewood Cliffs, N. J.: Prentice-Hall, 1973.

THE DENVER ARTICULATION SCREENING EXAMINATION (DASE)

Amelia F. Drumwright

University of Colorado Medical Center, 1971, distributed by Ladoca Project and Publishing Foundation, Inc.

Cost Reference manual, $2.50; manual/workbook, $3.25; picture cards (per set), $ .60; test forms (per 25), $ .50; 1-hour training and proficiency film, $250.00; 1-hour training and proficiency video cassette, $100.00; 20-minute proficiency film, $100.00; rental of training and proficiency film (per week), $25.00; rental of training and proficiency video cassette, $25.00

Time 5 minutes, administration

Jay R. Jensen *Utah State University*

Purpose The primary purpose of the Denver Articulation Screening Examination is to detect articulation disorders in children 2.5 to 6 years of age.

Administration, scoring, and interpretation The administration of the test is extremely easy and can be accomplished by professionals, aides, parent groups, or lay personnel with a minimum of training. The technique of administration is primarily the imitative method; that is, the child is instructed to say what the examiner says. However, for the difficult-to-test child, simple line drawings are provided to assist the examiner in eliciting responses.

To score the response, the examiner is to circle the sound elements correctly produced in the child's response and then total the correct sounds produced over the 30 sound elements elicited. Additionally, the examiner is to make a judgment of intelligibility on a 4-point scale with 1 being "easy to understand," 2 "understandable half of the time," 3 "not understandable, and 4 "can't evaluate."

Interpretation of findings is made relatively simple. The raw score (total number of correct responses) is determined and is used to enter a percentile table provided on the back of the score sheet. The raw score is then matched with the column denoting the child's age, and the value given there is the child's percentile rank for articulation. The cutoff differentiating abnormal from normal is the 15th percentile. An intelligibility score is obtained from a simple matrix based upon age and whether or not a child is easy to understand, understandable one-half of the time, or not understandable.

The total result of this test is expressed as "normal" or "abnormal" and is determined from a composite articulation and intelligibility score. A child who scores normal (above 15th percentile) on articulation and normal on intelligibility would be ranked *normal*. A child who scored as abnormal on DASE and/or intelligibility would be ranked *abnormal*.

Evaluation of test adequacy The test is constructed from 34 sound elements that had been correctly articulated by 85 percent of six-year-old children studied by Templin (1957). Normative data on the sounds were then obtained from a sample of Anglo, black, and Hispano preschoolers in Denver, Colorado ($N = 1450$). The children were between ages 2 years 4 months and 6 years 3 months and were equally divided by sex. Since no significant differences were found between cultural groups or sexes, the data were combined to form the percentile chart provided with the score sheet.

Validation and reliability are reported, both of which are moderately high. Validation studies between the DASE and Hejna Developmental Articulation Test (qv) yielded copositivity scores of .88 and .92 and conegativity scores of .91 and .97. This essentially means that there is concurrent validity between DASE and the criterion measure, the Hejna test. However, it should be noted that the criterion test itself is supported by no published validity or reliability studies. Since the DASE purports to be only a screening examination, some predictive validity studies would seem to be in order. A test–retest reliability coefficient of .95 was obtained from test–retest administrations to 110 of the subjects.

The test manual provides interesting data on three cultural groups. Although these data did not discriminate between culture or sex, they are of interest and may provide a basis for additional research on phonological differences between cultures.

The cards provided for illustration seem almost an afterthought, and no directions for their use are provided. For the most part, the drawings are good but are awkward to use in presenting visual stimuli to the child. Pictures are printed on both sides of a card (approximately 3" X 5") and are fastened together in one corner by a rivet. The cards are not durable enough to withstand heavy usage.

Summary This screening test for articulatory proficiency of children age 2.5 to 6 years is a quick, easy-to-use screening measure. It will identify children with articulatory problems for whom more definite testing is needed. While the validity of the test is still in need of further investigation, the DASE offers a way for skilled and unskilled examiners to identify children whose articulatory proficiency is disordered sufficiently to warrant further evaluation.

References

Hejna, R. F. *Developmental Articulation Test.* Madison: American Printing and Publishing, 1959.

Templin, M. C. *Certain Language Skills in Children.* Minneapolis: University of Minnesota Press, 1957.

DEVELOPMENTAL ARTICULATION TEST

Robert F. Hejna

Speech Materials, 1968
Cost $3.00
Manual, 1 page; score sheet, 1 page
Time 15-20 minutes, administration and scoring

Ralph R. Leutenegger *University of Wisconsin—Milwaukee*

Purpose The presumed uniqueness of the Developmental Articulation Test at the time it was published lay in the arrangement of the scoring blank according to "developmental age level." The test constructor defined this as "the age by which 90 percent or more of children have acquired the sound. . .the developmental age levels are approximate and are based on normative data bearing on this subject." The sources of such data are not presented in the single-page instruction sheet.

Administration, scoring, and interpretation Consonant sounds are tested in initial, medial, and final word positions by having the child name the objects pictured on 4½" X 6" cards. Most of the cards contain three pen and ink drawings. The "blend" cards contain four or five. The /ʒ/ and /hw/ sounds are omitted: 14 "blends," in which /l/, /r/, and /s/ are clustered with other consonants, are included. Medial and final /r/ sounds are tested with pictures to elicit "barn" and "car."

On a few items stimulus questions are included for use when the child is unable to identify the given picture. For other stimuli not identified, the examiner is advised to name the picture and score the child's repetition of the name.

In administering the test, the examiner asks the child to identify the pictures. The examiner indicates in the appropriate initial–medial–final column the nature of the misarticulation (if any), i.e., substitution, omission, or distortion. In a fourth column the examiner indicates whether or not the child could produce the sound in isolation. An additional blank column is used to record any "comments" deemed of value.

Evaluation of test adequacy No validity or reliability information is available nor any other information to indicate validation of the test as a standardized measurement tool.

In general, the pictures can be assumed suitable for eliciting the words desired. Possibly ambiguous exceptions are the pictures of "potato" and "jump rope." One might question the value of designating as containing examples of medial sounds the underlined sound elements in too<u>th</u>brush, orange <u>j</u>uice, dog<u>h</u>ouse, spider <u>w</u>eb, and thank <u>y</u>ou.

The colors brown, orange, green, red, blue, and yellow are utilized on white cards. No given card contains more than one color of ink. The basis for color selection is not apparent; it indicates neither place nor manner of production nor developmental age level.

Summary The test constructor maintains that after testing is completed, one can tell at a glance on which sounds the child is "within normal limits of articulatory development." He further notes that the results "will clarify which sounds should be worked with first in certain cases." The reviewer believes this test to be of primarily historical interest.

THE FISHER–LOGEMANN TEST OF ARTICULATION COMPETENCE

**Hilda A. Fisher and
Jerilyn A. Logemann**

Houghton Mifflin Company, 1971

Cost $18.50

Therapist's Manual, 38 pages; two scoring forms: picture version, sentence version

Time Picture form, 20–45 minutes; sentence form, 8–10 minutes, administration; 10–20 minutes, scoring

John V. Irwin *Memphis State University*

Purpose As set forth in the therapist's manual that accompanies the test, "The Fisher–Logemann Test of Articulation Competence is designed (1) to implement the examination of the test subject's phonological system in an orderly framework; (2) to provide ease in recording and analyzing phonetic notations of articulation; and (3) to facilitate accurate and complete analysis and categorization of articulatory errors." The test is designed to be used in either diagnostic examination of articulatory deficiencies or in research in developmental phonology.

Administration, scoring, and interpretation

The Picture Version The picture version consists of 109 colorful line drawings arranged in patterns of two to five stimuli on each of 35 8½" X 11" hardboard cards. A spiral binding facilitates easy presentation. Eleven of the cards are tab-indexed for screening test applications. Each picture is designed to elicit a spontaneous single-word response. The words have been selected so that each test word satisfies the following four criteria: (1) the stimulus word contains the phoneme being tested, in conformity with the phonology of standard dialects; (2) the occurrence of the phoneme in stimulus words is systematized on the basis of syllabic function; (3) test words are common to the vocabulary of a person in the age range being tested; and (4) the picture stimuli should elicit the test words spontaneously. In general, these criteria are relevant and are satisfied by the test.

The test phonemes are 25 consonants, 21 consonant blends (seven blends of /s/ plus another consonant in prevocalic position; eight blends of prevocalic /r/ preceded by all possible consonants; six blends of prevocalic /l/ preceded by all possible consonants); final syllabic /l/; 12 vowels; and the four phonemic diphthongs.

Scoring and analysis of individual picture test data are accomplished by using two sides of an 8½" X 11" scoring form. Side one is used for the 25 singleton consonants; side two, for consonant blends, vowels, and diphthongs. The procedure is designed to record not only (1) instances in which the subject produces the phonemes of English acceptably by adult standards but also (2) an analysis of the nature of the misarticulations. Consonant phonemes are analyzed on the basis of a three-feature system: place of articulation (bilabial, labio-dental, tip-dental, tip-alveolar, blade-alveolar, blade-prepalatal, front-palatal, central-palatal, back-velar, and glottal); manner of articulation (stop, fricative, affricate, glide, lateral, and nasal); and voicing (voiced and voiceless). Vowel phonemes are analyzed on the basis of a four-feature system: place of articulation (front, central, and back); height of tongue (high, mid, and low); tension (tense, lax); and lip rounding (rounded, unrounded).

Data from the 11 consonants tested in the screening test are recorded on the consonant record forms; the 11 screening consonants are conveniently identified on the form by a heavy border.

Detailed instructions for administration of the test are given. Treated are such items as appropriate test environment, optional use of a tape recorder, identification techniques, cueing for items not spontaneously recognized, and methods of scoring. For singleton consonants and vowels, it is recommended that only errors be scored. For the blends, it is suggested that both acceptable and deviant productions be recorded in order to facilitate the analyses of phonetic context.

Suggested techniques for the recording of omissions and of standard substitutions are conventional; that is, it is suggested that the examiner use (−) for an omitted sound and a phonetic symbol if one phoneme is substituted for another. But distortions should be recorded by using the simplest allophonic variation that will be meaningful in subsequent analysis of the subject's misarticulations. For consonants, a convenient list of allophonic symbols and modifiers arranged by phoneme is provided. References for additional reading are cited. For vowels, a list of modifiers to use with each standard symbol is suggested.

The effect of dialects on the phonological performance of individuals is noted. The distinction is carefully drawn that misarticulation consists of phonetic disagreement with the speaker's native dialect and not with an idealized set of English phonemes. A table of gross native dialect patterns by selected geographic regions and for Negro dialect is given. A table for foreign dialects is also presented.

Two basic advantages of distinctive feature analysis to articulatory therapy are offered. First, it is suggested that the identification through feature analysis of the nature of the faulty production of a phoneme provides a meaningful target in the correction of the error phoneme. Second, it is suggested that the identification of feature violations common to several phonemes facilitates speech therapy in that (1) it reveals the minimal basis for achieving a distinction between two phonemes that are not adequately differentiated in the subject's speech and (2) the acquisition of the feature in one phoneme can be transferred to other phonemes in which the violation had previously occurred.

The Sentence Version   The sentence test consists of 15 sentences. It is printed in large, legible type on a single card. It tests every singleton consonant in all syllabic functions consistent with English phonology and every vowel phoneme of English.

Three criteria governed the selection of stimulus words in the sentence test. As in the picture test, criteria one and two were concerned with securing a representative phonological sample that is systematized on the basis of syllabic function. The third criterion stipulated that the words must be common to the reading vocabulary of the person being tested. The printed form is reported to have been used successfully with children as early as the third grade.

Although a separate recording form is provided, the system of notation and analysis is the same as that employed in the picture test. Dialectal treatment is also similar to that in the picture test.

Detailed instructions for administration of the sentence test are offered. Such factors as lighting, use of tape recorder, dialectal identification, and reading one sentence at a time are described. As in the picture test, distortions should be recorded as exactly as possible by the use of allophonic symbols and modifiers.

Evaluation of test adequacy The development of both versions of the test is described in detail in the manual. Of interest is the pilot testing accomplished in the Chicago area by 30 speech therapists with some 500 children. Ages, sociolinguistic backgrounds, and existence of handicapping conditions are described generally. Some feel for the kinds of reactions received and the kinds of changes made is given.

Unfortunately, no quantitative expression of the reliability of either version is presented. Such information would have been particularly helpful in view of the allophone-modifiers system of notation introduced. The comparability of the two versions is not reported quantitatively but, in fairness, it should be pointed out that the two versions are not presented as equivalents. No quantitative relationship between the screening form of the picture version and the full picture version is expressed.

Data from the Fisher–Logemann Test are to be interpreted as a sample of phonological behavior for English-speaking subjects. If content validity may be judged by the sampling adequacy of the content of an instrument (Kerlinger 1973), the Fisher–Logemann Test satisfies many criteria. Thus in the complete picture version all phonemes and several crucial blends are sampled in carefully constructed one-word contexts. In the sentence version, all vowels are sampled and each singleton consonant is tested in the syllabic functions consistent with English phonology. Phonetic rather than morphologic contexts are emphasized. Whether either or both of these samples are adequately representative of a nonstructured, conversational sampling is, at the moment, a matter of judgment (Winitz 1975). But compared with the content validity of other structured samples, the Fisher–Logemann Test does very well.

No measures of criterion-related or construct validity (Kerlinger 1973) are reported. Norms by age, sociolinguistic background, or handicapping condition are not available in the manual. Interpretation must be made by each clinician on the basis of his or her individual standards.

Summary The Fisher–Logemann Test of Articulation Competence is an extremely useful test. The linguistic basis is thorough. The physical realization is excellent: pictures are large, colorful, and generally identifiable; the sentence stimuli are clearly presented; and the forms are well printed.

The handling of distortions is innovative, although the phonetic notation is possibly beyond the scope of some users. The distinctive feature system, which is limited and not compatible with many current systems (Singh 1976), is articulation-based and offers the clinician traditionally useful information. Information on reliability and validity is limited. But, despite its emphasis on structured context, the test has high face validity. It adds many new dimensions to articulatory testing.

References

Kerlinger, F. N. *Foundations of Behavioral Research* (2d ed.). New York: Holt, Rinehart and Winston, 1973.

Singh, S. *Distinctive Features: Theory and Validation.* Baltimore: University Park Press, 1976.

Winitz, H. *From Syllable to Conversation.* Baltimore: University Park Press, 1975.

GOLDMAN–FRISTOE TEST OF ARTICULATION (GFTA)

Ronald Goldman and Macalyne Fristoe

American Guidance Service, Inc., 1969, 1972
Cost $22.60
Examiner's manual, 27 pages; 50 response forms, 2 pages
Time 45 minutes, administration and scoring

Merlin J. Mecham *University of Utah*

Purpose The purpose of the Goldman–Fristoe Test of Articulation as set forth by its authors is to provide a systematic method for locating and recording articulation errors as an aid in defining problems and providing a guide for effective remedial service. Although it is designed primarily to test for consonant errors, most vowels can also be observed and evaluated. The test is designed to facilitate elicitation of spontaneous production of English consonant sounds in single words in their most common positions as well as 11 consonant blends; it also helps elicit production of most consonant sounds within the context of sentences or phrases through use of picture stories that are presented to examinees for them to tell back to the examiner. It enables the examiner to assess the examinees' ability to produce misarticulated phonemes correctly when given maximum audiovisual stimulation.

Administration, scoring, and interpretation General instructions include suggestions for optimal lighting, sound environment, and proper seating. Scoring instructions provide equivalent procedures across subtests and suggest two possible levels for making scoring judgments: (1) judging for presence or absence of error in production of each sound being sampled (instructions imply that "untrained" examiners should use this level only); and (2) judging for types of errors observed in the subject's responses (to be used only by persons trained and qualified in speech pathology). Scoring symbols are specified for various types of judgments concerning production and may be recorded on the score sheet. A filmstrip version of the GFTA is also optionally available. Each of the subtests has its own more specific instructions.

The Sounds-in-Words Subtest is given by presenting 36 large colored line-drawn picture cards mounted on a flip-type easel (cards are presented one at a time). Instructions for stimuli presentation and scoring criteria are printed on the backs of the cards on the side of the easel facing the examiner; only the pictures are made visible to the child. As the child names the pictures, the examiner records judgments concerning nature and extent of any errors made by the examinee on sounds (phonemes) specified for each card. Each card (stimulus word) assesses more than a single phoneme. Responses elicited from the examinee are to be spontaneous, so care is taken to avoid the possibility of imitational responses.

Scores on the Sounds-in-Words Subtest (total errors only) and Stimulability Subtest (syllabic portion) can be interpreted by use of percentile norms which are given in the manual. Normative data are not presented for the word or sentence portions of the Stimulability Subtest, the Sounds-in-Words Subtest, or for the various positions (initial, medial, final) for the Sounds-in-Words Subtest.

The Sounds-in-Sentences Subtest consists of two narrative stories read by the examiner and is illustrated by nine line-drawn colored picture cards. The first story is read by the examiner from the back of the easel kit as the first five picture cards are being shown to the child. The examiner tells the story then goes back and presents the pictures one at a time and asks the child to retell the story, using the pictures as cues. As the child retells the story, the examiner listens for any phonemic errors and records them on the portion of the score sheet devoted to the Sounds-in-Sentences Subtest and makes the proper entries. The second story of this subtest is presented to the child using the remaining four Sounds-in-Sentences Subtest picture cards, and the child is asked to retell the story as the examiner goes back and presents each card again. Errors produced by the subject for the second story are noted in the places provided for them on the score sheet. The portion of the score sheet provided for this subtest has two different places for noting errors: (1) The key word section, on the left hand side, has key words listed in the order in which they would appear in the story; the examiner records the manner in which each phoneme was produced by the child immediately above the number assigned to it. The response codings used are the same for all subtests and have been described under general scoring procedures above (except in the Sounds-in-Sentences Subtest, the unelicited words are left blank). (2) Specific errors matrix, on the right hand side, has spaces in which the errors can be transferred after the entire subtest is completed.

The Stimulability Subtest is given to determine the extent to which the child can correctly imitate the sounds on which he or she made spontaneous production errors in the first two subtests. Stimulability is checked at each of three complexity levels, i.e., syllabic, words, and sentences.

Interpretation of test results are made in terms of classification of types of errors made and norms are available for comparative interpretation on the Sounds-in-Words Subtest and the syllabic portion of the Stimulability Subtest.

Evaluation of test adequacy One of the early criticisms of the Goldman–Fristoe Test of Articulation was its relative lack of standardization (Byrne 1972). In the 1972 revision, norm-referencing data for two of the subtests (Sounds-in-Words and Stimulability) are tabulated in percentile tables. These were based on data collected in a national survey of 38,884 children from grades one through twelve, collected over all nine census divisions in the United States. Although the norm-referencing group appears to be nationally representative, no breakdown is actually given in the manual as to the number of boys and girls at each of the age breakdowns.

Also, the 1972 edition reports temporal and interjudge reliability estimates for portions of the Sound-in-Words Subtest and Sounds-in-Sentences Subtest. Acceptable interjudge reliability has also been established for the Stimulability Subtest. No reliability estimates are given for various age levels, even though age levels are the basis for the presentation of norms. One would suspect that reliability for older age levels would be greater than for younger age categories, but there is no way of knowing what that discrepancy might be. Also, means and standard deviations for various age groups are lacking; it is therefore impossible to make a comparison of the age groups in terms of expected standard error of measurement.

For all one can tell from the manual, most of the children might have been fifth graders. (Examination of the standardizing survey, Hull et al. 1971, however, reveals that the sample was fairly representative in terms of age, sex, and population densities.)

The content validity of the Sounds-in-Words Subtest appears to be adequate, since it samples all consonant phonemes except one; the Stimulability Subtest includes all sounds that have been erroneously produced by the child. The content validity of the Sounds-in-Sentences Subtest, which assesses sounds presumably most often found in error in children, is subject to question since types of errors tend to vary from one etiological group to another and are certain to vary from one child to another. No concurrent validity evidence is reported in the manual. An attempt was made to evaluate construct validity by comparing the scores of 37 children on the Sounds-in-Words Subtest and the Sounds-in-Sentences Subtest to verify the assumption that their scores would differ since they are measuring differing levels of complexity of behavior; the resulting differences (scores on the sentences were lower) tended to support this assumption. No other evidence of validity is available at the present time.

Clinical application of this test as a norm-referenced instrument should be restricted to children who are six years or above in chronological age. Any use below that age should be criterion-referenced rather than normative since norms are not available below age six.

Its major strength as a clinical tool appears to be its ability to classify the types and severity of various articulation errors; such information is useful for grouping children for intervention, for planning therapeutic objectives, and for measuring progress in therapy. Its major weakness is its cumbersomeness in scoring; this is compounded by the inclusion of a nonstandardized subtest (Sounds-in-Sentences Subtest) that is time consuming and requires relatively complicated scoring procedures.

Summary Although the Sounds-in-Sentences Subtest may be considered by many speech–language pathologists to be the most important subtest, it is still the weakest subtest in terms of standardization and any interpretations of the results of the test should be made cautiously. It would be more appropriate to have appended this test and labeled it clearly as a "domain-referenced" rather than a norm-referenced subtest; its interpretation should likewise be presented separately from the interpretation of the other subtests.

Probably the greatest weakness of this test, in terms of current views of phonology, is one that still generally pervades the area of articulation testing; that is, it emphasizes the *motor* production errors and does not adequately assess phonological errors made by children. It gives only a superficial picture of how children violate such rules as *sound duration* or *position, complex clustering*, etc. Most articulation tests need to make a substantial shift in emphasis to include phonological error assessment in addition to *motor* production.

References

Byrne, M. C. Goldman–Fristoe Test of Articulation: Review #952. In O. K. Buros (ed.), *The Seventh Mental Measurement Yearbook.* Highland Park, N. J.: Gryphon Press, 1972.

Hull, F. M., P. W. Mielke, R. J. Timmons, and J. A. Willeford The national speech and hearing survey: preliminary results. *Asha* 13: 501-509, 1971.

Shelton, R. L. Goldman–Fristoe Test of Articulation: Review #953. In O. K. Buros (ed.), *The Seventh Mental Measurement Yearbook.* Highland Park, N. J.: Gryphon Press, 1972.

INTEGRATED ARTICULATION TEST

Orvis C. Irwin

Published in Orvis C. Irwin, *Communication Variables of Cerebral Palsied and Mentally Retarded Children.* Springfield, Ill.: Charles C Thomas, 1972
Two equivalent forms, Part Tests A through E and Alternate Part Tests A through E

Cost $20.75
Manual and test forms are not available except as a part of the book

Ruth M. Lencione *University of California at Los Angeles*

Purpose The Integrated Articulation Test represents one component in a series of comprehensive research studies conducted by Irwin over a 13-year period dealing with the communication skills of children with cerebral palsy. The results of this pioneer work are collected in his book *Communication Variables of Cerebral Palsied and Mentally Retarded Children* (1972). When the author began his studies in the mid 1950s, there were no articulation tests standardized specifically on children with cerebral palsy.

Administration, scoring, and interpretation The Integrated Articulation Test and its alternate form consist of five parts—four consonant tests and one vowel test for ages three to 16 years. The "part tests" range from 15 to 18 words each and were especially designed to accommodate, as Irwin states, "the child with cerebral palsy who usually has a short attention span and who fatigues easily." The part tests are intended to be administered on several different days and consist of 87 phonemes of which 76 are consonant sounds in the initial, medial, and final positions in words, and 11 vowels. The test stimuli are verbal and require the child to imitate words, one at a time, as spoken by the examiner. The individual record sheets contain a list of the stimulus words in random order. Opposite each word, the position of the consonant or vowel is indicated by dashes. Tabulation of responses may be recorded in six categories: (1) correct, (2) substitution, (3) omitted, (4) distorted, (5) no response, and (6) neutral. The examiner may transcribe the responses at the time of the examination, or the responses may be tape recorded for later analysis and tabulation. In scoring the tests, the sums derived for each of the six categories provide a numerical score on each part test and on the test as a whole. The test, originally published by Irwin in *Cerebral Palsy Review* in 1961, included a manual and individual record sheets but is no longer available in this form. Individuals wanting to use the Irwin test format and procedures will need to write to the publisher of the book to obtain permission to use the materials. In addition to the Integrated Articulation Test, Irwin developed and standardized a separate Short Diphthong Test which contains five diphthongs in three positions in words.

The Integrated Articulation Test was designed primarily as a diagnostic instrument to measure and evaluate the status of cerebral-palsied children's ability to articulate sounds over the whole spectrum of speech sounds. All five parts of the test are concerned with only one ability, namely that of phonetic articulation of 87 phonemes in the three positions in words. Within this format, the test yields two kinds of information about the child's articulation: a quantitative score of articulatory errors and deficits that can be systematically identified and recorded providing a numerical score on each part test and on the test as a whole; and a qualitative assessment about the improvement of particular sounds in the three positions and new misarticulations. Overall, the test provides a means of test–retest evaluation that enables the speech–language pathologist to develop specific therapy procedures to match the child's needs.

Evaluation of test adequacy   No discussion of Irwin's validation of the Integrated Articulation Test would be complete without a brief overview of the studies that preceded the standardization of the integrated test. Through the development of the original four short consonant tests and the vowel test, reliability and validity of each test was obtained; difficulty ranges of the items in each test were calculated; age progression in the scores was determined; and the discriminating power and uniqueness of the items were found. Each part test was standardized on a different sample resulting in a total of 1155 children with cerebral palsy from 80 public schools and centers in 44 states.

For the standardization of the whole test, parallel form reliability was calculated, observer agreement was determined, and internal consistency was applied to the sounds in the initial, medial, and final positions in words. The standardization group consisted of two samples of children. One sample contained 147 children from speech centers, public schools, and hospitals in seven states, primarily north central; the other consisted of 118 children in eight western and midwestern states.

Parallel form reliability was .98; observer agreement averaged 90 percent. Comparison of the two samples indicated the following: (1) Means of the first and second groups did not differ significantly, and the variances were homogeneous. (2) Differences between the means of the two groups of boys and two groups of girls were not significant. (3) Reliability of consonant sounds in initial, medial, and final positions was similar for the two groups. For the groups combined, reliability coefficients ranged from .92 to .97. (4) Reliability of vowels was similar for the two groups, and for the groups combined was .89 and .91 for initial and medial positions, respectively. (5) There were no significant differences between means of the spastics, athetoids, quadriplegics, hemiplegics, and paraplegics in the two groups.

The external criteria for validity were a medical diagnosis of mild or severe paralytic involvement and speech–language pathologists' ratings of very good or very poor speech intelligibility and general language facility. For both comparisons, differences between extreme groups were significant with children diagnosed as mildly involved or rated very good in general language having significantly better articulation scores.

The Integrated Articulation Test was standardized, also, for use with retarded children. The standardization group consisted of 162 children from five states. They were from three to 16 years old with a mean CA of 10-7 and a mean MA of 6-7.

Reliability of the test sounds in initial, medial, and final positions was fairly high, but it was low for final consonants. Validity was determined by comparing scores of the educable (IQ 51-80) and trainable (IQ 25-50) children. The mean score for the educable group was significantly higher than the mean for the trainable group, but the trainable group was more variable. Irwin concluded that the integrated test is not as precise with retarded children as with children with cerebral palsy and that results of the test used with retarded children should be interpreted with caution.

Summary   Irwin's contribution to the body of knowledge concerning the communication skills of cerebral-palsied children is inestimable. At the time he began his pioneer studies, there was little valid and objective information about the abilities and disabilities of this group of speech-handicapped children. He was among the first to break down the communication process into its basic elements and to develop and construct quantitative measuring instruments. The primary purpose of his work in the area of articulation was to provide a diagnostic tool to evaluate the child's ability to articulate speech sounds in various positions in words. The emphasis in therapy at that time was to help cerebral-palsied children develop expressive language skills, and within that context, the Integrated Articulation Test provided the speech–language pathologist with an objective test from which to develop speech strategies and to assess progress. Irwin's research and tests provided a theory for organizing, integrating, and interpreting the variables of articulation and treating them as independent components. Since that time, the contribution of linguists and psycholinguists and a greater understanding of language and speech acquisition have changed the approach to the assessment and management of children with neurological deficits considerably. Notwithstanding these changes, Irwin's historic work is a landmark in the evolution of sound, reliable, quantitative research and was a forerunner of subsequent test procedures.

References

Irwin, O. C. A manual of articulation testing for use with children with cerebral palsy. *Cerebral Palsy Rev.* 22: 1–20, 1961.

Irwin, O. C. *Communication Variables of Cerebral Palsied and Mentally Retarded Children.* Springfield, Ill.: Charles C Thomas, 1972.

PHOTO ARTICULATION TEST (PAT)

Kathleen Pendergast, Stanley E. Dickey, John W. Selmar, and Anton L. Soder

Interstate Printers and Publishers, Inc., 1969
Short and long forms available

Cost $14.75
Manual, 19 pages; score sheet, 1 page

Time 5 minutes or less, administration and scoring

Donald Mowrer *Arizona State University*

Purpose Although the authors do not specifiy the purpose of the Photo Articulation Test, it is obvious that the instrument was designed to provide the speech-language pathologist with a means of rapidly assessing the articulation skills of children.

Administration, scoring, and interpretation The test consists of 72 color photographs of objects familiar to most young children. The child is asked to name each picture as the clinician evaluates the adequacy of the target sound being tested and records the response on a score sheet. Twenty-three consonants are tested in initital, medial, and final positions. Eighteen vowels are also tested. Omissions, substitutions, three levels of distortions, and ability to correctly imitate sounds are noted on the score sheet. Three pictures are used to help evoke a story so that connected speech can be evaluated. Scoring is accomplished by totaling the numbers of errors made on tongue sounds, lip sounds, and vowel sounds. The examiner is referred to age norms compiled from testing 684 children ages 3 to 12. Both short and long forms of the test are available. Additional test words are also provided to give the clinician more detailed information about articulation skills.

Evaluation of test adequacy This test includes a brief but well written manual, an easy to follow score sheet, and well prepared stimulus materials as well as information concerning reliability and validity. One hundred children were used for reliability and validity tests. A coefficient of .991 was found using the test-retest method. To determine validity the test results were compared with results on the Bryngelson-Glaspey and Templin-Darley Articulation Tests (qv). Validity coefficients were .984 and .975, respectively. These reliability and validity coefficients are certainly respectable even though sample size was rather small and only two other articulation tests were used.

Although there was no statistical treatment of data comparing the short and long forms, it was reported that of 1000 children tested, less than 1 percent of the total sound errors were missed when the short form was used. It seems strange that the authors would even bother to use the long form, the only difference being omission of testing in the medial position of words in the short-form version.

The norms included in the test provide the clinician with little information of real value. For example, two children with quite different sound error patterns may obtain identical scores on the test. Although the age norms would appear to suggest how many years a child would be retarded in articulation, such global information is of little value in diagnosing the problem or in planning therapy.

The strength of this test is that it provides a means of quickly assessing the general nature of a child's articulation ability. The test is easy to administer, simple to score, and easy to transport. The only additional item required is a pen or pencil. It was not designed to provide the clinician with a means of intensive diagnosis or as a tool to help plan and execute therapy.

The pages tend to tear out of the test booklet with repeated use, but decks of the photographs published as individual cards are available if desired. A few of the picture cards could be updated or improved upon (lamp, teeth, vacuum cleaner, and witch) but for the most part, they appear to be appropriate, well photographed items.

One other limitation is that only limited samples of connected speech are obtained during the test. The speech sample is restricted chiefly to monosyllabic utterances. Most diagnosticians today require a much more detailed picture of a child's articulation skills than simply a three-position test. But then again, this test was not designed to yield a detailed picture.

Summary   This test appears to accomplish the purpose for which it was designed, that is, to provide the clinician with a quick overview of a child's articulation skill. It is not intended to provide detailed diagnostic information or guidelines for therapy. The norms provided are probably of little value. I would recommend the use of this test provided the clinician realizes that it is best used only as an articulation survey instrument.

PREDICTIVE SCREENING TEST OF ARTICULATION (PSTA)

Charles Van Riper and Robert L. Erickson

Western Michigan University, Continuing Education Office, Third Edition, 1973

Cost $1.00

Manual, 18 pages; score sheet, 5 pages

Time 7–8 minutes, administration and scoring

Gordon M. Low *Brigham Young University*

Purpose

". . .the basic purpose for which the Predictive Screening Test of Articulation has been devised is to differentiate children who will master their misarticulations without speech therapy from those who, without therapy, may persist in their errors. More specifically, the PSTA is used to identify, among primary school age children who have functional misarticulations at the first grade level, those children who will—and those who will not—have acquired normal, mature articulation by the time they reach the third grade level" (Manual, p. 1).

Administration, scoring, and interpretation The PSTA is administered to children at the first grade level during the first ten weeks of their school enrollment. Total time for administering and scoring the PSTA typically is about seven minutes. The test is administered following brief conversation with a child. All 47 items, except number 46, are presented as words, sentences, sounds syllables, and hand clapping for the child to imitate. Item 46 requires the child to discriminate between a correct and incorrect production of the word *finger*. The examiner scores the response correct in the various speech imitation items if the child produces the target sound correctly and in the hand clapping if the rhythm and number of claps are accurate. Total score equals the number of items correct.

Results are interpreted in terms of normative data that indicate the percentage of children who may be expected to acquire normal articulation at the third grade level without speech therapy when they obtained a particular score on the PSTA administered to them in the first grade. The authors recommend that the final selection of a cutoff score be decided in terms of the needs and orientation of the clinician as well as the nature of the clinician's program and add, "The clinician should regard the recommended cut-off score of 34 as a tentative one until he has demonstrated it to be an optimal cut-off score in his own situation" (Manual, p. 5). It can be determined from the normative data tables what the consequence will be of using a higher or lower score than the recommended cutoff score of 34. Using a higher score to decide which children will be enrolled for therapy will neglect more children (false negative errors) who will not acquire normal articulation without therapy whereas using a higher cutoff score will include more children (false positive errors) in therapy who would not have required it.

Evaluation of test adequacy Examiner qualifications for administering the PSTA include the ability to make judgments as to correct or incorrect articulation of speech sounds.

The brief manual of the PSTA contains a rationale, a description of the construction of the test and its validity, and instructions as to scoring and variations in score interpretation that may be appropriate. Data from studies in which the PSTA has been used are provided to assist the examiner in deciding which cutoff score to apply in selecting clients for enrollment in speech therapy. The authors acknowledge that using the recommended cutoff score of 34/47 results in some false positive referrals and some false negative referrals. Their suggestion is that users of the test study the data and determine for themselves how they might reduce inappropriate decisions.

The PSTA was standardized on children, users of middle-American standard English, during the first ten weeks of their enrollment in first grade. Use of the test with children whose spoken language varies in dialect from middle-American standard English is not appropriate. The test also is not intended to predict from first grade results the articulatory status of children other than at the third grade level.

Criterion-related validity of the PSTA is relatively clearly indicated, both in the description of the test construction and in subsequent studies. In the several studies in which the PSTA was administered to children at first grade and again at third grade level, percentages of correct prediction ranged from 72 to 92 percent of those children who have functional defective articulation in the first grade (Barrett and Welsh 1975; Carr and Stover undated; Kibbey 1970; Marks 1973). Those who have used the PSTA as its purpose is defined have concluded that it has useful prognostic value.

With relation to construct validity, the PSTA measures not only behavior that may be associated with speech articulation, the spontaneous improvement of which the test is intended to predict, but it also uses actual articulation behavior as the predominant attribute to be measured. In reducing the original 111 items to 47, the authors have developed a brief screening test whose items are related to spontaneous articulatory improvement, a prediction that apparently cannot be made through a simple count of the number of phonemes misarticulated at the first grade level.

A product–moment correlation coefficient of .81 was obtained between scores of the original 293 cross validation subjects on two randomly selected halves of the PSTA. Correlations between examiners ranged from .90 to .99. There was no signigicant difference between boys' and girls' PSTA scores at the first grade level, and boys did not differ from girls in the frequency with which they acquired normal articulation.

It is apparent, and acknowledged by the authors, that further use of the PSTA will extend the confidence with which it can be used for populations other than those on which it was standardized. The authors also suggest further refinement of the test so that those items which may be associated with the identification of false positive and false negative referrals, for example, may be considered in avoiding over- or under-referral.

Summary It is interesting, in light of results of studies reported here, that Winitz (1975) observes, "Without reviewing all of the evidence, it is now clear that articulation tests predict and diagnose very poorly. As a point of fact, their only reliable function is that of assessing phonetic proficiency, the results of which are used to index incorrect sound productions." Barrett and Welsh, Carr and Stover, Marks, and Kibbey, on the other hand, agree that the PSTA may be an effective predictive screening test of articulation of first grade children. The PSTA is not as comprehensive an assessment of articulation behavior as are some traditional articulation tests. It thus, perhaps, does not have as great face validity as some articulation tests. However, it has sufficient criterion-related validity to be useful in priority selection of clients having communication disorders—a responsibility speech–language pathologists must assume.

References

Barrett, M. D. and J. W. Welsh   Predictive articulation screening. *Language, Speech and Hearing Services in Schools* 6: 91–95, 1975.

Carr, V. and J. Stover   A report on use of Van Riper's Predictive Screening of Articulation: a three year study. Unpublished paper, Rochester, New York, undated.

Kibbey, S. G.   A Validation Study of the Predictive Screening Test of Articulation. Unpublished masters thesis, Central Washington State College, 1970.

Marks, A. R.   The Validity of the Van Riper Predictive Test of Articulation. Unpublished masters thesis, Illinois State University, Bloomington, Illinois, 1973.

McDonald, E. T.   *A Screening Test of Articulation.* Pittsburgh: Stanwix House, 1968.

Winitz, H.   *From Syllable to Conversation.* Baltimore: University Park Press, 1975.

SCREENING SPEECH ARTICULATION TEST (SSAT)

Merlin J. Mecham, J. Lorin Jex,
and J. Dean Jones

Communication Research Associates, Inc., 1970

Cost· Manual, 30 pages, $3.00; score sheets, $1.50 for pad of 25

Test booklet, 30 pages

Estimated time for administration and scoring: Picture portion: 5 to 8 minutes; consonants in sentences: 3 to 5 minutes; vowels in sentences: 2 minutes; blends in words: 1 minute

Marvin L. Hanson *University of Utah*

Purpose   A screening test for articulation disorders.

Administration, scoring, and interpretation   There are 66 black-and-white line drawings for testing consonants in the initial, medial, and final positions. The examiner asks the child to name each picture as it is pointed to. If the word called for in the test is not produced, the examiner gives the child a choice between two words, one being the desired word. Test sentences in the latter part of the booklet may be either read or repeated by the child. The examiner records the errors, using "D" for "distorted," "O" for "omitted," and the substitute sound when a substitution error is made.

Evaluation of test adequacy   The simplicity of this test and the nature of its purpose make it inappropriate to apply standards for psychological test construction. With an occasional prompting from the clinician, most children produce the wanted response to most of the stimuli in the test. In this sense, it is a "valid" instrument.

Strengths   The test serves to determine quickly whether or not a subject has defective articulation. The test booklet is lightweight. The spiral binder is convenient. Most pictures are clear and simple and elicit the proper words. Sounds tested are presented in general developmental sequence. The scoring is simple. Most test sentences included contain familiar words. The test may be used with readers or nonreaders.

Weaknesses   The paper cover and pages are neither durable nor washable. Artwork is not of high quality, and some of the pictures are dated. A few words, such as "bucket" and "horseshoe," are forthcoming only with help from the examiner. One or two sentences such as "Zebra dolls are easy to squeeze" and "Let's make a gay cake" may draw a smile from more mature readers.

   The scoring system as explained does not provide for degrees of types of errors. Clinicians, of course, can use their own scoring system if they prefer.

Summary   This is a fairly typical screening test of articulation, simple to administer and suitable for its purpose. I would recommend that some pictures be modernized, but in its present form it is acceptable.

SOUTHWESTERN SPANISH ARTICULATION TEST (SSAT)	Academic Tests, Inc., 1977
	Cost $8.95
	Examiner's manual and test stimuli together, 55
Allen S. Toronto	pages; assessment sheet, 1 page
	Time 15 minutes, administration and scoring

Parley W. Newman *Brigham Young University*

Purpose The purpose of the Southwestern Spanish Articulation Test is to assess rapidly articulation of Spanish consonants in single words.

Administration, scoring, and interpretation Forty-seven simple line drawings are presented to a child who is asked to name them. Each elicited word contains a target phoneme in its initial, medial, or final position in the word. Notation is made on an assessment sheet of the type of error produced by the child. One item consists of the printed word *pronto*, which must be presented to the child orally for repetition if the child cannot read. No appropriate picture could be found which consistently elicited the *pr-* cluster.

No attempt is made to account for variations in Spanish dialect beyond suggesting that the examiner be a native speaker of the dialect spoken by the child. The author briefly discusses aspects of testing in Spanish by examiners who have been trained in English. In addition to recognizing vocabulary differences among Spanish-speaking communities, he discusses the bases for dialectic variations in both English and Spanish and problems of allophonic variation due to differing phonemic contexts. This information may be useful to a speech–language pathologist in interpreting the results of the test.

Evaluation of test adequacy The SSAT is adequate for its stated purpose. It is intended to serve as an informal assessment tool and is supported by no standardized data. The test was field-tested in central Texas to assure the adequacy of the pictures. However, vocabulary and dialect vary considerably among ethnic and geographical groups, and some of the items will probably not be appropriate for Spanish speakers outside of central Texas. The author suggests that the speech–language pathologist produce original stimuli to replace the inappropriate items. The words selected for the test are generally known in most dialects.

Assessment of a child's contextual speech is necessary for a complete evaluation of articulation. The SSAT provides no means for this type of assessment, and the author suggests that in addition to the test, the speech–language pathologist complete his or her own informal analysis of the child's spontaneous speech. This simply points out the fact that successful articulation assessment lies more with the listening skills of the examiner than with the structure of a test.

THE TEMPLIN–DARLEY TESTS OF ARTICULATION, SECOND EDITION

Mildred C. Templin and
Frederic L. Darley

University of Iowa Bureau of Educational Research and Service, Sound edition, 1969

Cost $5.00

Manual, 38 pages, Appendix A, test words, Appendix B, test sentences, 57 stimulus cards with 141 colored drawings and starter sentences; reusable overlays for scoring, $ .50 set of nine; test response forms, 4 pages, $ .60 each; specimen set, $5.40 postpaid

Time Variable; no time limit

Dorothy D. Craven *University of Hawaii*

Purpose This second edition represents a revision of the 1960 Templin–Darley Screening and Diagnostic Tests of Articulation, which consisted of a 176-item Diagnostic Test and a 50-item Screening Test. The test was revised to provide a "somewhat shorter (141 items), more flexible test with colored rather than black-and-white stimulus pictures." The authors have stated three purposes in testing articulation:

(1) . . .to assess the general accuracy of articulation, in which case a screening test is used. . .The test need include only those sounds and sound clusters which are associated with significant progress in development of articulation; (2) . . .to know whether, and with what consistency, the child can produce speech elements of a given type; for example, consonants requiring substantial intraoral breath pressure for their efficient production, or clusters of consonants involving a given phoneme; and (3) . . .to obtain a detailed description and analysis of a child's articulation . . .which may assist in deciding whether the child needs speech therapy, but more often to aid in prescribing the nature of the speech therapy.

To fulfill these purposes, the present 141-item Diagnostic Test has been divided and organized into nine overlapping subjects: the 50-item Screening Test indicates general articulation adequacy; the 43-item Iowa Pressure Articulation Test assesses the adequacy of speech sounds requiring greater oral breath pressure and, by inference, the adequacy of palatopharyngeal closure; the other subtests (a 42-item grouping of initial and final consonant singles, 31 two- and three-phoneme /r/ and /ə/ clusters, 18 two- and three-phoneme /l/ clusters, 17 two- and three-phoneme /s/ clusters, nine miscellaneous two-phoneme clusters, 11 vowels, and six diphthong and combination items) provide information about articulation of specific phonemes.

Admininstration, scoring, and interpretation The authors suggest that a child's production of speech sound elements should be tested first in a series of single words; then those sounds misarticulated should be presented in isolation, in syllable, in words for imitation; and finally intelligibility of conversational speech should be evaluated. For nonreaders, picture stimuli are used to evoke a spontaneous response. Starter questions and sentences to elicit the desired response are provided to be used as necessary. If time or other pressures require it, examiners may ask the child to repeat test words after them, thus obtaining imitative rather than spontaneous responses.

For older children who can read, test sentences containing two test words for each sound element are provided. Imitative tasks for misarticulated sounds and evaluation of conversational speech are identical to procedures used with nonreaders.

The child's responses are recorded on the four-page test form according to a provided code so that errors and correct sounds are clearly identifiable. An overlay for each subtest facilitates determining the child's score.

The first step in interpreting a child's performance on the test is to compare the child's score with appropriate norms. Norms provided for each subtest as well as the complete Diagnostic Test are based on data from Templin's (1957) study of language development in children. The norms are presented in 14 tables, each of which presents mean scores by age (3, 3.5, 4, 4.5, 5, 6, 7, 8) for boys, girls, sexes combined, and upper and lower socioeconomic groups. Each group is further identified by the number studied and the standard deviation. In using these norms the speech–language pathologist should recall that Templin's subjects were "all white, monolingual singletons of normal intelligence with no gross evidence of hearing loss, enrolled in 14 public schools and 21 nursery schools in Minneapolis and St. Paul."

On the Diagnostic Test, in addition to comparing the child's score with the norm, it is recommended that errors be analyzed according to type of error, consistency, and stimulability. A discussion of the interpretation and implication of these analyses is provided.

In addition to norms, the Screening Test provides a cutoff score at each age level that separates adequate from inadequate performance and thus identifies the child who needs further study of his or her speech sound articulation.

The Iowa Pressure Articulation Test (IPAT), which utilizes 43 items, was developed by Morris, Spriestersbach, and Darley (1961) to assess the adequacy of oral breath pressure for speech sound production and thus inferentially the adequacy of palatopharyngeal closure. Selection of items was based on study of 50 cleft-palate children (25 designated as good closure group, 25 inadequate). However, interpretation of scores on IPAT must be made recognizing that the norms provided are for Templin's normal subjects selected without regard to palatopharyngeal adequacy.

The groupings of consonant clusters provide subtest scores that may be compared to norms, but more importantly they provide information on the pattern of a child's inconsistency. The manual quotes findings of several research studies that may be used in interpreting inconsistency patterns in various clinical groups.

Evaluation of test adequacy

Test Construction   The second edition of the Templin–Darley Tests of Articulation represents both an expansion and a revision of the 1960 edition, but its basic format, the model of disordered articulation that it represents, and the interpretation of its findings present a traditional view of articulation testing.

The manual has been expanded to include more precise directions for administration, scoring, and interpretation of the test. Research data have been added to give further support to the authors' views, particularly in the presentation of the stimulus words and interpretation of results. The discussions in the manual clearly state some of the conflicting and unresolved problems in articulation testing prevalent at the time of publication (such as imitative vs. spontaneous stimulus presentation).

The validity of the test, that is, " its ability to predict through its scores on small samples of highly structured speech, the impact on listeners of the articulation characteristics of children's contextual speech," has been established by the work of Jordan (1960). Winitz (1969), while acknowledging that this is one way of defining validity, questions whether a more appropriate criterion for validation would be articulatory change or proficiency.

More recent criticisms of the Templin–Darley Tests have reflected the contemporary viewpoint that articulation is a subsystem of oral language (Irwin 1972). Children's misarticulations are seen as an expression of their phonological rules, and distinctive feature analysis of error patterns is recommended. Tests such as the Templin–Darley, which provide a quantitative measure of errors but do not provide information about the underlying rules, are judged inadequate or insufficient.

Ingram (1976) stressed the need for linguistics in construction of an adequate diagnostic test. His criticism of the Templin–Darley Tests is based in part on his presumption that it is a purely imitative test, but he is also critical of tests utilizing picture naming since they use words in isolation. He further criticized the use of a single test word for each sound. As Irwin (1972) states,

> Conventional picture stimulus tests such as Templin–Darley are criticized because they sample isolated words and may not represent a valid measure of contextual articulation.

Singh (1976) reported on studies by Kelly and Singh in which they investigated the relationship between the Templin–Darley test scores and distinctive feature scores. They concluded that their seven distinctive features could be used to predict performance on the Templin–Darley with a high degree of reliability. After further analysis, Singh concluded that the Templin–Darley is a unitary measure of the child's performance, but the distinctive feature score is a measure of differential skill on a number of parameters reflecting the child's underlying competence.

Clinical Usefulness Although the earlier Templin–Darley Tests of Articulation had been identified as one of the two most widely used commercially available diagnostic tests (Powers 1971; Ingram 1976), its clinical usefulness has been enhanced by changes evident in the second edition. The rearrangement of test items, including the renumbering of the 50 screening items, the shortening of the Diagnostic Test by 35 items, the addition of color and modification of stimulus pictures, provision of scoring overlays, and expansion of the norms increased the flexibility and convenience of the test.

Winitz (1969) has criticized screening tests such as the Templin–Darley which provide a statistical norm to sort out children whose performances are deviant. Ingram (1976), on the other hand, believes that although a numerical score tells nothing about a child's language system, it may be useful for comparative purposes. Irwin (1972) pointed out that screening procedures are usually preliminary to dismissal or further testing. Templin and Darley have indicated that identification of a child who does or does not need more complete study of his or her speech sound articulation is an important function of the cutoff scores.

Winitz (1969) suggested that although the recommended diagnostic uses of the test appeared to have value, they needed experimental validation. After examining these premises, he concluded that the "test approaches but does not reach the goal of a diagnostic instrument."

The Iowa Pressure Test of Articulation has been used by Van Demark et al. (1975) and found to be a reliable predictor of palatopharyngeal competence. Clinical usefulness as well as research potential appears to be established.

Summary The Templin–Darley Tests of Articulation are inexpensive, compact, traditional tests of articulation that are widely used by practicing speech–language pathologists. The test manual gives detailed information about the administration, scoring, and interpretation of the results, so that even an inexperienced student may follow standardized procedures. Of the subtests, the Iowa Pressure Test of Articulation deserves special comment because of its demonstrated usefulness in predicting palatopharyngeal competence. The reliability of these tests, as with all tests, is dependent on the presumed competence of the examiner. Critics who reflect current interest in studying misarticulations as expressions of phonological rules have raised questions about validity. Although their questions are provocative and theories promising, at the present time no new testing procedures have been validated. For the speech–language pathologist whose purposes match those of the authors and whose population is similar to the normative group, these tests will continue to be useful.

References

Ingram, D. *Phonological Disability in Children.* New York: Elsevier, 1976.

Irwin, J. V. *Disorders of Articulation.* Indianapolis: Bobbs-Merrill, 1972.

Jordan, E. P. Articulation test measures and listener ratings of articulation defectiveness. *J. Speech Hearing Res.* 3: 303–319, 1960.

Morris, H. L., D. C. Spriestersbach, and F. L. Darley An articulation test for assessing competency of velopharyngeal closure. *J. Speech Hearing Res.* 4: 48–55, 1961.

Powers, M. H. Clinical and educational procedures in functional disorders of articulation. Chapter 34 in L. E. Travis (ed.), *Handbook of Speech Pathology and Audiology.* New York: Appleton-Century-Crofts, 1971.

Singh, S. *Distinctive Feature Theory and Validation.* Baltimore: University Park Press, 1976.

Templin, M. C. *Certain Language Skills in Children.* Minneapolis: University of Minnesota Press, 1957.

Van Demark, D. R., D. P. Kuehn, and R. F. Thorp Prediction of velopharyngeal competence. *Cleft Palate Journal* 12: 5–11, 1975.

Winitz, H. *Articulatory Acquisition and Behavior.* New York: Appleton-Century-Crofts, 1969.

Part III
Appraisal of
Language Perception

Introduction

The popularity of tests purporting to tap such perceptual functions as auditory attention, sound discrimination, sequential analysis, short-term memory, and audition in noise dates from two early works by Travis and his associates. Travis and Davis (1927) administered some of the Seashore Measures of Musical Talent to college freshmen of mixed speaking abilities. The inferior group, which included various types of speech defectives, did less well than the other groups. Travis and Rasmus (1931) developed a test for speech–sound discrimination which they gave to college students, one group of whom was comprised of those having "functional articulatory defects." Because the articulatory-defective group did less well than the good speakers, the authors concluded that inferior sound discrimination ability is an important etiological factor in articulation disorders. Tests of auditory memory span probably came to the profession as digit-span protocols borrowed from other psychometric instruments. Later, however, Anderson (1939) developed a test employing speech sounds as a measure of auditory memory span. He found no relationship between auditory and memory span and either pitch discrimination or auditory acuity, but did find a relationship with ability in learning a foreign language.

These and other "relationships" were too often projected to a status of "causation," as in the case of the alleged capability of the Travis–Rasmus Test of uncovering an important etiological factor in articulation disorders. Not surprisingly, therefore, in the next decade Mase (1946) recommended tests of auditory acuity, auditory articulation discrimination, and auditory memory span (among others) in order to establish the etiology of articulation defects.

This proclivity of the test creators to attribute causation when only relationships have been established must rank as the most serious criticism of the early instruments. Unfortunately, it remains very much with us today. For example, the publisher's brochure for one of the most widely used auditory discrimination tests currently on the market states flatly: "Research has demonstrated the test's usefulness in determining the cause of specific learning disabilities, especially when used in conjunction with [two other tests by the same publisher]." The "research" in question is elusive to say the least. According to Bloom and Lahey (1978), research has not yet demonstrated the value of determining whether a language-disordered child is able to distinguish the sounds of the language—that is, whether words such as "pat" and "bat" sound the same to the child. They argue further that the value of testing for such abilities or deficits has not been established.

Just when (or how) the instruments designed to show relationships between auditory processing and articulatory skills broadened their capabilities to encompass the vast areas of language and learning disabilities cannot be specified by this writer. A prime candidate for the expansion rationale would nevertheless have to be the influence of Orton's work (1937, p. 144 ff). Orton linked deficient auditory skills with disorders of developmental alexia, special disability in writing, developmental word deafness, motor speech delay, stuttering, and developmental apraxia. If nothing else, this linkage launched "auditory skills" into more central functions as the boundaries separating sensory, motor, and symbolic operations came tumbling down.

Today most tests of language perception are ostensibly developed for purposes of identifying and remediating specific abilities thought necessary for language processing. For the most part the theoretical bases on which these instruments are grounded are either unacknowledged or highly controversial (Rees 1973). The fact is that, although normal speech perception is a heavily researched field, how the mind extracts a message from an acoustic signal remains poorly understood. The process, according to Studdert-Kennedy's (1975) model, entails at least these stages of analysis: (1) auditory, (2) phonetic, (3) phonological, (4) lexical, syntactic, and semantic. All stages beyond the first are abstract, involving recognition of properties that do not inhere in the signal. Yet when the input is speech we cannot expect the auditory stage to function independently of the higher (linguistic) stages. Consider, for example, the verbal input units thus far defined in linguistic theory: distinctive features, phonemes, context-sensitive allophones, syllables, syntactically defined phrases, and context-sensitive semantic effects. The role or level of operation of these various input units cannot be decisively settled on the basis of currently available information (Bond 1976; Broadbent 1977). Clearly, if researchers in speech perception have yet to resolve the many issues involved in their field, we must assume that assessment instruments purporting to measure specific abilities or deficits in perception have vastly overstepped their grounding in theory and research.

Some of the reviewers of tests included within this section have addressed these and other theoretical issues concerned with the underpinnings of the given test under review. Others, to avoid redundancies, have not. Nevertheless, the user is strongly encouraged to consult all of the reviews of a given test type in order to get information about these matters as well as for cross-comparisons among tests.

Finally, it should be recognized that evaluative alternatives are available for assessing language perception. One such approach is the analysis of spontaneous speech as undertaken by Bloom and Lahey (1978). A language intervention program can then be custom-designed on the basis of the child's observed linguistic behavior. Such an approach circumvents assumptions about specific abilities or deficits.

Warren H. Fay

References

Anderson, V. A. Auditory memory span as tested by speech sounds. *Amer. J. Psychol.* 52: 95-99, 1939.

Bloom, L. and M. Lahey *Language Development and Language Disorders.* New York: Wiley, 1978.

Bond, Z. S. On the specification of input units in speech perception. *Brain and Language* 3: 72–87, 1976.

Broadbent, D. E. The hidden preattentive processes. *Amer. Psychol.* **32**: 109–118, 1977.

Mase, D. J. Etiology of articulatory speech defects. *Teach. Coll. Contr. Educ.*, No. 921. New York: Teachers College, Columbia University, 1946.

Orton, S. T. *Reading, Writing, and Speech Problems in Children.* New York: W. W. Norton, 1937.

Rees, N. S. Auditory processing factors in language disorders: the view from Procrustes' bed, *J. Speech Hearing Dis.* **38**: 304–315, 1973.

Studdert-Kennedy, M. The perception of speech. In T. A. Sebeok (ed.), *Current Trends in Linguistics* **XII**, pp. 2349–2385. The Hague: Mouton, 1975.

Travis, L. E. and M. G. Davis The relation between faulty speech and the lack of certain musical talents. *Psychol. Monogr.* **36**: 71–81, 1927.

Travis, L. E. and B. J. Rasmus The speech sound discrimination ability of cases with functional disorders of articulation. *Quart. J. Speech Educ.* **17**: 217–226, 1931.

AUDITORY DISCRIMINATION TEST (ADT)

Joseph M. Wepman

Language Research Associates, Inc., 1973

Two equivalent forms, IA and IIA

Cost Specimen sets (manual plus one copy each form), $3.15
Manual of directions, $2.10; Form IA (pads of 50), $8.40; Form IIA (pads of 50), $8.40

Time 5 minutes, administration and scoring

John L. Locke *University of Illinois at Urbana-Champaign*

Purpose The Auditory Discrimination Test (ADT), which first appeared in 1958, is said by its author to be "an easy to administer method of determining a child's ability to recognize the fine differences that exist between the phonemes used in English speech." The 1973 version, though revised in the literal sense of the term, in practice is the same as the earlier test. The more recent edition derives an accuracy score instead of an error score. The manual is longer but the instructions, test form, and items are the same.

Administration, scoring, and interpretation The manual tells how to give the test, how to score it, and—ostensibly—how to interpret the results. The actual test is a single sheet of paper containing 40 pairs of monosyllabic English words, Form IA. Should examiners wish to readminister the test, they are invited to use Form IIA which is similar in all major respects but contains different words. Though the test is said to take only "about five minutes to administer," the manual states, incongruously, that "some young children respond negatively to the test because of its length."

Some of the test words are among those a child would know, for example, *gum*. Many others lie outside the receptive vocabulary of most children and many adults (e.g., *lath*). These words, by operational definition, function as nonsense syllables. Apparently the author is aware of this for he advises the tester to "familiarize yourself with the words by reading them aloud before giving the test." Some of the words contain diacritical markings to aid the tester in correct pronunciation.

In the administration of the ADT, the manual directs the examiner to give the following instructions:

> I am going to read some words to you—two words at a time. I want you to tell me, or let me know in some way, whether I read the same word twice or two different words.
>
> Remember, if the two words are exactly the same, you say "yes" or "same"; if they are not exactly the same, you say "no" or "different."

The manual goes on to say that the examiner actually can use any instructional language as long as the child "understands what it is he is supposed to do." In practice, however, the precise wording could be important. One reason is that items such as *thief-sheaf* may not, to the child, be two *different* words. Just any instructional wording may not do, also, because none of the items—even the noncontrastive pairs—would genuinely be *the same* (i.e., physically identical) if presented in live-voice fashion. Should a child think that any difference, no matter how subtle or linguistically nonsignificant, is to be reported, the child properly could say "different" to *all* pairs.

Evaluation of test adequacy   Of the 40 pairs on each form, 30 involve two different words. In all cases these different words are minimal pairs, that is, words that differ at a single syllable position. Twenty-six items are consonantally contrastive, half in the syllable-initial position (e.g., *fie–thigh; guile–dial*), half in the syllable final position (e.g., *lāve–lāthe; sheaf–sheath*). The consonantal contrasts in all cases involve two phonemes whose production differs by just one phonetic feature, place-of-articulation. Why this particular feature was selected is not revealed; unfortunately, the fact of its selection invalidates the test. The ADT cannot claim to sample fairly the contrasts of English while systematically excluding those involving voicing, manner of articulation, or the multiple features identified by more contemporary schemes. Research shows, in fact, that the place feature is the most difficult one to discriminate (Miller and Nicely 1955). The other four pairs are vocalically contrastive (e.g., *shoal-shawl; bum-bomb).* The remaining ten items are phonemically noncontrastive (e.g., *wretch-wretch ;par-par*). In Form IA, the 15th through the 28th items all have the correct answer of "different"; whether children get nervous about giving the same answer 14 times in succession is not known.

When the child has completed the 40 items, the examiner is to subtract the number of errors on contrastive items from 30 (the total possible errors) and obtain, thereby, the child's number correct. This figure, the child's "score," then is to be compared against a set of norms of unspecified derivation. If the child is five-, six-, seven-, or eight-years-old, the child's level of achievement may be interpreted in accordance with these norms. A child of five with a score of 29 or 30 right is said to have "very good development." Should the child have scored 27 or 28 correct, this score would be an indication of a "positive but not yet fully developed ability." A still lower score of 24 to 26 suggests that this five-year-old has "an average ability"; however the child would be credited with only "a moderately low ability indicative of a continuing problem" should he or she get just 19 to 23 of the items correct. Anything worse than that is "below the level of the threshold of adequacy" which, according to the manual, implies the presence of "some pervasive pathology." Though this level of performance is to be "treated with full consideration," the manual suggests that there may be no effective treatment of auditory discrimination failure. The ADT, then, can give us a pathological child and a teacher with no training ideas or reason to be hopeful. What is the nature of the "full consideration" the teacher is, in lieu of effective training, encouraged to give? The reader/tester is not told.

The child, at any rate, has a way out. The examiner is not supposed to count the performance of a child who scores low enough (less than 10 correct). Also, the score of a child who says "different" to more than three of the ten noncontrastive pairs is similarly discarded.

The manual particularly recommends this test because, it says, auditory discrimination ability is relevant to articulation (and reading, and language). This is an interesting claim. If there is a relationship between speech production and speech perception, one could observe it only by examining a child's performance on the same contrasts in the same phonetic environments in both tests. This is because both perception and production vary with phonetic context. What sounds do children have trouble producing, and what sounds do they say in place of these sounds? Inventories such as Snow's (1963) show that children commonly substitute /b/ for /v/, /w/ for /r/, /θ/ for /s/, and so forth. The discrimination question, then, is can the children tell /b/ from /v/, /w/ from /r/, /θ/ from /s/.

But one finds none of *these sounds* in contrast on the ADT. To be sure, /b/ is on the test, but it is paired with /g/ in one case and /d/ in another. Children do not typically substitute /b/ for /d/ and /g/. According to Snow's data, if a child substitutes /b/ for anything, it will be for /v/. Now if a child does this, his or her speech may suggest an inability to tell /b/ from /v/, and the only appropriate /b/ item on the test would be /b/-/v/.

Let us assume that the ADT *had* been sensitive to children's speech difficulties and that the author had put /b/-/v/ on the test. The child at hand who says /b/ for /v/ will get one chance to reveal his or her discrimination of the target sound and the substitution sound. As a binary task, the child would have a 50-50 chance of being correct even if totally deaf. Should our /b/ for /v/ child respond correctly, the conclusion that the child discriminates /b/-/v/ would be no more accurate on logical grounds than the parallel assumption of clairvoyance were the child to call correctly one flip of a fair coin.

Too few opportunities to discriminate the relevant contrasts would, then, be one problem—if the relevant contrasts were on the test, and they are not. But if there were a /b/-/v/ on the ADT, this would be helpful only to the clinicians of "Master Everychild," a statistical average of all children. It would not be relevant to the particular child who might, for example, say /f/ for /v/. If the child might not be able to tell /f/ from /v/, why test the child on /b/ and /v/? Or what if the child says /v/ correctly? Should the examiner go ahead and test the child's ability to discriminate /v/ from sounds the child never says in place of /v/? If so, how will the performance be valued? Should the child get the contrast right, it will confirm what the clinician already knows, that the child does not confuse /v/ with other sounds. If the child gets the item wrong, the clinician is in an interesting quandary. First, why doesn't this child substitute /f/ for /v/—or /v/ for /f/—if unable to tell them apart? That the child says /f/ and /v/ appropriately, or at least does not say one for the other, suggests that he or she has two different targets to shoot for. How did the child come by these different targets except by efficient speech perception? Lip reading cannot handle this. Second, since the child probably was brought into the clinic because of a *speaking* problem (or characteristic), should the clinician work on the child's discrimination failure when it is demonstrably not relevant to the child's speech?

Of the 36 most common phonemic confusions in child speech (Snow 1963), 22 involve differences in voicing (e.g., s/z) or manner of articulation (e.g., b/v). Since the ADT for unstated reasons includes only place contrasts, 61 percent of the test is immediately irrelevant to child problems of articulation. Of the remaining 12 items, only six are on the ADT. A child who appeared with all 36 of these confusions in speech output, and was able to discriminate *none of the error sounds* could still get a score of 24 on the ADT, demonstrating "average ability."

If the ADT has just six of the 36 most common error contrasts, what does it have in their place? In their place it has speech-irrelevant contrasts such as *moon–noon* which none of Snow's (1963) 438 first graders confused in their speech, since none of them ever misproduced syllable-initial /m/ and /n/. (In fairness to the ADT, we should add that all of the popular discrimination tests suffer—more or less equally—from the problem of phonemic irrelevance and insufficient trials.)

Finally, let us return to the matter of validity. Earlier we commented that the ADT probably was invalid purely because it makes no effort to sample evenly the featural contrasts of English. The ADT also would be invalid if its results did not agree with another important measure of speech discrimination—children's speech *differentiation*. A study by Beving and Eblen (1973) shows that children who did not say "different" to the contrastive pairs on a same-different test were able to say the syllables correctly when, on another occasion, they were asked to imitate them. In fact, four-year-old children had the same good differential production of the syllable pairs as children at the age of eight. The only thing that observably changed, with age, was discrimination *test scores*. It is possible, then, for a child to have good speech discrimination and still do poorly on a test like the ADT.

Summary   There is nothing one reasonably could think of as evidence, in the manual or anywhere else, that the ability tested by the ADT is more than coincidentally relevant to reading or to articulation or to language. But the author only makes his ADT available; individual clinicians may decide for themselves, as they always have, whether they wish to use the test in the service of their clients.

References

Beving, B. and R. E. Eblen   "Same" and "different" concepts and children's performance on speech sound discrimination. *J. Speech Hearing Res.* **16**: 513-517, 1973.

Miller, G. A. and P. E. Nicely   An analysis of perceptual confusions among some English consonants. *J. Acoust. Soc. Amer.* **27**: 338-352, 1955.

Snow, K.   A detailed analysis of articulation responses of "normal" first grade children. *J. Speech Hearing Res.* **6**: 277-290, 1963.

AUDITORY MEMORY SPAN TEST

Joseph M. Wepman and
Anne Morency

Language Research Associates, Inc., 1973
Two alternate Forms, I and II

Cost $9.50
Manual, 8 pages; Form I, 1 page; Form II, 1 page

Time 5 minutes, administration and scoring

Laurence B. Leonard *Memphis State University*

Purpose As its name implies, the Auditory Memory Span Test is a measure of a child's span of auditory recall. According to Wepman and Morency, auditory memory span unites with auditory discrimination and auditory sequencing to form the auditory perceptual process. Presumably this process, in conjunction with other sensory processes, is central in enabling the child to gain a conceptual grasp of the world.

The Auditory Memory Span Test measures a child's ability to recall single-syllable spoken words in progressively increasing series. Two alternate forms are available, each with 15 series ranging from two to six words in length. Three series are used for each length. Each word series consists of primarily single-syllable nouns taken from the frequency count data of Wepman and Haas (1969).

Administration, scoring, and interpretation The administration of the test involves instructing the child to repeat the words read by the examiner. After the child is presented with one or, if necessary, two practice items, the examiner presents the test items, proceeding without comment to word series of increasing length. All 15 series are presented unless the child fails all three series of any given length. At such a point, testing is discontinued.

A child who repeats all of the words of a series, in any order, without adding words, is credited with a correct response. The numerical credit that any given correct response receives is equal to the number of words in that particular series. A child's test score is the total number of credits. For the age span of five to eight years, a child's test performance can be compared with that of the child's peers by referring to standardization data in the test manual. For each one-year span, test scores are divided into five ratings ranging from −2 (at or below the 15th percentile) to +2 (at or above the 85th percentile).

Evaluation of test adequacy There are several criteria by which the Auditory Memory Span Test can be evaluated. One criterion is the extent to which it may be said to measure a particular theoretical construct. According to Wepman and Morency, the construct involved in this test is auditory memory span. In referring to the importance of auditory memory span, Wepman and Morency state: "In language development as the span increases two words are put together, later three and so on, as more words become incorporated into the child's vocabulary." (Manual, p. 1). Thus the assumption seems to be that a developing auditory memory span is necessary for language to develop. The question that must be asked, however, is whether this is true for the type of auditory memory span assessed in this test.

An inspection of the test standardization data reveals that as age increases, a generally corresponding increase is seen in test scores. However, these data are limited to children between the ages of five and eight years. It is important to point out that the bulk of language development occurs prior to five years of age (Dale 1976). Further development takes place after this period, primarily involving attainments such as handling surface and deep structure mismatches (Cromer 1970), changes in pronominal reference (Maratsos 1973), and the use of complex sentences involving subordination where they were previously limited to simple conjoining (Ingram 1975). However, most of these attainments do not result in increases in the length of utterances produced by children, a state of affairs seemingly related to Shriner's (1969) observation that utterance length beyond age five is not a good index of linguistic development.

Wepman and Morency's case might have been stronger if they had found a close relationship between Auditory Memory Span Test performance and age for children ranging from two to four years of age, the ages during which the greatest amount of language development is seen and the greatest increases in utterance length are evidenced. However, such an examination was not made, apparently because children younger than five years (and, in fact, a number of five-year-olds) could not "take the test successfully" (p. 4). It is not clear whether this was due to younger children's unwillingness or inability to follow the instructions, or simply to the fact that children of this age perform poorly on this type of task. Surely the latter would weaken Wepman and Morency's case that the auditory memory span abilities assessed in their test are important for language development.

Another means by which the test can be evaluated is to examine its effectiveness in predicting certain presumably related abilities in children. Wepman and Morency examined the relationship between first grade children's performance on the Auditory Memory Span Test and their performance on various subtests of the Metropolitan Achievement Tests during the third, fourth, fifth, and sixth grades. A number of the coefficients were statistically significant, particularly those pertaining to third grade Metropolitan Achievement Test performance. However, all correlations were low; no correlation exceeded .32 and most were under .30. Wepman and Morency also assessed how closely second graders' performance on the Auditory Memory Span Test related to their reading performance on the subscales of the Wide Range Metropolitan Reading Achievement Test. The observed correlations were low, none exceeding .28. Thus it must be concluded that the Auditory Memory Span Test is not a good predictor of academic achievement, at least as it is measured by these particular tests.

Given their theoretical position, it is somewhat surprising that Wepman and Morency did not examine the relationship between children's performance on the Auditory Memory Span Test and their performance on various tests of speech and language. A number of available speech and language tests are standardized on children between five and eight years of age. Without this information, it cannot be assumed that children's performance on this test relates at all to their speech and language abilities.

The Auditory Memory Span Test manual contains little information concerning reliability. The authors report a high correlation for alternate form reliability (.92). It is usually preferable to use item-to-item percentages of agreement rather than correlation coefficients in order to provide a more accurate assessment of reliability. Item-to-item agreement is more difficult to assess with alternate forms. However, given that each form contains three series for each of the five lengths and that the corresponding series appear in the same order on the two forms, this type of computation might have been appropriate. No attempt was made to assess the inter- and intraexaminer reliability involved in scoring children's responses. Wepman and Morency also did not assess the internal consistency of the Auditory Memory Span Test, which might have been done by performing a split-third reliability analysis of the word series of each length.

Summary The Auditory Memory Span Test is an easily administered test which takes little time to score and interpret. Children's performance on this test increases with age, at least for the span of five to eight years. It is conceivable that a clinician might wish to assess a child's performance on this test if she or he has questions about a child's auditory perceptual skills. Before making use of this test, however, two major cautions should be borne in mind. First, it is not at all clear that the auditory memory span abilities tapped on this test are related to those necessary for the child to acquire language. They also do not appear highly related to academic success. Second, a large amount of validity and reliability information about this test is lacking. Therefore, at this time at least, the Auditory Memory Span Test should probably be used only as a supplementary measure to gain an informal impression of a child's auditory retention skills. Major diagnostic decisions should not hinge on the child's performance on this test.

References

Cromer, R. "Children are nice to understand": surface structure clues for the recovery of a deep structure. *British Journal of Psychology* 61: 397–408, 1970.

Dale, P. *Language Development.* New York: Holt, Rinehart and Winston, 1976.

Ingram, D. If and when transformations are acquired by children. In D. Dato (ed.), *Georgetown University Round Table on Language and Linguistics.* Washington, D. C.: Georgetown University Press, 1975.

Maratsos, M. The effects of stress on the understanding of pronominal reference in children. *J. Psycholing. Res.* 2: 1–8, 1973.

Shriner, T. H. A review of mean length of response as a measure of expressive language development in children. *J. Speech Hearing Dis.* 34: 61–68, 1969.

Wepman, J. and W. Haas *A Spoken Word Count: Children 5, 6, and 7.* Chicago: Language Research Associates, 1969.

AUDITORY POINTING TEST

Janet B. Fudala, LuVern H. Kunze, and John D. Ross

Academic Therapy Publications, 1974
Two equivalent forms, A and B

Cost $17.50 for complete test package
Manual, 66 pages; test form, 4 pages

Time No allotment of time for test administration is suggested

Norma S. Rees *City University of New York*

Purpose The stated purpose of the Auditory Pointing Test is to measure children's short-term memory in terms of both span and sequencing abilities. The age range for which the test is intended is 5–0 to 10–11. In order to be specifically applicable to children with "oral" speech and language problems (presumably those with production deficits), the test is designed so that pointing is the only response expected of the subject. The manual indicates that scores from this test may be used to develop training programs specific to either or both of the two allegedly separable skills of memory span and sequencing. Therefore, the Auditory Pointing Test also has the purpose of providing a basis for the design of remediation.

Administration, scoring, and interpretation The test is administered to children individually. The examiner places a card in front of the child and instructs the child to point to the picture(s) named in the order mentioned. The pictures are black-and-white line drawings and most are unambiguous. Following a number of demonstration items that include also an optional vocabulary check, 23 stimulus series increasing in length from two to ten items are presented. The examiner ends the test when the child has omitted or added items in three consecutive series. A shortened version for sampling purposes is also offered. All items are picturable monosyllabic nouns. Scoring instructions, which are simple, allow the examiner to distinguish between items remembered in the correct order and items remembered regardless of order of recall.

Percentile scores are given. Recommendations for interpreting scores in terms of three diagnostic patterns are offered. The manual includes a section on suggestions for remediation for deficits in short-term memory identified by this test, together with a brief annotated bibliography of remediation programs.

Evaluation of test adequacy The test was standardized on normal children from kindergarten through fifth grade in the Seattle schools. Reasonable precautions were taken to ensure the adequacy of the standardization population. Reliability was tested and found adequate. Two forms, A and B, were developed and found to be equivalent. Measures of validity were provided by computing correlations with chronological age, mental age, and with similar tests such as relevant subtests of the Illinois Test of Psycholinguistic Abilities (Auditory Sequential Memory) and the Wechsler Intelligence Scale for Children (Digit Span). All correlations were satisfactory.

The Auditory Pointing Test is based on a number of assumptions that have been attractive to many persons responsible for the assessment and remediation of children with language and/or learning disabilities. These assumptions have, however, by no means been universally accepted. The notion that auditory memory abilities as measured by word-units are implicated in the development of normal language or in language/learning disabilities has been challenged by Rees (1973), Sanders (1977), Bloom and Lahey (1978), and Rees (1978). Sanders (1977), for example, questions the assumption that the auditory processing of spoken language is an independent function at all, suggesting instead that the complexities of linguistic processing cannot be reduced to a "combination of discrete auditory skills feeding information to a language system for linguistic analysis and interpretation." Studdert-Kennedy (1976) describes with persuasive lucidity how the perception of speech depends on interlocking processes at the auditory, phonetic, phonological, lexical, syntactic, and semantic levels of analysis. These and other comprehensive accounts of what goes on when the listener analyzes a segment of spoken language render any approach to clinical assessment that identifies discrete abilities such as auditory memory span or auditory sequencing ability of extremely dubious validity.

Other serious questions have been raised about the basis for selecting any given unit, such as the monosyllabic word as used in the Auditory Pointing Test, for the purpose of measuring auditory memory (Jenkins 1974). No satisfactory rationale exists for selecting the monosyllabic over the polysyllabic word, nor the nonsense syllable, multiword phrase, or the sentence itself, as the correct unit for measuring auditory memory. If one unit is as good or as poor as another in terms of any notion of psychological reality (see Foss and Swinney [1973] for an interesting review of some of this research), it is difficult to assign any meaning to the results of tests that measure children's memory span in wordlike units.

An underlying assumption of the Auditory Pointing Test is that, in order to understand sentences, children have to remember the individual word units in the order given, an assumption that fails the test of careful research and ignores the complexity of the process whereby listeners assign meaning to the sentences they hear.

The test also assumes that measuring the child's short-term memory in terms of series of monosyllabic words will reveal a strength or deficit of crucial importance to learning and language comprehension. The relationship between short-term memory and language/learning is, unfortunately, not as simple as the test manual suggests. Olson (1973), for example, concludes from his analysis that an increasing memory span is not a prerequisite but a concomitant of the child's maturing ability to handle verbal information. If that is so, measuring auditory memory span is unnecessary because it adds nothing to what we already know about children with language deficits. It is also well known that recall for word sequences is improved when these sequences constitute meaningful sentences, suggesting that information about a child's memory span for unrelated words says little or nothing about ability to comprehend sentences or to relate the meaning of what the child hears to a learning task.

One of the stated purposes of the Auditory Pointing Test is to provide a basis for specific remediation programs. The authors offer as a strength of their test that it allows the clinician to decide whether to remediate memory span, or sequencing, or both. The foregoing discussion leads to the conclusion that no rationale exists for measuring auditory memory for unrelated words in the first place; it follows, therefore, that there exists no rationale for remediating it, either as a whole or in its separable components. A similar conclusion is reached by Bloom and Lahey (1978). Indeed Hammill and Larsen (1974) found no conclusive evidence that remediation programs designed on such a basis were effective in improving children's discrete auditory skills (among other "psycholinguistic" skills) nor in improving children's ability to handle language in communication.

Summary It must be pointed out that the above comments, while relating to the Auditory Pointing Test, are by no means limited to that test alone. Rather, they should be understood as this reviewer's conclusion about this and other tests purporting to measure discrete auditory abilities (including speech sound discrimination, auditory memory span, auditory sequencing, speech perception in noise, and auditory reception) with the intention of providing diagnostic or baseline information about children's language or learning skills. This test is not recommended for standard clinical or educational use as described by the authors.

References

Bloom, L. and M. Lahey *Language Development and Language Disorders.* New York: Wiley, 1978.

Foss, D. J. and D. A. Swinney On the psychological reality of the phoneme; perception, identification, and consciousness. *J. Verb. Learn. Verb. Behav.* **12**: 246–257, 1973.

Hammill, D. D. and S. C. Larsen The effectiveness of psycholinguistic training. *Exceptional Children* **41**: 5–14, 1974.

Jenkins, J. J. Remember that old theory of memory? Well, forget it! *American Psychologist* **29**: 785–795, 1974.

Olson, G. M. Developmental changes in memory and the acquisition of language. In T. E. Moore (ed.), *Cognitive Development and the Acquisition of Language.* New York: Academic Press, 1973.

Rees, N. S. Auditory processing factors in language disorders: the view from Procrustes' bed. *J. Speech Hearing Dis.* **38**: 304–315, 1973.

—— Art and science of diagnosis in speech and hearing. In S. Singh and J. Lynch (eds.), *Diagnostic Procedures in Hearing, Language, and Speech.* Baltimore: University Park Press, 1978.

Sanders, D. A. *Auditory Perception of Speech: An Introduction to Principles and Problems.* Englewood Cliffs, N.J.: Prentice-Hall, 1977.

Studdert-Kennedy, M. Speech perception. Chapter 8 in N. Lass (ed.), *Contemporary Issues in Experimental Phonetics.* New York: Academic Press, 1976.

THE AUDITORY SEQUENTIAL MEMORY TEST

Joseph M. Wepman and Anne Morency

Language Research Associates, Inc., 1975
Two equivalent forms, I and II

Cost Manual, $2.10; pack of 50 forms (I or II), $8.40
Manual, 6 pages; Form I, 1 page; Form II, 1 page

Time Estimate for administration and scoring: less than 5 minutes

Elizabeth M. Prather *Phoenix (Arizona) Union High School System*

Purpose The purpose of the Auditory Sequential Memory Test as set forth by the authors is to study the ability of children to recall the exact order of an auditory stimulus. Though no documentation is presented, sequential memory skills are purported to be important in speech accuracy, language usage (especially syntactic phrasing), phonic reading, written language, and every mathematical process.

Administration, scoring, and interpretation Digit sequences, presented at a rate of two per second, are used in the test. Each of the two forms of the test includes 14 digit sequences, two each at the seven levels from two- to eight-digit strings. A ceiling is reached when the child fails both strings at a given level.

A scoring table for children at each year level from ages five to eight is provided. According to the authors, "Normative data are not reported for ages over 8 years since this perceptual process has reached its ceiling of development in normal children by the time they reach their 9th birthday" (Manual, p. 2). Raw scores are converted to a five-point Rating Scale Index based on cumulative frequencies. The scale ranges from +2 to −2, the lowest level including the low 15 percent of the scores for each age category and defined as "below the level of the threshold of adequacy."

Evaluation of test adequacy No description is given of the selection criteria nor of the number of subjects used in the standardization study. Test item construction is not described. Percentile ranges can be inferred from the scoring table in the manual, but group means and standard deviations are not included. On page 5 of the manual a table shows raw score means and standard deviations at yearly levels from five through eight obtained "by using the present test . . . in one study." The study cited, however, is not included in the test reference list and thus cannot be located for clarification. A test-retest reliability coefficient based upon administration of the two forms of the test is reported (.82), but no information concerning the reliability study is provided (number and ages of subjects and length of time between administration of the two forms).

Several suggestions given by the authors are excellent, including the importance of (1) retesting children who score poorly to reduce possible effects of inattention, distraction, or unfamiliarity with the task, and (2) the study of other auditory functions, and the auditory modality as a whole, when auditory sequential memory seems poor.

Summary Use of this test cannot be recommended because basic information concerning its construction and standardization is not reported. The test itself is short and easy to score. It might be used as a simple screening test of auditory sequential memory. Children who perform poorly could be retested with better documented tests.

THE BOSTON UNIVERSITY SPEECH SOUND DISCRIMINATION TEST

Wilbert Pronovost

Go-Mo Products, 1953
Two forms, short and long

Cost $19.95
Instruction manual/data; 36 picture card sets, 75 screening forms, 35 test forms, note-folio binder case

Time Not specified; no time limit

William T. Stephenson, Jr. *Oakland Schools, Pontiac, Michigan*

Purpose The instruction pamphlet states that the Boston University Speech Sound Discrimination Test is intended for use with young children as a means of identifying children with auditory discrimination problems. The test purports "to assess a young child's abilities in auditory discrimination of acoustically similar consonant and vowel sounds."

Administration, scoring, and interpretation The test consists of 36 picture cards with three pairs of pictures on each card. The line drawings are clear and readily recognizable. Two of the pairs on each card contain pictures of identical objects while the third portrays objects whose names differ by one phoneme, i.e., Cat-Cat, Bat-Bat, Cat-Bat.

The test format requires the child to discriminate whether the pairs named by the examiner are the "same" or "different." The child provides a nonverbal response, pointing to the stimulus pair of pictures.

The test has a short and a long form. The author suggests that the short form be given first, with the long form administered to children receiving low scores on the short form. The long form utilizes each set of 36 pictures twice for a total presentation of 72 items.

The standardization of the test was conducted on 700 middle-class kindergarten and first grade children from the suburbs of Boston. The mean score obtained was 65.5 with a standard deviation of 6.55. The standardization of the 26-item short form test on 300 kindergarten children of middle-class families in suburban Boston revealed a mean score of 20.5 and a standard deviation of 3.5. Normative data have not been obtained on children younger than five years of age.

Evaluation of test adequacy Although the most current printing of this test was in 1974, the construct has remained unchanged since its initial publication in 1953. At that time speech-sound discrimination tests employed a paired-comparison context, and this test allowed small children to point to same and different paired word stimuli.

The potential consumer might question what information can be derived from evaluating a child's responses to the "different" discrimination tasks presented on the short form of this test, i.e., Cone-Comb, Clown-Crown, Rock-Lock, Mouse-Mouth, Knot-Nut, Cat-Bat, Chip-Ship, Pen-Pin, Pan-Pen, Log-Lock, Wash-Watch, Vase-Face, Cap-Cat. Also, the subject's familiarity with the vocabulary on paired-comparison tests such as this is of concern.

In the years since the introduction of this test, a considerable body of information has developed in psychoacoustics and psycholinguistics. The paired stimuli used in this test fail to reflect consideration of this information. For example, the test does not attend to distinctive feature theory. In addition, paired-comparison tests of auditory discrimination incorporate the phonological and semantic components of language but do not include syntactic nor pragmatic considerations. Children, however, appear to use the latter components when making sound discrimination judgments. These concerns are relevant to the construct of the Boston University Speech Sound Discrimination Picture Test.

It is anticipated that future developments in speech sound discrimination testing will incorporate recent findings so that the scores derived from them may be used as a basis for treatment planning.

Summary   This test, developed in 1953, is of questionable utility inasmuch as it fails to reflect modern research on the subject of sound discrimination and its relative importance to the speech act.

DETROIT TESTS OF LEARNING APTITUDE (DTLA) SUBTESTS: AUDITORY ATTENTION SPAN FOR UNRELATED WORDS; AUDITORY ATTENTION SPAN FOR RELATED SYLLABLES; ORAL COMMISSIONS

Harry J. Baker and Bernice Leland

The Bobbs-Merrill Company, Inc., 1967

Cost $10.80

Examiner's handbook, 139 pages; pupil's record book, 14 pages

Time 7 to 12 minutes per subtest

Mary Gordon *Portland State University*

Purpose The Auditory Attention Span for Unrelated Words Test (Test 6), the Auditory Attention Span for Related Syllables Test (Test 13), and the Oral Commissions Test (Test 7) are three subtests of the Detroit Tests of Learning Aptitude (DTLA). The authors do not explicitly set forth the purpose for the test battery or the subtests; however, they state that the DTLA is "offered to meet the demand of psychologists whose task it is to solve children's learning problems in practical ways. . . . Strengths and weaknesses in the psychological constitution are disclosed." They further indicate that these three tests assess the "mental faculty" of "auditory attentive ability." According to the authors, the Oral Commissions Test additionally evaluates "practical judgment," "number ability," and "motor ability."

Administration, scoring, and interpretation The Auditory Attention Span for Unrelated Words Test is administered by instructing the child to repeat sets of unrelated words in the same order as presented. The words in each set are presented at the rate of one per second, the number of words ranging from two to eight. Two types of scores are given: (1) *simple score* in which one point is awarded for each word recalled in any order, and (2) *weighted score* in which the number of words correct in each set is multiplied by the number of words in the span.

The Auditory Attention Span for Related Syllables Test seems to be misnamed as it in effect evaluates auditory memory for sentences. The child is instructed to repeat 43 sentences ranging in length from five words (six syllables) to 22 words (27 syllables). The score for each sentence ranges from 0 to 3 depending on the number of errors, i.e., omitted, added, and substituted words.

The Oral Commissions Test is administered by instructing the child to carry out a series of commands, the units increasing in number from one to four, e.g., "Walk to the door; then bring me that book." One point is given for each command correctly executed in the correct order.

Each test score is converted to a mental age (MA) via a normative table; each MA is then recorded on a profile. Generally, the performance levels can be interpreted to reveal "auditory attentive ability."

The tests, with only one test form, were published initially in 1935, with revisions in 1959 and 1967. Although the manual merely alludes to the purpose of the tests, it provides clear administration and scoring procedures. The authors emphasize that the tester must adhere to these directions. Interpretations are described as to possible relationships of test scores to success or failure in learning school subjects, especially relative to low scores and probable deficiencies. Six illustrative case studies aid in interpretation of test scores. The manual specifies the age levels and handicapping conditions (e.g., deaf, orthopedic defects, and impaired speech) for which the individual tests are appropriate. The authors state that "only those persons who are fully equipped by training to administer and interpret psychological tests can expect to obtain reliable and consistent results."

Evaluation of test adequacy Although the authors describe what scores on various subtests might mean in terms of school performance, no statistical analysis or research results are reported in support of such interpretations. The rationale for the proposed interpretations relative to abilities is not specified. Logically these three subtests seem to assess "auditory attentive ability"; however, it is unclear to this reviewer why the Oral Commissions subtest also evaluates "practical judgment" and "number ability." Baker and Leland report that the results of one study of over 4000 cases showed the DTLA to be suitable for examination of mentally retarded students as well as for average students; however, the design and statistical analysis are unclearly and incompletely described. The DTLA has been administered to over 75,000 individuals in the Psychological Clinic of Detroit Public Schools, most of whom were candidates for classes for the mentally retarded.

Test–retest reliability measures reportedly were .959 for 48 subjects with an interval of five months between testings and .675 on 792 subjects with a testing interval of two to three years. The latter measures were for mentally retarded, delinquent, and emotionally unstable subjects. The reliability samples and measures are not described adequately. No reliability measures for individual subtests are reported.

The majority of correlations between subtests range from .20 to .40, but specific intrasubtest correlations are not presented.

Norms are published for each subtest. The normative sample was comprised of Detroit Public School students who were in the normal grade for age and who had IQ's from 90 to 110, with 150 students at each age level (three-month intervals from 3–0 to 19–0 years). Neither standard scores nor percentiles are presented; thus, distribution of scores is not reflected.

Evaluation of short-term auditory memory skills may provide useful information for clinical management of clients with language and articulation deficiencies (Emerick and Hatten 1974; Wepman 1973; and Wiig and Semel, 1976). Among others, Emerick and Hatten (1974), Johnson and Myklebust (1967), and Wiig and Semel (1976) have suggested the use of Auditory Attention Span for Unrelated Words and Auditory Attention Span for Related Syllables (sentences) tests for evaluating short-term memory span.

Evaluation of short-term auditory memory through more than one stimulus mode seems to provide useful clinical information (Burford 1976; Johnson and Myklebust 1967; and Wepman and Morency 1973). The DTLA tests being reviewed, therefore, would be potentially helpful in supplementing the frequently used digit span tests.

The ability to follow commands intuitively seems necessary to functioning in many daily activities. Evaluation of this ability is recommended for language/learning disordered individuals. Oral commissions-type items are included on several tests, e.g., Utah Test of Language Development (Mecham, Jex, and Jones 1967) (qv) and the

Sequenced Inventory for Communication Development (Hedrick, Prather, and Tobin 1975) (qv); however, oftentimes the items are scattered throughout the test. In the DTLA the format is to present oral commissions sequentially.

A primary advantage to the DTLA is that individual subtests can be administered selectively without administering the entire test battery. Additionally, normative data are available for each individual test. The administration and scoring directions are sufficiently clear so that, in this reviewer's opinion, most special education professionals can capably and reliably administer the subtests. Administration time is relatively short. None of the three subtests requires expensive or uncommon materials.

The primary limitation of the three subtests is the absence of normative data for variability of performance. Provision of standard deviations, percentiles, or standard scores would have allowed comparison of each testee with the testee's age level group in addition to assignment of an MA for each subtest. In the Auditory Attention Span for Related Syllables test, the sentences are not controlled for syntactical complexity, a factor known to influence sentence recall (Wiig and Semel 1976).

Summary Scoring and administrative procedures are standardized and clearly described. The normative sample seems to be adequate in size. Validity research has been minimal and reliability studies are described inadequately. Normative data are provided for each subtest, but variability of performance for each age level is not reported. Logically, these tests seem to evaluate short-term auditory memory skills (i.e., "auditory attentive ability") in differing stimulus modes which provide clinical information about children with language and articulation deviancies. This reviewer recommends use of these subtests, especially the Oral Commissions and Auditory Attention Span for Related Syllables (sentences) tests.

References

Burford, S. Auditory short-term memory span and sequence of five different stimulus types. Master's thesis, Portland State University, 1976.

Emerick, L. and J. Hatten *Diagnosis and Evaluation in Speech Pathology.* Englewood Cliffs, N.J.: Prentice-Hall, 1974.

Hedrick, D. L., E. M. Prather, and A. Tobin *Sequenced Inventory of Communication Development.* Seattle: University of Washington Press, 1975.

Johnson, D. and H. Myklebust *Learning Disabilities Educational Principles and Practices.* New York: Grune and Stratton, 1967.

Mecham, M. J., J. L. Jex, and J. D. Jones *Utah Test of Language Development* (2nd ed.). Salt Lake City: Communication Research Associates, 1967.

Wepman, J. M. and A. Morency *Auditory Sequential Memory Test.* Chicago: Language Research Associates, 1973.

——— *Auditory Memory Span Test.* Los Angeles: Western Psychological Services, 1973.

Wiig, E. and E. Semel *Learning Disabilities in Children and Adolescents.* Columbus: Charles E. Merrill, 1976.

DIFFERENTIATION OF AUDITORY PERCEPTION SKILLS (DAPS)

Cora Lee Reagan and
Susanne A. Cunningham

Communication Skill Builders, Experimental Edition, 1976

Cost $30.00
Manual, 7 pages; 3 noisemakers in cloth bag; individual student booklet, 16 pages, pack of 25; storage box

Time 10 minutes, administration and scoring

Belle Ruth Witkin *Alameda County Office of Education, Hayward, California*

Purpose According to the examiner's manual, Differentiation of Auditory Perception Skills is a screening instrument designed to determine selected aspects of auditory perception, defined as "the act of recognizing sensation through the medium of the ear, retaining the image and relating it to previous experiences."

Administration, scoring, and interpretation DAPS is administered individually to children between five and eight years of age. It consists of five subtests, each with ten items. Time required is five to ten minutes. Stimuli are noises made by three noisemakers—a hammer, rattle, and clapper—or words, sounds, or sentences produced by the examiner. Responses are oral or motor repetition or performance of a task or sequence of tasks. The examiner records responses as right (+) or wrong (−) in an individual test booklet. Total possible score for the test is 50. The examiner may also record observations about the child's behavior during the test and make recommendations for specific activities to remediate deficiencies uncovered during testing.

Subtest I, Auditory Cadence, requires the child to reproduce patterns of hand claps, taps, and syllable and sentence stress, and recognize whether or not two or more words rhyme. If the child does not understand the meaning of "rhyme," he or she is to tell if the words sound the same or different.

Subtest II, Auditory Distinction, relates to the ability to discriminate among sounds. The task is to recognize whether pairs of words and sentences are the same or different. The differences in half the pairs are primarily in juncture (example: *ice cream* and *I scream*).

Subtest III, Auditory Imagery, includes reproducing patterns of hand claps and noisemakers, repetition of digits forwards and backwards, and repetition in sequence of series of syllables with short and long vowels.

Subtest IV, Syllable Completion, requires that the child respond to directions in sentences varying from three to 14 words in which one or more initial or medial consonants are omitted from the sentence.

Subtest V, Auditory Reasoning, pertains to "the ability to relate heard information to previously heard (stored) information." It consists of sentence completion tasks, most of which require reasoning by analogy (e.g., "A boy is to a man as a girl is to a _____").

Evaluation of test adequacy There is confusion in most of the subtests as to precisely what perceptual abilities are being assessed. The terms "same and different" are used to indicate responses to both rhyming and auditory discrimination/juncture tasks. The syllable completion test is actually a test of auditory closure complicated by memory for multistage directions. The test of auditory reasoning is a sentence completion test.

Directions to the examiner are brief and allow for considerable variation in administration of the items. There is no indication, for example, of the duration of time between digits or syllables in the auditory imagery task. There are few practice items, and these are left largely to the discretion of the examiner. The reliability of the test could be seriously weakened by subtests in which considerable examiner variability is likely to occur, as in Subtests II, III, and IV.

DAPS was normed on 80 children, 20 in each group, by teachers in a southern California school district. The children were enrolled in regular classes and had no known disabilities. No other characteristics of the norming population are provided.

No information is given on how the test was developed, the rationale for the subtests, nor the specifications followed in writing items. It is assumed that all the items within a subtest measure the same ability, but content examination shows that in most subtests, two and sometimes three different types of auditory processing are required.

Interpretation of test scores is left to the examiner. The authors point out that the test is more difficult for younger than for older children but that the differences in means across all subtests between ages six and seven are small and nonsignificant.

The strengths of the DAPS are that it is brief and relatively easy to administer, the manual and booklets are easy to read, format is clear, and scoring is simple. The test could give the trained speech-language pathologist or psychologist some qualitative indications of auditory perceptual functioning. Its weaknesses are that the subtests are misnamed, there is no indication that they measure what they purport to measure, presentation mode and timing are not controlled, there are no guidelines for interpretation of scores, and there is no discussion relating the skills tested to a model of auditory perception or to remediation of deficits. The authors state only that the skills chosen are "presumed to be among those skills that have significant influence upon speech perception and language learning. . . ."

Summary This test is an experimental edition. It might be a useful tool in primary grades to screen out children with gross auditory perceptual disabilities and to indicate the general type of problem(s) presented. Care must be taken in interpreting the meaning of the subtests, however, and it should be recognized that in several of them the items are too few or too disparate to constitute a valid subtest. More work needs to be done on construct validity, and the test should be tried with children from different language backgrounds and with learning or language disabilities. Until more information is gathered that would guide cutoff points for screening and implications for remediation of patterns of responses, the test should be used with caution.

FLOWERS AUDITORY TEST OF SELECTIVE ATTENTION (FATSA), EXPERIMENTAL EDITION

Arthur Flowers

Perceptual Learning Systems, 1975

Cost Not yet specified

Available in reel-to-reel or cassette audiotape Manual, 17 pages, in loose-leaf binder with pouch for audiotape; test booklet, 12 pages including identification page, three practice items, and 32 test items, seven line drawings per item. Intensity Calibration System with speakers available

Time 45 minutes, administration and scoring time for screening 12 individuals

Reinhardt J. Heuer *Temple University*

Purpose The Flowers Auditory Test of Selective Attention, subtitled "A Test of Auditory Vigilance," is considered by the author to be a test of auditory attention span for school-age children. Flowers states in the manual that the skills tested are specific selective attention skills requiring continuous auditory watchkeeping and specific verbal signal monitoring.

Administration, scoring, and interpretation The skills above are tested by having the individual listen to a test audiotape and put a mark on one or more of the seven pictures provided for each item in the test. The testee must hear the name of that picture preceded by the word "George" before being allowed to make a mark. There is a variety of distractors that increase in number and complexity as the test proceeds through 32 items. The first 21 items include the following: picture names not preceded by George; nonpictured nouns; picture names preceded by other proper names, such as Jack, John, etc.; repetitions of proper names; picture words preceded by proper names similar to George, such as, Georgette, Georgia, Georgiana; nonsense words; changes in speaking rate by the voice on the tape; pauses; changes in emphasis and melody by the speaker; changes in intensity of the sound on the tape; and filtering of the signal. Items 23 and 24 add white noise to the other distractors. Items 25 through 27 introduce electronic tones and music overlaid on the speech the individual under test is to listen to, and items 28 through 32 introduce overlaid verbal material such as counting, stories, the reading of an article on tennis and admonishments of "Don't listen to me!" Thus, auditory watchkeeping and specific verbal monitoring skills are defined and tested by the individual's ability to listen for "George + picture name" and to mark the appropriate picture out of a series of seven in the presence of a variety of distractors and signal distortions.

Although the FATSA can be administered to a single individual or up to 35 children, Flowers recommends testing groups of 12 individuals. Norms are available only for groups of 12 children of school age. Children with untreated hearing loss are excluded. Instructions are given in the manual for arranging the seats of the children to be tested. A calibration tone, test instructions, practice items, and the test are all presented via audiotape. An electronic intensity calibration system and special speakers may be purchased; otherwise a sound pressure level meter must be available to calibrate the intensity of the taped presentation. This equipment specification would seem to present a major obstacle to standardized administration in the classroom given the costs and skills involved.

Test booklets are provided in groups of 12. The pages are color-coded to assist the examiner in knowing if the individuals under test are on the appropriate page. Line drawings of bike, cow, cup, fish, ball, dog, and clock are provided for the children for marking each of the 32 items in the test. Three practice items are included, and more than one pass-through on the practice items is allowed if one or more of the children under test are confused.

The entire testing procedure should take from between 24 and 30 minutes depending on whether the individuals under test require more than one pass-through on the three practice items. There is a break between items 19 and 20 necessitated by the need to turn the tape over. The testees are allowed to stretch and relax during this interval.

Scoring is extremely simple. The examiner need only check each item's group of pictures. An item may be scored correct only if the exact pictures are marked as indicated on the score sheet. There are no partial scores; the item is either correct or incorrect. The raw score is the total number of correct items.

Currently tables are available indicating selected percentile midyear scores for regular class children with chronological ages 6.1 to 12.0, for children referred by their regular classroom teachers for special testing, for mildly retarded students, and for students in special education classes for educable mentally handicapped children. (See references.)

Training programs (primary and advanced vigilance training programs) are available for use with children falling below the 25th percentile on the FATSA. These should be useful for those who use the test as a prescriptive diagnostic tool.

Evaluation of test adequacy   The manual for the FATSA is well written, inclusive, and, above all, honest. Flowers repeatedly indicates that the FATSA is experimental and that currently no validity data are available. Unfortunately there is no discussion of the selection of the type or frequency of the distractors used in the test or of where auditory vigilance may fit into the auditory process. Obviously it is too early in the development of the test to have the results of predictive studies.

The test appears, however, to have some face validity in attempting to screen and identify individuals who may be easily distracted by distorted, similar, or competing messages in an atmosphere in which auditory attention is required for success.

The manual reports Kuder–Richardson estimates of internal consistency of .69 and .82 for mixed groups of grades one and two, and grades two and three students, respectively. Group sizes ranged from 56 to 60.

The normative tables are based on average numbers of individuals as follows: normal pupils, 46.2 subjects; referred for special testing, 60 subjects; mildly retarded pupils, 36 pupils; educable retarded pupils, 16.2 subjects, per age group. No criteria are given for the selection of subjects in the manual.

Summary   The FATSA should currently be considered an experimental test yielding data on a specific problem of auditory inattention. It may be of some value as a screening test for isolating students possibly having difficulty in the typical educational setting due to "auditory inattention" and who may need training in these skills. The instructions and test format are perhaps difficult for some younger children or children from "inner-city" settings. These children may require additional training or help with knowing which item number is currently being presented. Because of the electronic sophistication of the taped format, the test is not readily adaptable for children whose primary language is not English unless the originator of the test provides additional versions of the test. The test is a screening tool dependent on specific scored calibration or measuring equipment that may have a "future" as more data are gathered and as more information is obtained in regard to central auditory processing and disruptions.

References

Flowers, A. *FATSA Test Manual.* Dearborn, Mich.: Perceptual Learning Systems, 1975.

Small, V. Results of central auditory abilities (CAA) and language testing for children with learning problems, grades one–three in a "diagnostic-prescriptive" setting. Rockville, Md.: Montgomery County Schools, 1974.

Tavalsky, E. *FATSA* test norms for educable mentally handicapped children. Special Research Report. Jamestown, N.Y.: Jamestown Public Schools, 1973.

Vorobey, N. Group auditory perceptual testing (CAA of mentally handicapped, mildly retarded children). Special Research Report. Fairfax, Va.: Fairfax Public Schools, 1975.

FLOWERS–COSTELLO TEST OF CENTRAL AUDITORY ABILITIES

Arthur Flowers, Mary R. Costello, and Victor Small

Perceptual Learning Systems, 1970

Cost $69.50

Manual, 53 pages; two picture booklets 24 pages/booklet; scoring sheets

Time Not stated

Lloyd E. Augustine *University of Oregon*

Purpose The Flowers–Costello Test of Central Auditory Abilities was designed to be used by various professionals (educators, psychologists, physicians) to identify those young children whose auditory perceptual deficits interfere with their ability to acquire normal language facility and with their ability to learn academically. According to the authors, the test can be used at the kindergarten level to identify children with general central auditory abilities (CAA) dysfunction and to establish probabilities for future success in reading.

At grades one through six, its use is reported as follows:

1 In identifying children with general CAA dysfunction

2 In identifying, among the low achievers, those children whose low CAA scores indicate specific learning disabilities, which may be interfering with the child's programs in school

3 To assist professionals in making educational judgments regarding ways to remediate CAA disabilities, i.e., proper program planning for children with auditory disabilities

Administration, scoring, and interpretation The test is so designed that any school, hospital, or clinical professional persons can administer it. They need only to familiarize themselves with the test and its administration. Paraprofessionals can also give the test under supervision. The test must be given in a "relatively quiet" room in the school, and all subjects must be exposed to a routine audiometric screening test before testing. All test stimuli are tape recorded to control for loudness level. The manual stresses calibrating the test for loudness level; however, the equipment to do this is no longer provided with the test, and the manual has not been corrected accordingly. The audiotape presents to the child all directions, practice items (nine in number) and test stimuli (sentences). According to the authors, because all information is audiotaped ". . . very little preparation of the child for testing is required."

Two subtests are administered: A Low Pass Filter Speech Test (LPFS) and a Competing Message Test (CM). The two subtests are similar in that each contains 24 sentences in which the appropriate words are either distorted or eliminated at the end of each sentence. The child is required to select from pictorial choices the deleted or distorted words. The two tests differ in that only the target words in the LPFS are subjected to low-pass filtering, whereas all of the sentences in the CM subtest are presented against a competing background of an interesting story.

Scoring is based on the "wrong" score approach. A wrong score results from pointing to the incorrect picture in the picture booklets. The sum of these errors is ubtracted from the total of 24 to obtain the raw score for each subtest. For kindergarten children the raw score can be converted into a stanine score. This score is purportedly used to predict future difficulty in reading and to indicate the need for a special CAA remedial program. For diagnostic-type testing of children above kindergarten (grades 1–6), percentile scores are used.

Evaluation of test adequacy   Although the authors maintain that little preparation of the child is necessary for administration, this is probably not the case if the child has a significant language or learning problem. Children with such problems would undoubtedly have difficulty following the rather laborious instructions delivered by tape.

The test has been normed on children from kindergarten through the sixth grade. However, beyond third grade its sensitivity decreases, and a ceiling is reached at grade five. The appropriateness of the test beyond grade three is questionable, inasmuch as the internal reliability changes from .87 at the kindergarten level to .60 and .37 for grades three and four respectively. Values for grades five and six were below .30. It is important to note that there are no validity data available for CAA scores reported above kindergarten level. The authors suggest that local norms be developed and used for interpretation.

The authors discuss at length the critical importance of intelligibility in central auditory processing. They point out that the test should be calibrated with an "Electronic Intensity Calibration System" to ensure standardized presentation of the message. Their arguments regarding the need to control intensity–intelligibility when dealing with CAA testing are quite convincing, yet they have subsequently eliminated the calibration system from the test package. If the authors are sincere in their statements regarding the need for standardization and control of intensity–intelligibility, then the removal of the calibration system for whatever reasons seriously weakens the value of the test.

Research by Flowers (1946) and Flowers and Costello (1965) reportedly indicates that LPFS and CM differentiate normal and low reading achievement. Wiig and Semel (1976), however, suggest that the test ". . . may tap semantic–cognitive and convergent production abilities . . ." They state that identification of the target words may be facilitated by context and structure of the carrier phrases used to introduce the target words. Wiig and Semel further point out that accurate selection of the target words may be facilitated by such factors as syllable length (duration) because the duration of the target words frequently differs considerably from the duration of the foils.

Summary   There is a need for the development of tests to evaluate the central auditory processing abilities of children (Bocca and Calearo 1963). The Flowers-Costello Test is an attempt in this direction. Administering, scoring, and interpretation are rather straightforward. There are, however, several concerns that should be addressed before using this instrument. First, without the "Electronic Intensity Calibration System" recommended by the authors, standardized message presentation is in doubt. Second, the cost of the test without the calibration system is not high ($69.50), but with the endorsed system included it rises sharply ($300-$400). Third, the appropriateness of the test beyond grade three is questionable because a marked decrease in internal reliability occurs from third grade through grade six. In light of the above, the test must still be considered experimental in nature. Much more extensive research and careful validation are needed before it can be accepted as adequate to its task.

References

Bocca, E. and C. Calearo Central hearing process. In J. Jerger (ed.), *Modern Developments in Audiology*. New York: Academic Press, 1963, pp. 337–368.

Flowers, A. *Central Auditory Abilities of Normal and Lower Group Readers*. Cooperative Research Project No. 5-076. State University of New York, 1964.

—— and M. R. Costello *The Resistance to Distortion Factor in Auditory Perception and Its Relationship to Specific Phonetic Abilities*. Technical Research Report N. K001, Office of Research and Evaluation, Oak Park, Mich.: Oak Park Schools, 1965.

Wiig, E. H. and E. M. Semel *Language Disabilities in Children and Adolescents*. Columbus: Charles E. Merrill, 1976.

GOLDMAN–FRISTOE–WOODCOCK AUDITORY SELECTIVE ATTENTION TEST

Ronald Goldman, Macalyne Fristoe, and Richard W. Woodcock

American Guidance Service, Inc., 1976

Cost $21.00

Manual, response forms (package of 25), test tape (cassette) or 5" open reel, all contained in an Easel-Kit

Time Approximately 20 minutes

Edwin A. Leach *University of Nebraska Medical Center*

Purpose The Goldman-Fristoe-Woodcock Auditory Selective Attention Test measures an individual's ability to attend to a listening task in the presence of competing noise that is systematically varied in intensity (signal to noise ratio) and type (fanlike, cafeteria noise, and voice). According to the authors, the intent for use of these three forms of background noise is systematically to introduce three factors of distraction: intensity (shift of signal-to-noise ratio), variability (cafeteria noise), and meaningfulness (voice). This test development, like the total G–F–W Battery development, is largely the result of an increasing concern by special educators, speech–language pathologists, and classroom teachers with auditory difficulties beyond simple acuity problems. In recent years terminology such as auditory processing problem and central auditory disorder has become much more popular to describe apparent problems of many children. The G–F–W Battery, including the Auditory Selective Attention Test, is a clinical procedure attempting to measure this important area of auditory ability.

Administration, scoring, and interpretation All auditory stimuli are presented by means of prerecorded tape via earphone presentation. During the test the subject's task is to point to one of a set of four pictures as instructed by recorded voice. Prior to the beginning of the actual test, there are 15 training items for ample preparation of the subject's responses. The Auditory Selective Attention Test comprises 110 items, divided into four subtests.

The first 11 items, the Quiet Subtest, are presented without background noise. The next 33 items are the Fan-like Noise Subtest, the next 33 the Cafeteria Noise Subtest, and the final 33 items the Voice Subtest. Noise intensity is a factor in three subtests. As each subtest progresses, the signal-to-noise ratio shifts from a positive value (approximately +12 dB) to a negative value (approximately −10 dB) thus increasing the background noise from a level below the stimuli to a level which is of greater intensity than the stimuli.

The performance of subjects on the G–F–W Auditory Selective Attention Test is scored as either correct or incorrect for each of the four subtests (Quiet, Fan-like, Cafeteria Noise, and Voice) and for all 110 items. The raw score performance on each subtest may be translated into both age equivalency and percentile rank for comparisons of relative performance. This test together with the four subtests is combined with the results of the 12 tests to form a profile for each subject. Administration time for the Selective Attention Test is estimated at 20 minutes although this will vary considerably from subject to subject.

Evaluation of test adequacy The norming data were gathered from several locations in the states of California, Florida, Maine, and Minnesota. The norming study obtained data from subjects ranging in age from three to 80 years. However, most of these data concentrated in the range of three to 12 years since this was the range of greatest interest. Both normal subjects and clinical subjects participated in the norming study. Internal consistency reliability coefficients are presented for both groups of subjects, normals and clinical samples, by age range and by the G–F–W Battery test.

Content validity is discussed by comparing the Selective Attention Test in terms of its similarities and differences with the G–F–W Auditory Discrimination Test and with other tests not included in the battery. Construct validity is reported in terms of the intercorrelations among the various tests of the battery for three selected age ranges, three to eight years, nine to 18 years, and over 19 years. Reliability estimates for test–retest reliability are not presented.

The strength of this test lies in its very nature. Auditory retention, especially for school age children, is critical for the educational process. If children who have attending problems can be identified, then appropriate remedial planning can be initiated. Also of value is the fact that this test, like the other 11 tests in the G–F–W Battery, can be used independently providing percentile ranking and age equivalency scores. Since the total battery is quite time consuming, the utility of single tests in the battery is valuable. Many speech–language pathologists will find this quite advantageous.

In terms of weaknesses, a primary concern of clinicians and researchers alike will be focused on the reliability of this test as well as the whole battery. No test–retest reliability information is provided to allow the examiner to make an estimate of this procedure's utility in that regard. Presumably, the test–retest reliability would vary at least as a function of age.

A second concern, especially for speech–language pathologists, involves the applicability of the information from this test. Assuming the test would identify areas of proficiency as well as areas of deficiency, the clinician will be interested in applying this information to a remedial plan. This test will not provide help either in sequencing remedial objectives or in placing priorities upon specific deficits especially in the case of a profile of all 12 tests. This important phase of remedial planning, i.e., sequencing and priority placement, must still rest largely with the judgment of the clinician. Finally, the validity of this test, as well as the validity of the total battery, is yet an open question. The authors present some preliminary validity data that suggest that the instrument is sensitive to some types of communication problems. However, the validity of the instrument is still in question until sufficient numbers of clinicians and sufficient research data establish it as a sensitive index for auditory selectivity problems. These data are yet to be collected.

Summary The Goldman–Fristoe–Woodcock Selective Attention Test measures an individual's ability to attend to a listening task in the presence of competing noise. It can be administered singly or as part of the G–F–W Battery of diagnostic skills covering a wide range of auditory skills of both children and adults. Presumably problems of auditory inattention can be singled out for remedial intervention, although just how one applies this information to a remedial plan remains problematical. Validity and reliability of the instrument remain in doubt.

GOLDMAN–FRISTOE– WOODCOCK AUDITORY MEMORY TESTS

Ronald Goldman, Macalyne Fristoe, and Richard W. Woodcock

American Guidance Service, Inc., 1974

Cost Manual, 23 pages, and test tape (cassette or 5" open reel), $26.50; response forms (package of 25), $4.10; test tape (cassette or open reel), $6.75

Time Estimated time to administer and score: one hour; however, administration time will vary depending on the amount of time spent on pretraining

Louise R. Kent *University of Pittsburgh*

Purpose The purpose of the Goldman–Fristoe–Woodcock Auditory Memory Tests, as stated by the authors, is to identify children or adults who are deficient in short-term auditory memory (STAM) skills and to describe these deficiencies.

Administration, scoring, and interpretation The G–F–W Auditory Memory Tests consist of three separate tests presented serially to the subject. The tests are individually administered by an examiner using recorded auditory test stimuli (cassette or open-reel); earphones are recommended but not required. Each test is preceded by pretraining designed to ensure that the subject understands the task and to minimize the influence of prior vocabulary. On each test the subject's raw score is the sum of the correct responses. The raw score for each test is converted to percentile rank, age equivalent, standard score, and stanine by means of tables provided within the test. Resulting scores are recorded and plotted on a profile provided in the test booklet. A subject's performance can be compared with that of others in the same age group by means of percentile ranks, or performance can be reported as an age-equivalent score. Further interpretation of results depends on the availability of other information and test results on the subject.

Test 1 is entitled Recognition Memory and assesses the ability to recognize whether or not a given word has been heard in the immediate past. The test consists of 110 recorded words divided into five lists of 22 words each, each word occurring twice within a list. The separation of the first and second presentations of a word ranges from a minimum of zero intervening words during a three-second time span to a maximum of eight intervening words during a 24-second time span. The subject is expected to respond to each word by indicating, with a "yes" or a "no," whether or not that word has been presented previously in the list.

Test 2 is entitled Memory for Content. It requires the subject first to listen to a recorded list of words. Immediately after the last item is named, the subject is shown a set of pictures including all of those that were named plus two that were not named. The subject is expected to point to the two pictures that were not named in the list. Credit is given for each of the two pictures identified correctly, one point each. There are 16 lists which range in length from two words (with four pictures on the response page) to nine words (with 11 pictures). Words within a list are presented at the rate of one word every two seconds.

Test 3 is entitled Memory for Sequence. The subject first listens to a recorded list of words and then is shown a set of picture cards representing the list of words just presented. The subject's task is to put the cards into the same order as the list of words just heard. Credit is given for correctly placing the first and last card and for any sequencing of two cards that corresponds to the order of a continuous pair of words in the list. The 14 lists progress in length from two to eight words. Words within a list are presented at the rate of one every two seconds.

Evaluation of test adequacy   The test, the self-contained manual, the record forms, and the recorded tape are compactly and attractively packaged; instructions for administration and scoring are simple and clear. Administration requires a minimum of preparation and training for the examiner. A 23-page manual is packaged with the test. In addition to describing administration and scoring, it describes the rationale of the tests and provides tables for estimating raw scores and converting raw scores to percentile ranks for subjects from three years ten months to 85 years of age. Also included are tables, age-equivalence standard scores, and stanine tables.

A 36-page technical manual for the complete G-F-W Battery is available but must be ordered separately at extra charge. This manual includes descriptive data on the norming sample, discussion regarding validity and reliability, and data to support claims of validity and reliability. The authors state that the tests are appropriate for subjects from ages three to 85 who display communicative difficulties. It is clear that the intent for use with respect to children is for those displaying communicative difficulties in the areas of language, articulation, listening, reading, spelling, or writing in an effort to identify STAM deficits that are independent of auditory acuity deficits. The authors are not specific about the adult populations for whom the test might be useful. There is no discussion of how the identification and description of the deficit(s) might be used to remediate their deleterious effects.

There is no question that the tests do test aspects of STAM; however, Test 1 and Test 2 also involve negation, which makes the directions somewhat complex for all subjects and which may make pretraining to criterion difficult if not impossible for young children whose language development has not progressed to the mastery of negation. The latter would be especially true for a clinical population of young children.

The authors present data to support their inference that each of the tests measures a different STAM ability and that these abilities are also independent of a variety of other language-related auditory skills tested in other parts of the G-F-W Auditory Skills Test Battery. References are offered to support the position that auditory memory is related to articulation, language, reading, learning disabilities, mental retardation, and auditory analysis of sound blending.

The implication is that if all people in the United States from the age of three to 85 were tested on these tests, those doing poorly would also display—to some criterion on some proper measures—identifiable difficulties across a broad range of language-related tasks which involve STAM. The authors present data to support such predictive validity. For example, two groups of clinical subjects were shown to do less well on the tasks than normal subjects. Although the data reported support predictive validity, they are unable to establish it.

One cannot be sure whether the norming sample was large enough for the intended purpose or whether it was sufficiently representative of the population at large. The norming sample on the three tests included 352, 335, and 293 normal subjects, respectively, and 123, 127, and 115 subjects from two clinical populations—mildly dysfunctional and moderately to severely dysfunctional. Those with mild speech and learning difficulties were, or recently had been, among the case loads of speech or learning clinicians in the public schools who were seeing children in regular classroom settings. The subjects with severe learning difficulties were educable and trainable mentally retarded persons attending special classes or schools. In the norming sample on the three tests there were 56, 55, and 51 subjects, respectively, in the "mild" group and 67, 72, and 64 in the "severe" group.

The norming sample is described by age, race, and geographical location but not by sex. Age is relatively well described for subjects 18 and under, but not for those 19 and over. This lack weakens the interpretations based on percentile ranks for subjects over 18. Although the tests purport to be useful for subjects from three to 85, the number of subjects in the norming sample for the three tests who were 19 and over ranged from only 16 to 22 percent; this fact weakens interpretations based on the percentile rank tables which are roughly broken into 15 age intervals between the ages of 17 and 86.

The authors state that the norming sample concentrated on subjects between three and 12 years of age because the most rapid development of auditory skills takes place during that time. No data are presented to support this statement nor is it clear that the statement, if true, affords a rationale for the extent to which the norming sample is age biased.

The racial mix of the norming sample for these tests ranged from 86 to 87.6 percent white, 7.4 to 9.1 percent black, and 4.9 to 5 percent other. No data are presented that allow one to know the age ranges, membership in the subpopulations (normal versus clinical), or test performance relative to race.

Information regarding geographical representation is limited to lists of schools or institutions in Minnesota, Maine, California, and Florida, suggesting that most of the subjects were from Minnesota. Data relating locale to number of subjects, age, sex, race, or subpopulation are not reported.

There is no discussion of the importance of local norms or description of methods for their calculation. No data are reported regarding how the adult subjects were secured or what criteria were used for their selection.

Split-half reliability data are reported for each test for three age groups, 3-8, 9-18, and 19+. Correlations were uniformly high (.95, .93, and .95) on Test 3, but low for the middle age group on Tests 1 and 2 (.62 and .48, respectively). Caution is therefore suggested in using these two tests for estimating total raw scores from data on subjects for whom administration of the entire test(s) is discontinued due to poor performance. No data are reported to support the estimation of total raw scores from incomplete performance data.

No test–retest data are provided for any age group. One would not expect scores for children to be stable over time; however, relative stability would be expected in the age range from 15 to 40.

There are no reports of the clinical usefulness of these tests. Of the three, the Memory for Sequence test appears to be the strongest. The other two are limited by the nature of the tasks and the complexity of the instructions. The relatively small number of subjects in the norming sample in the adult age group is a severe limitation for interpretation of results with adults.

Summary Within the stated limitations, this reviewer would recommend the use of these tests for short-term auditory memory in conjunction with others such as the ITPA Auditory Sequential Memory Subtest (qv) (Kirk, McCarthy, and Kirk 1968). Caution should be used with respect to interpretations based on percentile ranks, particularly for adults. Data obtained on individual subjects may be most useful if used descriptively.

Reference

Kirk, S. A., J. J. McCarthy, and W. D. Kirk   *The Illinois Test of Psycholinguistic Abilities.* Urbana, Ill.: University of Illinois Press, 1968.

GOLDMAN–FRISTOE–WOODCOCK SOUND–SYMBOL TESTS (G–F–W SOUND–SYMBOL)

Ronald Goldman, Macalyne Fristoe, and Richard W. Woodcock

American Guidance Service, Inc., 1974

Cost Technical manual, $2.75; test kit with casette *or* 5″ open reel, $21.75; examiner's manual, 33 pages; response form, 9 pages

Time Not indicated

Kenneth W. Burk *Wichita State University*

Purpose The Goldman–Fristoe–Woodcock Sound–Symbol Tests are one component of the more comprehensive Goldman–Fristoe–Woodcock Auditory Skills Test Battery (1974a). According to the authors (1974b), The G–F–W Sound–Symbol are tests " . . . designed to measure several basic abilities which are prerequisite to advanced language skills, including reading and spelling" (p. 203). Test results are regarded to be of use to a variety of specialists, including the speech–language pathologist, school psychologist, and those who work with the learning disabled. Normative data are available for the age range of three to more than 80 years, although the major data are for those in the three- through 12-year age range. The authors (1974a) report this as the age range of greatest emphasis, ". . . because the most rapid development of auditory skills takes place during that time" (p. 19).

Administration, scoring, and interpretation The seven tests comprising the G–F–W Sound–Symbol assessment of auditory comprehension skills are described by the authors (1974b, pp. 203–204) in the following manner:

Test 1—*Sound Mimicry* measures the ability to imitate nonsense syllables immediately after auditory presentation (involves discrimination and echoic memory).

Test 2—*Sound Recognition* measures the ability to recognize isolated sounds comprising a word (involves hypothesis testing, sound analysis and/or synthesis).

Test 3—*Sound Analysis* measures the ability to identify component sounds of nonsense syllables.

Test 4—*Sound Blending* measures the ability to synthesize isolated sounds into meaningful words.

Test 5—*Sound–Symbol Association* measures the ability to learn associations between unfamiliar auditory and visual symbols.

Test 6—*Reading of Symbols* measures the ability to make grapheme-to-phoneme translations (involves phonic and structural analysis skills). Errors can be plotted in the Reading Error Inventory for diagnostic evaluation.

Test 7—*Spelling of Sounds* measures the ability to make phoneme-to-grapheme translations.

Test administration is on an individual basis. Through use of the Easel-Kit, the examiner is provided test instructions and training procedures for each test, in addition to test stimuli for the Sound Recognition and Association tests.

Stimuli for Sound Mimicry, Recognition, Analysis, Blending, and Spelling tests are presented using a professional quality cassette or reel-to-reel tape recording, requiring that the examiner monitor the test tape. These tests are intended to be administered over earphones, and it was by this procedure that the normative data were obtained. The test manual in the Easel-Kit provides information on rationale for the tests, description of test materials and procedures, and information on scoring and interpretation of the tests. In this manual the authors advise that the tests may be expected to differentiate with greater precision among degrees of defective than of normal functioning. They advise also that care should be taken in interpretation of high error scores on the Sound Mimicry, Analysis, Blending, and Reading of Symbols tests when the individual being tested presents an articulation disorder. Use of percentiles is regarded by the authors as the most useful procedure for interpreting findings; however, age equivalent, standard score, and stanine information is given, in addition to a table for transforming percentile ranks into equivalent standard scores and stanines. Grade equivalent values are available for Reading of Symbols. Figures are provided illustrating the interquartile range of performance on each test across the age range of the norming sample. Finally, information is given on the Performance Profile that permits a graphic representation on the Response Form of the results across all tests. It is based on the ten- to 50-year age range of the sample used in norming.

Evaluation of test adequacy Information on construction of the G–F–W Sound–Symbol Tests is presented in the technical manual for the Goldman–Fristoe–Woodcock Auditory Skills Test Battery (1974a). The reader interested in the background and rationale for the battery, criteria employed in its design, and test development and technical data should consult this resource. Norming data were obtained from public and parochial schools and other institutions from the states of California, Florida, Maine, and Minnesota. An attempt was made to obtain representative data from ages three to 80, but with an emphasis on the three- through 12-year time period. The authors caution that these data are cross sectional rather than longitudinal and must be interpreted with this in mind. Considering only the norming data for six of the G–F–W Sound–Symbol Tests (excluding Reading of Symbols), the average number of subjects was approximately 550, with a range of 405 (Spelling of Sounds) to 705 (Sound–Symbol Association), with the greatest number of these subjects in the nine- to 18-year age range compared to three to eight years, and with the lesser number in the 19 years and over age category. Approximately 88 percent of subjects were white, with black subjects the next most numerous in terms of racial distribution. Separate normative data for the Reading of Symbols Test were drawn from results on the Word Attack Test of the Woodcock Reading Mastery Tests (1973), with approximately 4790 in the sample. Norms for this test consider only school-aged subjects. Data are reported for two additional groups: subjects with mild speech and learning difficulties, and those with severe learning difficulties. The greatest representation in the mild clinical group is in the 7- to 12-year category, there being a range of 48–60 subjects for any one test across the three age categories. The greatest number of subjects in the severe learning difficulty group fell in the 11- to 16-year range, with the total sample across age groups ranging from 48 to 60, excluding the small representation in the tests Reading of Symbols and Spelling of Sounds. Subjects in this category were educable and trainable mentally retarded individuals.

As reported in the technical manual (1974a), data analysis was performed utilizing the calibration and scaling procedures based upon the Rasch model. Test reliability was evaluated for normal and clinical groups, and for normal subjects combining all age groups, utilizing a split-half procedure and application of the Spearman–Brown correction. The median and range of coefficients across the seven tests, by age group for normal subjects, are as follows: 3–8 years (.92, .81–.97); 9–19 years (.86, .73–.96); and 19 years and over (.92, .87–.97). The authors regard these coefficients as conservative estimates of internal consistency. The maximum estimates, obtained by combining all normal subjects, yielded coefficients ranging from .89 to .98, with a median value of .96. Coefficients for the mild speech and learning difficulty group range from .74 to .98, with a median of .88. Comparable values for the severe clinical group for five tests are .93 to .97, the median being .93.

Information on validity of the G–F–W Sound–Symbol is presented in the technical manual (1974a) in terms of content (face) validity and construct validity. Intercorrelations among the tests of the battery, analyzed at three age levels (3–8, 9–18, and 19 years and older), were interpreted inferentially to indicate that each test in the battery is measuring a different skill. Using the same age groups, the correlation between test scores and age became progressively less with increasing age. This was interpreted by the authors as evidence of a hypothesized "... age-related growth and decline of auditory skills" (p. 27). An analysis of variance comparison of mean scores of normal subjects and those of the mild and severe clinical groups revealed a significant differentiation of normal subjects from those with severe difficulties. Most of the normal vs. mild clinical group comparisons were significant, with age-within-group often being a more significant source of variance than subject grouping.

Summary Test materials for the G–F–W Sound–Symbol Test are prepared in a professionally usable package, and ease in handling is facilitated by the Easel-Kit. Instructions for administering and scoring the tests are clear and to the point. The visual test stimuli for the Sound Recognition and Association tests are carefully prepared and attractive. When used with a playback system of the quality specified by the authors, there should be no difficulty in the presentation of the acoustic stimuli using the professionally prepared audiotapes. Estimates of reliability and validity are regarded as being of a magnitude sufficient to warrant satisfaction with the clinical application of these tests, so long as it is kept in mind that the strongest normative data are for individuals three through 12 years of age.

References

Goldman, R., M. Fristoe, and R. W. Woodcock *Technical Manual for Goldman–Fristoe–Woodcock Auditory Skills Test Battery.* Circle Pines, Minnesota: American Guidance Service, 1974a.

——— *Goldman–Fristoe–Woodcock Auditory Skills Text Battery: Sound–Symbol Tests.* Circle Pines, Minnesota: American Guidance Service, 1974b.

Woodcock, R. W. *Woodcock Reading Mastery Tests.* Circle Pines, Minnesota: American Guidance Service, 1973.

GOLDMAN-FRISTOE-WOODCOCK TEST OF AUDITORY DISCRIMINATION (G-F-W TAD)

Ronald Goldman, Macalyne Fristoe, and Richard W. Woodcock

American Guidance Service, Inc., 1970

Cost Kit containing test plates, manual, cassette test tape and 50 response forms—$23.00; optional large training plates, $4.20; 50 response forms, $3.50

Manual, 31 pages; response forms, 1 page

Time Training procedure, 5 minutes to administer; test tape, 7.5 minutes to administer

Delores Kluppel Vetter   *University of Wisconsin—Madison*

Purpose The Goldman-Fristoe-Woodcock Test of Auditory Discrimination was designed to measure speech-sound discrimination under conditions of ideal listening as well as in the presence of controlled background noise. It can be used for individuals aged 3 years 8 months to 70 years and older.

Administration, scoring, and interpretation The test consists of three parts: a Training Procedure, a Quiet Subtest, and a Noise Subtest. It also has an optional set of large training plates for use with groups of subjects to reduce the time required for the Training Procedure.

The Training Procedure is designed to acquaint the subject with the pictures and associated words used during the two subtests. There are 16 plates with four pictures on each consisting of line drawings of familiar subject matter. The associated words are all one syllable in length and are consonant–vowel–consonant or consonant–vowel when spoken. The examiner reads instructions asking the subject to point to one of four pictures on the first plate; then asks the subject to point to a second picture. Whenever an error occurs, the correct information is given verbally or gesturally. The examiner repeats this procedure until the subject has responded to two pictures on each of the 16 plates. The examiner then returns to the first plate and asks the subject to point to the remaining two pictures on each plate. When all combinations of words and pictures have been tested, the examiner retests the word–picture associations in error on the first training trial. Training is repeated for any errors on this review. The criterion for completion of training is the correct identification of each picture on the training plates or three attempts to match words with pictures. A record is kept of the word–picture associations not trained.

After the Training Procedure is completed the test tape containing a calibration tone and the two subtests is presented. It is recommended that a high-quality tape player be used and that testing take place through high-fidelity earphones or through speakers in a very quiet or sound-treated room. The calibration tone may be used by the examiner to set a comfortable listening level for the subject, or, if appropriate equipment is available, to establish the volume setting required for 60–70 dB SPL at the subject's ear level. Unfortunately differences in listening level may introduce variability in a subject's performance.

The instructions for each subtest are contained on the tape, and the examiner manipulates the test plates and records the subject's responses to one of four pictures on each plate. The Quiet Subtest has no background noise on the tape. The Noise Subtest has background noise which is 9 dB less intense than the signal superimposed on the tape. The background noise was obtained by recording the environmental noise in a busy school cafeteria and then amplitude-compressing it to produce semi-intelligible noise at a relatively constant amplitude. The 9 dB difference was chosen because it was the point at which normal subjects showed a marked decrease in discrimination performance.

The authors suggest two levels of scoring a subject's performance. The more general scoring procedure is to count the total number of errors made on each subtest. These values may be transformed into percentile or standard scores for comparison with normative tables. A second level of scoring recommended only for research or clinical exploration classifies the errors into a speech–sound matrix.

Three normative tables are presented in the manual. In one the total errors on the subtest are converted to percentile ranks calculated to the midpoint of each raw score interval. A second converts the raw scores into normalized T-scores with a mean of 50 and a standard deviation of 10. The third, which the authors recommend for clinical use, calculates the percentile rank calculated to the upper limit of each raw score interval. The values from this table indicate the percentage of the standardization sample that made the same number or more errors on the subtest. A comparison of the subject's performance on the Quiet Subtest and the Noise Subtest may yield additional information useful in planning an appropriate remediation program for individuals with poor auditory discrimination.

Evaluation of test adequacy   The manual which accompanies the test is explicit in describing the nature of the construction of the test, the requirements of the examiner and testing facilities, and the precise administration procedure. There are difficulties for the reader, however, in understanding and keeping track of the various samples for which standardization data are presented. The authors state that a standardization sample of 745 subjects ranging in age from three years to 84 years was tested. Kindergarten and school-age children were drawn from schools while preschool children and adult-aged subjects were obtained by personal contact. There was no attempt made to select subjects according to their auditory discrimination ability, but subjects with known moderate or severe hearing losses were excluded. Additional clinical groups, e.g., mental retardation, speech and language impairments, were selected to provide descriptive data on reliability and validity. The means, standard deviations, and cell sample sizes are presented for each subtest by age of the subject for the ages 3 years 5 months to 86 years. It is not clear why these ages differ from those reported in the text for the standardization sample.

An analysis of variance evaluating age, sex, and subtest was conducted on a sub-sample of the standardization sample (50–149 months). It yielded significant main effects and significant second-order interactions between subtest and age and subtest and sex. Sex had not been predicted to be a significant source of variance, and the authors state that after a study of the interaction, separate tables by sex were not warranted.

Although there was a significant interaction between age and subtest in the analysis of variance of the subsample (50–149 months), the authors chose multiple t-tests to evaluate differences between adjacent age levels (4 years to 60+ years) from the standardization sample. These indicated that, in general, performance tended to improve until age ten years on the Quiet Subtest and to the 13-24 year age level on the Noise Subtest with degradation of performance after age 25 years on both subtests. The conclusion was drawn from the post hoc testing and from the table of means of the total standardization sample that auditory discrimination continues to develop until age 20 to 30 years, after which there is increasingly poorer performance. It is difficult to evaluate this conclusion given the use of multiple *t*-tests and the lack of an analysis on the subsample aged four years to 60+ years. It would be more conservative for an examiner to use the tabled means and standard deviations from the total standardization sample as reference or to interpret the significant differences between age levels with extreme caution.

The proportions of errors for speech-sound categories for three age groupings (5-9 years, 10-20 years, and 21-60 years, $N = 703$) were calculated. They indicate that nasals account for the largest proportion of errors on the Quiet Subtest and nasals and voiced continuants on the Noise Subtest. As age increases, nasals account for an increasing proportion of the errors while errors on voiceless plosives decrease with age. Voiced plosives and continuants and voiceless continuants tended to be stable over age.

Internal consistency of the test was determined on a combined group of several clinical samples ($N = 242$) and for several age levels from the standardization sample. Split-half reliabilities were calculated and corrected by the Spearman-Brown formula. Direct comparisons of the reliability coefficients and standard errors of measurement for the clinical sample and the standardization sample are not possible because the statistics were calculated on different age groups of subjects. The composite clinical sample was divided into groups from 4-6 years, 7-9 years, and 10-12 years. The standardization sample was divided into groups from 3-6 years, 7-11 years, and 12-70+ years. It appears that the split-half reliabilities are slightly less for the standardization sample on each subtest than for the combined clinical sample while standard errors of measurement were larger for the clinical sample. The authors acknowledge that the reliability coefficients are low ($r = .51-.88$) when compared to values obtained on other tests of psychological abilities, but they suggest that this is due in part to the length of the test even though the Spearman-Brown correction was used. It was suggested that the lower reliabilities for the standardization sample are a function of the narrow range of performance for normal subjects and that the G-F-W TAD is not the test to use to discriminate among normally functioning individuals.

The G-F-W TAD was administered and readministered two weeks later to 17 speech handicapped preschool children. The test-retest correlation was .87 for the Quiet Subtest and .81 for the Noise Subtest. The sample chosen for test-retest reliability is very small and clinically deviant. It would be helpful to have additional test-retest reliability determined for a larger normal population. When the Quiet Subtest and Noise Subtest are intercorrelated as two independent measures of auditory discrimination, the correlations are substantially lower ($r = .32-.62$) than the test-retest reliabilities.

The authors reiterate the rationale behind the construction of the G-F-W TAD as the basis for assuming the content or face validity of the test. It appears that the G-F-W TAD tests auditory discrimination through the use of a simple pointing response reflecting recognition memory. The Training Procedure is designed to build word-picture associations if they are lacking, and the manual contains a difficulty index for each word–picture combination. The Quiet Subtest and the Noise Subtest permit auditory discrimination under ideal listening conditions as well as under more real-life listening conditions. In general the test appears to have content or face validity.

Correlations between clinical judgments of "good" and "bad" discriminators and *t*-scores from the G–F–W TAD subtests were calculated. A point-biserial correlation of .68 was found between the clinical judgments and the Quiet Subtest and .72 with the Noise Subtest. The magnitude of these validity coefficients indicates a moderate relationship between the G–F–W TAD and clinical judgments.

The authors suggest that there is evidence from three sources for the construct validity of the test. First, there are consistent changes in performance with age which are typical of a developmental trait. Second, performance of certain selected clinical samples, e.g., hard-of-hearing, mentally retarded, speech and language impairments, are consistently poorer on the G–F–W TAD than the performance of the standardization sample. Finally, it is argued that relatively low correlations between the G–F–W TAD and other psychological measures not tapping auditory discrimination are indicative of construct validity. This final argument is most difficult to accept since low correlations between the G–F–W TAD and nonmeasures of auditory discrimination may be a function of many variables including the reliability of the G–F–W TAD.

Relatively few published investigations have evaluated the G–F–W TAD. Finkenbinder (1973) studied correlations between the G–F–W TAD and CA, MA, and selected reading variables for primary school children. The internal consistency and test-retest reliability of the G–F–W TAD were not substantial, and correlations predicting reading achievement were questionable. Finkenbinder suggested that further research was necessary to make the G–F–W TAD more discriminatory.

Mangan (1972) compared the G–F–W TAD with the Modified Rhyme Test (House, et al. 1963) and found correlations of .72 with the Quiet Subtest and .46 with the Noise Subtest. He also found higher correlations for subjects with hearing losses than for those with normal hearing.

The G–F–W TAD has had widespread use in a number of clinics and schools. Its value as a clinical tool lies in its ease of administration and the extremely short presentation time. Other clinical data should be collected and published so that the test can be better evaluated.

Summary The G–F–W TAD is a brief, nicely packaged test of auditory discrimination for persons aged 3 years 8 months to 70+ years. The Training Procedure is a process provided to ensure that errors in responding on the subtests are due to problems in auditory discrimination and not to a lack of word–picture associations. The subtests have some face validity based on the test construction, but there are no correlations presented between the G–F–W TAD and other measures of auditory discrimination. The values correlating the G–F–W TAD and clinical judgment are moderate; there is need for other validity data on the G–F–W TAD. Split-half reliabilities and test–retest reliabilities are relatively low. Because of the difficulty of interpreting the data presented on the standardization samples, its present use should be restricted to further research exploration. If it is used as a test of an individual subject's auditory discrimination ability, interpretation should be made with caution.

References

Finkenbinder, R. L.   A descriptive study of the Goldman–Fristoe–Woodcock Test of Auditory Discrimination and selected reading variables with primary school children. *Journal of Special Education* 7: 125–131, 1973.

House, A. S., C. E. Williams, M. H. L. Hecker, and K. D. Kryter   *Psycho-acoustic Speech Tests: A Modified Rhyme Test.* U.S. Air Force Systems Command, Hanscom Field, Electronics System Division, Tech. Doc. Report SED-TDR-63-403, 1963.

Mangan, J. E.   Comparison of the Goldman–Fristoe–Woodcock and Modified Rhyme Tests of Auditory Discrimination. Master's Thesis, University of Montana, 1972.

THE ILLINOIS TEST OF PSYCHOLINGUISTIC ABILITIES (ITPA), REVISED EDITION

Samuel A. Kirk, James J. McCarthy, and Winifred D. Kirk

University of Illinois Press (rev. ed.), 1968

Cost $43.50 (includes manual, test materials, 25 record forms and carrying case)

Time 45–50 minutes, administration; 15 minutes, scoring

Carol A. Prutting *University of California, Santa Barbara*

Purpose In 1957 Osgood described a model of communication which formed the basis upon which the Illinois Test of Psycholinguistic Abilities was designed. The model, as described in the manual, consists of three different dimensions of cognitive abilities: channels of communication, psycholinguistic processes, and levels of organization. The 12 subtests which make up the content of the ITPA tap various aspects of the model. The ITPA, therefore, is an attempt to separate and measure various modalities (auditory–vocal, auditory–motor, visual–motor, visual–vocal) psycholinguistic processes (expressive and receptive) and organizational components (representational and automatic levels). The assessment profile obtained from the ITPA provides guidelines for selection and remedial programming.

Administration, scoring, and interpretation All of the ITPA tests are untimed except for the Visual Closure Subtest. The average administration time is about 45–50 minutes. Each examiner is instructed to administer and score a minimum of 10 tests before becoming a qualified examiner. Each of the 12 subtests has individualized administration and scoring procedures and all are presented in a specified order.

The subtests are as follows:

Representational Level—Six tests access the child's ability to comprehend, produce, and internally manipulate auditory and visual symbols:

Auditory Reception (50 items) The child's ability to comprehend the spoken word is assessed.

Visual Reception (40 items) The child's ability to comprehend pictures is assessed.

Auditory Association (42 items) The test assesses the child's ability to relate concepts presented orally.

Visual Association (42 items) The test assesses the child's ability to relate concepts presented visually.

Verbal Expression (4 items) The test assesses the child's ability to express concepts verbally.

Manual Expression (15 items) The child is asked to demonstrate knowledge of the use of objects pictured.

Automatic Level—Six tests measure the child's ability to perform "nonsymbolic tasks":

Grammatic Closure (33 items) The child is asked to say the grammatical form to complete a statement.

Visual Closure (4 items) The child is asked to point to particular fragmentary objects within a specified time limit.

Auditory Closure (30 items) This is an optional test. The child is asked to complete a word of which the child hears fragments.

Sound Blending (32 items) This is an optional test. Child is asked to synthesize into words syllables spoken at half-second intervals.

Auditory Sequential Memory (28 items) The child is asked to produce from memory sequences of from two to eight digits presented at half-second intervals.

Visual Sequential Memory (25 items) The child is shown geometric forms in various sequences. The lengths are from two to eight figures and the child has five seconds to duplicate the pattern.

Scoring procedures are presented by basal levels and ceilings and vary across subtests. For each individual subtest a scaled score or an age score can be obtained. An overall psycholinguistic age can be obtained from the total raw score.

Kirk and Kirk (1971) have devoted a book to interpretation and remediation using the ITPA. They advocate studying the intraindividual differences, that is, comparing the child's subtest scores with each other. Specific areas of deficit which require remediation are delineated. In addition the strong areas are noted in order to use these abilities to develop parallel abilities in the deficit areas. Kirk and Kirk (1978) have cautioned against the interpretation of "scores and labels without their relationship to other information."

Evaluation of test adequacy There are many favorable points which can be stated about the ITPA. Only some of the main issues will be dealt with in this critique. First, the general purpose of the ITPA was to delineate specific language areas so that this assessment tool could reveal areas requiring remediation in a given child. This is an ambitious and important purpose since a valid remedial program is determined by the strength of the assessment procedure.

Another plus for this particular test is that the statistical information on the development, reliability, and psychometric characteristics of the test is exhaustive. Few tests have been constructed, tested out, and standardized in this careful manner (Paraskevopoulos and Kirk 1969).

In addition, the authors have provided detailed instructions as to the administration, scoring, and interpretation of the ITPA. They suggest that only those qualified to administer individual intelligence tests should administer the ITPA. They have provided a film demonstrating the ITPA.

At present, there exists a substantial body of research relating the ITPA to other tests, general academic achievement, reading, ethnic differences, and various clinical problems. This type of information provides the clinician with information about the ITPA in regard to other assessment procedures measuring similar abilities and comparisons of psycholinguistic abilities to general academic abilities (Kirk and Kirk 1978).

There are some aspects of the test which can be critiqued as weaknesses. The first is that the authors describe the purpose of the test being to "isolate defects." While this point was previously mentioned as a strength (that is, we as clinicians have a need for this type of information), it is doubtful that the cognitive–language–communicative system operates in this manner and therefore doubtful that we can extrapolate this type of information. Many scholars have discussed the part–whole question. Lashley (1951) stated:

> Input is never into a quiescent or static system, but always into a system which is already actively excited or organized. In the intact organism, behavior is the result of interaction of this background of excitation and input from any designated stimulus. Only when we can state the general characteristics of this background of excitation, can we understand the effects of a given input.

Watts (1963) wrote, "It becomes suddenly clear that things are joined together by the boundaries we ordinarily take to separate them." This statement was made in the context of how human beings, both past and present, operate under perceptual constraints and as a consequence have perceived and investigated natural phenomena in a linear and singular manner. More recently, R. Buckminster Fuller (1975) stated that investigation of natural phenomena takes place by investigating whole systems, that is, by perceiving and investigating synergistic systems. Fuller defines synergy as "the behavior of whole systems unpredicted by the behavior of their parts taken separately." Restated, the behavior of any components or subsystems is not equal to, or does not predict, the behavior of whole systems.

The assertion that Kirk, McCarthy, and Kirk separate out and measure subprocesses, as reflected in their subtests, is problematic. A test by definition is valuable only if it measures what it purports to measure. There is no clear evidence that psycholinguistic abilities, as defined by the authors, can be separated and measured. The validity of this assumption, at this time, is questionable. The evidence the authors present is in the form of a model, which has not yet been tested. The model forming the basis for the construction of the ITPA is an explanatory model; however, there has not been an adequate connection between theoretical statements and data. The correctness of the predictions has yet to be determined.

A second area of concern is the content of the various subtests and the type of tasks which have been developed in order to measure various psycholinguistic abilities. There are now developmental data regarding the complexity of various aspects of psycholinguistic behaviors. For example, in the Grammatic Closure subtest, the first item is the plural of a noun while the fourth item is the present progressive form. According to Brown (1973) the present progressive form is simpler in terms of semantic-syntactic complexity and therefore would be learned earlier than the plural of the noun. When the content of the test was developed there was probably little information available regarding acquisition of specific structures. The ordering of various items in the subtests in terms of complexity would be an important consideration if a future revision were undertaken.

Some of the tasks on the ITPA are bothersome in that by their nature they may obscure responses. For instance, on the Verbal Expression subtest the child is asked to "Tell me all about this" and is shown four common objects. The child's productions are then scored on ten possible descriptive dimensions such as shape, composition, and function. If one wants to know whether the child knows various characteristics of these objects, it might be more clear-cut to ask such questions as "What is it made of?" or "What do you do with it?" As the subtest is given, a lack of responses from a child could mean that the child does not have the descriptive information, that he or she cannot code it linguistically, or that it is a case of what Labov (1970) has referred to as the "obviousness of the obvious." Given the context there may appear to be no need to communicate the information.

The rationale for inclusion of some subtests is questionable. For example, the authors justify inclusion of the Auditory Closure subtest because it taps a skill people need to have in order to understand foreign accents, poor telephone connections, or defective speakers. This seems to be a rather strange rationale for inclusion of a separate subtest.

One last comment about tasks concerns the Visual Closure subtest. The child is shown a picture of an object or objects to be found in a strip. The picture strip, with the object embedded in numerous places, is shown to the child, who is to point to as many of the objects as possible in 30 seconds. Scrutiny of the five Visual Closure picture strips shows that this is not a task one has to accomplish in everyday life. There is an apparent overload in terms of stimulus presentation, and one wonders what the correlates for this task might be in everyday life experiences.

In spite of the weaknesses discussed, the authors are to be commended for approaching the task of measuring psycholinguistic abilities. It has been a needed step. As Sidman (1960) has stated, ". . . Good data are notoriously fickle. They change their allegiance from theory to theory, and even maintain their importance in the presence of no theory at all." No doubt this is partially true of ITPA data. It is evident that there is a great deal more to be learned about the complex behaviors we assess. The authors of the ITPA were brave to assess psycholinguistic abilities and because of this we stand to learn more about these behaviors.

Summary   The ITPA has become one of the most widely used tests. Perhaps its best feature is that its purpose is assessment rather than classification. If used properly, the test profile can aid in the design of individualized remedial programs. This test should be used only as a supplement to accurate observations of any given child in a variety of communicative settings in which the need to communicate is maintained.

References

Brown, R.   *A First Language.* Cambridge, Mass.: Harvard University Press, 1973.

Fuller, R. B.   *Synergetics.* New York: Macmillan, 1975.

Kirk, S. A. and W. D. Kirk   *Psycholinguistic Learning Disabilities: Diagnosis and Remediation.* Urbana, Ill.: University of Illinois Press, 1971.

—— Uses and abuses of the ITPA. *J. Speech Hearing Dis.* 43: 58–75, 1978.

Labov, W.   Systematically misleading data from test questions. Lecture presented at the University of Michigan, Ann Arbor, 1970.

Lashley, K. S.   The problem of serial order in behavior. In L. A. Jeffress (ed.), *Cerebral Mechanisms in Behavior.* New York: Wiley, 1951.

Osgood, C. E.   A behavioristic analysis. In *Contemporary Approaches to Cognition.* Cambridge, Mass.: Harvard University Press, 1957.

—— Motivational dynamics of language behavior. In *Nebraska Symposium on Motivation.* Lincoln: University of Nebraska Press, 1957.

Paraskevopoulos, J. N. and S. A. Kirk   *The Development and Psychometric Characteristics of the Revised Illinois Test of Psycholinguistic Abilities.* Urbana, Ill.: University of Illinois Press, 1969.

Sidman, M.   *Tactics of Scientific Research.* New York: Basic Books, 1960.

Watts, A.   *The Two Hands of God.* New York: Collier Books, 1963.

LINDAMOOD AUDITORY CONCEPTUALIZATION TEST (LAC TEST)

Charles H. Lindamood and Patricia C. Lindamood

Teaching Resources Corp., 1971

Two Forms A and B

Cost $8.50

Preliminary manual, 38 pages; precheck card; pad of Forms A and B

Time 30 minutes, administration and scoring

John B. Burke *New York University*

Purpose The Lindamood Auditory Conceptualization Test is an individual test measuring auditory perception suitable for administration from preschool through adult levels. The auditory perceptual skill measured involves two related abilities: (1) the ability to discriminate one speech sound from another, and (2) the ability to perceive the number and order of sounds within a spoken pattern.

Administration, scoring, and interpretation The LAC test is untimed and requires no special training or preparation other than that the examiner be thoroughly familiar with the purposes and procedures of the test through its study, the use of the training tape provided with the kit, and by practice. Administration takes place in a well-lighted, quiet room free from materials other than the manual, 18 colored blocks (three each of red, yellow, green, white, blue, and black), and one individual record sheet (Form A or Form B).

The test begins with a precheck to assess the subject's familiarity with concepts of sameness and difference; number concepts to four; left to right order; and first/last concept. In Category I the subject manipulates colored blocks to indicate the number of sounds heard, whether the sounds are the same or different, and the order of the sounds. Through manipulation of the same colored blocks, Category II tests the subject's ability to track and represent changes that occur in syllable patterns as single sounds are added, substituted, omitted, shifted, or repeated.

The raw score (total number of correct responses) is converted on a simple grid printed on the individual record sheet, and then compared with grade-level recommended minimum scores. The authors suggest that failure to reach recommended minimum score for grade level be followed by an in-depth developmental or remedial program, such as their A.D.D. Program (Auditory Discrimination in Depth).

Evaluation of Test Adequacy The manual states that test–retest reliability between Form A and Form B is .96, but it does not detail the method used to derive the reliability coefficient. Moreover, the test manual does not demonstrate comparability of Forms A and B by reporting the means and variances of the two forms together with the coefficient of correlation between the two sets of scores. Finally, in an effort to encourage educational follow-up, the authors have made an upward adjustment of recommended minimum scores without detailing the method employed in arriving at the minimum scores.

While the LAC is easily administered and scored, its usefulness to the speech–language pathologist is limited for two reasons: recommended minimum scores are tied to academic grade level and not to level of speech/language development, and the test does not require the subject to make a motor speech response. Other standardized tests in which both receptive and expressive speech/language skills are assessed would be of more value in a diagnostic session.

Summary The LAC Test, which measures auditory perceptual skill through the ability of the test taker to discriminate one speech sound from another and the ability to perceive the number and order of sounds within a spoken pattern, is not recommended to the speech–language pathologist at this time for the following reasons: (1) the test measures only auditory perception without regard to speech–sound production; (2) recommended minimum test scores are tied to academic grade level without reference to the level of speech/language development; and (3) the authors' explanation of standardization procedures does not adequately demonstrate test–retest reliability, comparability of Forms "A" and "B," and the method used to arrive at recommended minimum test scores.

SCREENING TEST FOR AUDITORY PERCEPTION (STAP)

Geraldine M. Kimmell and
Jack Wahl

Academic Therapy Publications, 1969

Examiner's manual, 24 pages, $5.00; student answer sheets: set of 25, $3.75; set of 100, $12.00; scoring template, $1.00; cassette tape, $10.00

Time Approximately 45 minutes, administration; 5 minutes, scoring

Robert D. Hubbell *California State University, Sacramento*

Purpose The Screening Test for Auditory Perception is designed as a screening instrument for identifying weaknesses in aural perception.

Administration, scoring, and interpretation The test kit consists of a manual, score-sheets, and an overlay to aid in scoring. It is designed for use with children from second to sixth grades and in remedial classes. The test may be administered individually or to groups of children. In addition to the stimulus items, the manual contains directions for each subtest which are to be read aloud. A cassette audiotape of this material is also available. The test may be administered by classroom teachers or other examiners.

The test consists of five subtests. In the first, the child must determine whether the vowels in unisyllabic words are long or short, as in the words *hot, bet, note,* and *light.* In the second subtest, the task is to determine whether unisyllabic words begin with single consonants or consonant blends. Examples include *sat, clean, grate,* and *bone.* The third subtest deals with rhyming. One word is presented. Three more words are then presented, one of which rhymes with the original word. The child's response is to identify the word that rhymes by indicating its position in the sequence of three words. For example, *slip* is followed by *trap, hip, pep; much* is followed by *hush, lunch, touch.* The fourth subtest focuses on rhythmic sound patterns. Three sequences of from three to six taps, each sequence varying in rhythm, are presented to the child. One of these sequences is then repeated. The child is to identify the ordinal position of the repeated sequence among the original three. For example, the first three rhythms might be,

tap; tap, tap, tap
tap; tap, tap; tap
tap, tap; tap, tap

The child is then asked, "Which was this pattern:

tap; tap, tap; tap?"

No indications are given concerning speed of tapping or duration between sequences. The fifth subtest consists of a conventional auditory discrimination task in which the child must determine for each pair of words whether the examiner said the same word twice or two different words. Examples include *shop–chop, gum–glum, leaf–leave,* and *pace–face.* Each subtest contains 12 items except the fourth, which contains only six.

The child responds to all subtests with pencil on a response sheet. This sheet consists of squares, circles, and triangles, each colored yellow, orange, or gray. These figures are arranged in contrasting sets for each subtest. The child responds by marking one of these figures for each item. For example, in the fifth subtest, the child marks a yellow box if the two words are the same, and an orange box if the words are different. In subtest four, there are three circles in a row for each item. The child marks the first circle, which is yellow, the second, which is orange, or the third, gray, depending on which rhythmic pattern is the match.

Scoring consists of counting correct responses. Scoring is facilitiated by an overlay which comes with the test. The raw scores are converted to percentiles through tables in the manual. Directions for interpreting the test are not specific. It is stated that the test is a screening device and not intended to supplant other types of evaluation. It is suggested that children scoring in the lowest 25 percent be evaluated further.

Evaluation of test adequacy   This test has serious flaws in rationale, design, and statistical treatment. With regard to rationale, it is not clear why the particular tasks for the subtests were chosen or what they are intended to represent. The authors state that the five subtests are not designed to produce a differential diagnosis, but norms are presented for each subtest, and a place is provided on the score sheet to graph a child's profile among the subtests. There is no hint of what a particular profile might mean. Subtest four is particularly questionable. A child must retain three different rhythmic patterns of tapping in memory, hear a fourth pattern and compare it with the other three, and respond in terms of the temporal order of presentation of the first three. Further, the child's response is to mark one of three circles, which are arranged in a spatial order and are of different colors. A great deal of processing is required, much of it with auditory stimuli. One would be hard put to interpret a low score on this subtest. What does it mean relative to auditory processing? What are its implications for further evaluation, much less educational planning?

No mention of validity is made in the manual. It would seem that at least some comparison of the STAP with other substantial tests that sample aspects of auditory processing would be in order. Studies of predictive validity would be even more desirable. As Gains (1972) states, there is not even any indication of whether children who do poorly on the test manifest difficulties with reading or other learning, hearing loss, or other disabilities.

The authors' suggestions concerning interpretation are of little help in clarifying the meaning of the test. For example, after noting that many children do well on most subtests and that number four is the hardest, they state, ". . . a child who marks all the items but gets zero on the first, second, or fifth part is likely to succeed at the task, but it is obvious that he has not been able to retain directions given auditorily." There seems to be no point in using a test of auditory perception if poor performance on the test may be an *artifact* of a child's auditory skills or of the directions for the test which are presented through the auditory channel.

The construction of the test must also be faulted. The directions are complicated. The unique design of the response sheet, with its geometrical shapes of various colors, may be confusing for some children. The number of items in each subtest is small, perhaps too small to sample fairly a child's skill in that area. With regard to the auditory discrimination subtest for example, no other auditory discrimination test available consists of only 12 items. This factor is particularly obvious in subtest four. The difference between approximately the 50th and 25th percentiles is only one point out of a possible six points at a number of grade and age levels. Interpretation of such percentiles is impossible.

In addition, the reliability of the instrument is not well demonstrated. Thirty-seven first graders were retested in second grade, and 36 second graders were retested in third grade. Spearman rank order correlations for the younger and older children were .80 and .67, respectively. Immediately following the presentation of these data in the manual is a statement that the stability of auditory perception measures *increases* with age.

Problems with the normative data for the STAP have been discussed by both Bricker (1972) and Gains (1972). The norms were developed by testing children in three schools in a suburb of San Francisco. No mention is made of socioeconomic class, race, IQ, or other variables important in sample selection. The norms, consequently, are virtually uninterpretable. Further, as Gains (1972) points out, the authors are inconsistent in reporting how many children were in the normative sample. The total N is reported as 650, but when one adds up the totals reported for each grade level the total is 655; when the totals for each age are summed, the total is 543. Such discrepancies render the normative data further suspect. In addition, the N's for some of the subgroups are too small for conversion into percentiles. The N for seven-year-olds is only 16; for six-year-olds it is 30. Finally, means for the total test are presented for each age level. Standard deviations, however, are not given. Interpretation of the means is therefore difficult, particularly in view of the fact that the means for the older groups are very close. For ages four, five, and six, the means are 47, 48, and 49, respectively.

Summary   The STAP is designed as a screening test for auditory perception for children in elementary school. The test consists of five subtests representing various skills related to the processing of auditory input. The child responds to auditory stimuli by marking a special response sheet. Use of the test cannot be recommended. Important questions have been raised concerning its rationale, construction, norms, and interpretation. On the cover of the manual, copyright 1969, the STAP is subtitled, "Experimental Edition." It is past time to take it back to the drawing boards.

References

Bricker, A.   Review of the Screening Test for Auditory Perception. In O. K. Buros (ed.), *Mental Measurements Yearbook, Seventh Edition.* New Brunswick: Rutgers University Press, 1972.

Gains, R.   Review of the Screening Test for Auditory Perception. In O. K. Buros (ed.), *Mental Measurements Yearbook, Seventh Edition.* New Brunswick: Rutgers University Press, 1972.

SHORT TERM AUDITORY RETRIEVAL AND STORAGE TEST (STARS) (EXPERIMENTAL EDITION)

Arthur Flowers

Perceptual Learning Systems, 1972

Cost $49.50

Manual, 11 pages; test booklet, 13 pages; 240 pictures; audio cassette and reel-to-reel tapes

Time 25 minutes, administration; 5 minutes scoring

John M. Panagos *Kent State University*

Purpose The Short Term Auditory Retrieval and Storage test is designed to screen the "central auditory abilities" of normal school children (grades one through six) and selected groups of special education children.

Administration, scoring, and interpretation The test comes in a three-ring notebook containing a test manual, two stimulus tapes, and test booklet of pictures. It can be given in about 25 minutes by any professional who reads the manual. Entire class-rooms of children as well as individuals can be tested. Group administration requires a prescribed seating arrangement diagrammed in the manual. Test stimuli are recorded words played at a comfortable loudness level. There are 45 word pairs (e.g., *toothbrush–airplane*) and 10 three-word groups (e.g., *shoes–clown–eyes*).

Words vary in phonemic content and include compound, polysyllable, and mono-syllable items. On the stimulus tape words occur *simultaneously*. The child listens to the two or three words presented and marks in the test booklet the two or three pic-tures (line drawings) that correspond to them. For the two-word presentations, there are four pictures from which to choose; for the three-word presentations there are six pictures. One point is awarded for each correct word identification. A perfect score for the 120 test words is 120 points. Group norms (means, standard deviations, percen-tiles) for normal children (grades one through six), educable mentally retarded chil-dren (ages seven to 14 years), and learning-disabled children (grades one and two) are presented in tables. Children whose scores fall below the test norms are considered to be candidates for listening training.

Evaluation of test adequacy Favorable reliability estimates derived from the Kuder–Richardson formula have been established for the sample of normal children. Test validity has not been established.

Perhaps the fact that the STARS test is still "in its early stages of development" explains its obvious limitations. The construct of "central auditory abilities" is neither defined nor discussed in the manual. The method of presenting words simultaneously would appear to evaluate selective attention as much as retrieval and storage. The test also evaluates such factors as knowledge of word meanings stored in long-term memory, visual recognition of two-dimensional line drawings, word interpretation of pictures, matching words derived from two-input modalities, and motor encoding. Clearly, linguistic and cognitive abilities in addition to auditory ones are assessed by the STARS test. Recently, the construct validity of auditory perceptual tests has been challenged (Rees 1973).

The accuracy with which the STARS test measures the abilities assessed is also questionable. The vocal characteristics of the two male speakers are noticeably different in quality and intelligibility. Long words overlap shorter ones (e.g., *barber chair* vs. *reindeer*) and words vary in syllable, stress, and phoneme complexity (e.g., *school house* vs. *jar*). The last ten presentations are three-word combinations substantially increasing task complexity over the 45 two-word presentations. The influences of such factors (i.e., speaker characteristics, linguistic complexity, word familiarity, word length, short-term memory capacity) on the difficulty of individual test items and overall test results are not analyzed.

The questionable validity of the STARS test severely limits its educational applications. It is quick and easy to administer and can be given informally as a gross measure of information processing capacity. However, results should be compared with those of other language and perceptual tests that may well prove to be more accurate measures of the same abilities. Decisions to place children in remedial auditory training programs based solely on the results of the STARS test (suggested in the manual) should be avoided.

Summary The STARS is an easily administered test designed to screen "central auditory abilities" (an undefined construct) by presenting tape recorded words (pairs and triplets) simultaneously. The questionable accuracy of this method as well as the absence of demonstrated validity militate against its use as the sole measure for classifying children for remedial auditory training.

Reference

Rees, N. Auditory processing factors in language disorders: the view from Procrustes' bed. *J. Speech Hearing Dis.* **38**: 304–315, 1973.

SLINGERLAND SCREENING TESTS FOR IDENTIFYING CHILDREN WITH SPECIFIC LANGUAGE DISABILITY (1970 REVISED EDITION) Beth H. Slingerland	Educator's Publishing Service, Inc. (rev. ed.), 1970 **Cost** Specimen Set—One copy each of Forms A, B, and C and one Teacher's Manual, $3.00 Manual, 150 pages; test booklets, 15 pages **Time** Approximately one hour, administration and scoring

M. Irene Stephens *Northern Illinois University*

Purpose "The purpose of the Screening Tests is to screen from among a group of children those with potential language difficulties and those with already present specific language disabilities who are in need of special attention at the moment" (Teacher's Manual, p. xx).

Administration, scoring, and interpretation Three forms correspond to school grade levels: Form A for grades one and two; Form B for grades two and three; and Form C for grades three and four. The forms are said to differ mainly in vocabulary difficulty. In the manual the author refers to two other forms: Form D for grades five and six; and Pre-Reading Screening Procedures, which is suggested for use in place of Form A "in schools which contain disadvantaged populations" (p. 2).

There are eight subtests which are group-administered as well as a set of Individual Auditory Tests ". . . to be administered individually to the child who has exhibited difficulty in the last three subtests . . ." (p. 4). The child enters responses in a test booklet. The subtests are:

Subtest 1 Copying a brief story from a wall chart.
Subtest 2 Copying words and phrases and numbers from a sample in the test booklet.
Subtest 3 Memory for words, letters, and numbers. A stimulus is shown for approximately ten seconds and it is to be identified (circled) from an array of four items.
Subtest 4 Match to sample. Single words are underlined in the test booklet and the exact printed word appears in a column of four "words" and is to be underlined.
Subtest 5 Reproducing letters, numbers, and shapes after a brief exposure of the stimulus item.
Subtest 6 Sequences of letters, numbers, and short phrases which are presented orally are to be written in the appropriate space in the test booklet.
Subtest 7 Single words are presented orally and either the first or last sound of each word is to be identified with the corresponding letter.
Subtest 8 Words, numbers, or letter groups are presented orally which are to be identified (circled) from an array of four items.

There are specific directions for the room setting and for the group administration of the subtests. The scoring system uses three types of error counts: uncorrected errors, self-corrections, and poor formations. A Quick Analysis is made by summing these three categories. A Detailed Analysis involves 18 categories of errors such as insertion, reversal, mixed capitals and lower case, etc. Results are interpreted primarily by using a "break-off point" (a total of 12-15 errors on subtests 3-8 is considered a sign of probable disability), but the error totals are to be related to IQ, school achievement, family patterns, and developmental information supplied by the parents. A pattern of consistent error is said to be important because "in a disadvantaged population . . . children will make up to 20 errors without showing the consistent pattern that leads to suspicion of maturational lag or specific language disability" (pp. vi–vii).

Evaluation of test adequacy   There is no reference to the test's reliability. The determination of the "break-off point" is described as follows: "During the early years of experimentation and test construction, experience indicated that a total of 12-15 errors on subtests 3 to 8 could be considered a significant warning and might be considered the 'break-off' point. . . ." (p. vi).

Although the psychometric term validity is not used, there are generalizations made which relate to this concept such as: "Children who do well on the Screening Tests do well as they progress from grade to grade; children who do not do well and receive no help fall behind" (p. xiii); and "Children who performed well on the Screening Tests achieved well on the Metropolitan Achievement Tests according to their ability as shown on the Pintner–Cunningham Tests of General Ability. Children who exceeded the break-off point in number of errors did not achieve at grade level or as well as would have been expected on the basis of general ability" (p. vi). However, no correlations or actual scores or ranges are offered.

The concept of norms is discussed in some detail. The author states that no attempt has been made to establish standardized national norms because many sets of norms would have to be developed to cover the varying conditions of socioeconomic status, ethnic group, rural/suburban/city school population characteristics, etc. She stresses ". . . the development of local norms by the users of the Slingerland tests and the importance of individual evaluation of test performances that deviate from the overall performance of the peer group" (p. vi).

The only quantitative information given that relates to populations tested is in the form of percentages screened out. For example: "Our recent studies in suburban populations have confirmed earlier findings . . . that 20 to 30% of a group of middle-class, advantaged children will deviate from the norm of their peer group. We have found in other schools, schools with large numbers of deprived children, that the percentage will be greater—up to 50%" (p. xii).

The author's definition of "deviate from the norm of their peer group" is a puzzling, or, at least, idiosyncratic one. Since one standard deviation from the mean of a normal distribution encompasses 68 percent of the population, a 30 percent finding of disability in middle-class, advantaged children would place some children just outside this range, while a 50 percent finding of disability in deprived children would include many children within this range. It is difficult to see how as many as half the children could deviate from the norm of their own group. Traditional estimates of atypicality are usually much closer to two standard deviations.

The Individual Auditory Tests are probably of greater interest to the speech-language pathologist. These tests are covered in the manual beginning on p. 117. There are three tasks. The first requires the child to repeat a word or phrase several times; the second is a sentence completion task; and the third is a story retelling task. The evaluation of performance is quite global: "We may suspect either a maturational lag or a specific language disability in a child whose performance on the Individual Auditory Test is poor . . ." (p. 133). The examiner is encouraged to note behaviors such as sound substitutions within words, omission of syllables, sentence length, etc., but there is no scoring system nor any norms with which to compare the performance. For example, it is not known if the phrase "Nancy's pansy plant" becomes a tongue twister upon successive repetitions in children who display normal language abilities. Consequently, one would not know how to interpret an unsuccessful repetition on the part of a child suspected of specific language disability.

The eight subtests that form the core of the Slingerland Tests relate primarily to visual, auditory, and motor (hand) skills associated with reading and writing. The typical speech, hearing and language clinician would therefore be unlikely to use this test. However, a child might be referred to the clinician because of performance on the Slingerland Test and a certain familiarity with the test might be valuable. It is noteworthy that such a clinician may not be the receiver of the referral. For example, the statement "When a child manifests speech disorders to any degree, auditory acuity should be evaluated by a competent otologist" (p. 118) ignores the possibility that the school corporation may well have competent audiological testing or referral services.

Summary   At the present time, the information on the test's standardization is totally inadequate. The absence of reliability and validity checks greatly weakens the test's credibility. Emphasizing the need for local norms does not excuse a test developer from analyzing and reporting *some* normative data. Mention is made of large numbers of children who have been or are currently being screened by this device. These data need to be displayed in a psychometrically acceptable fashion.

SOUND DISCRIMINATION TEST	Not available commercially; published in Templin (1943, 1957) and as Appendix 3 in M. F. Berry and J. Eisenson, *Speech Disorders.* New York: Appleton-Century-Crofts, 1956 No manual or test blanks
Mildred C. Templin	
	Time No information available

Paul S. Weiner *University of Chicago*

Purpose The purpose of Templin's Sound Discrimination Test is implied in its title. It was devised to measure the ability of elementary school children to discriminate the speech sounds of English. Constructed to serve in a study of the development of *Certain Language Skills in Children* (1957), it was published in the report of that study and has never been made available commercially. As a consequence, there is no manual, and the norms consist simply of the means and standard deviations of the responses of the study sample. As befits a relatively minor portion of a study, the descriptions of the test, of its construction, and of its method of administration are brief.

Administration, scoring, and interpretation The Sound Discrimination Test consists of 50 pairs of nonsense syllables. Seven of these pairs involve identical syllables while the remaining pairs differ in one phoneme (e.g., āzh–āzh and sā–thā). In the administration of the test, the examiner reads each syllable pair in turn to the child, who must judge whether the syllables are the same or different. The score consists of the number of pairs judged correctly. The research sample which served as the basis for the "norms" consisted of 180 Minneapolis public school children with 60 at each of the age levels of six, seven, and eight years. (A picture sound discrimination test was used for the younger children in the study.) The group was equally divided according to sex. Thirty percent were designated as being upper and the remainder as being of lower socioeconomic status. No method of interpretation of individual test results is given as the interest of the author was in group rather than individual differences.

Neither reliability nor validity data are offered in the study. For applicable material, it is necessary to refer to an earlier study (Templin 1943) in which the original steps in the test's construction were taken. Templin first devised two tests, each containing 100 items; 32 of the pairs in each were the same and 68 different. The tests were essentially identical in content but the discriminative element or combination was placed in the initial position in one test and in the final or medial position in the other. As the author states, "As far as practicable nasals, plosives, semi-vowels, fricatives and combinations were included in the tests in the proportion that 103 preschool children had been found to make errors [in articulation] on these types of sounds in a previous study" (1943, p. 127). The combined test containing 200 items was used in a study of 301 elementary school children. On the basis of the results the 70 most discriminating items were selected. The test being evaluated here is a still shorter version containing the 50 most discriminating pairs. The correlation ratio for predicting scores on the 70-item test in terms of the 200-item test was .922. The relation of the final test to either of its precursors is unknown. The odd-even reliability coefficient of the 70-item test was .712, which Templin considered to be "not high."

Evaluation of test adequacy   If the Sound Discrimination Test is evaluated according to the *Standards for Educational and Psychological Tests* of the American Psychological Association (1974), it inevitably comes off poorly.

There is no manual. Norms are limited and derived from a rather small group of children who lived in a single geographical area. No attempt is made to provide guidelines for interpretation of results. Reliability and validity data specifically related to the 50-item test are lacking. Relevant data on the earlier short form of the test are also limited. In fact, no norms are given for the 70-item measure. The choice of sounds used in the test rests on grounds of uncertain acceptability. It is based in part upon a linguistic categorization and in part upon the nature of children's articulation errors. The former base would probably not be generally accepted as adequate today while the latter must be considered controversial. The use of nonsense syllables and of a "same–different" format may be criticized as tending to make the test too dependent on the verbal intelligence of the subjects. The relationship of the results on the test with vocabulary knowledge and with intelligence quotient ($r = .44–.58$) would seem to support this criticism.

As must be apparent, many of these criticisms result from the fact that the author prepared the test in another era and simply for research purposes. Some of the criticisms, particularly as they relate to inadequacies of standardization and the "same–different" format, are not peculiar to this test but can be made with reference to other currently popular tests of the same ability.

Summary   The potential value of the Sound Discrimination Test remains unknown. A careful analysis of the sounds used, the gathering of appropriate norms, and the determination of the test's reliability and validity would be necessary before a meaningful determination could be made. As matters stand, the test can be recommended only for research use.

References

American Psychological Association   *Standards for Educational and Psychological Tests.* Washington, D.C.: American Psychological Association, 1974.

Templin, M. C.   *Certain Language Skills in Children.* Minneapolis: University of Minnesota Press, 1957.

——   A study of sound discrimination ability of elementary school pupils. *J. Speech Dis.* **8**: 127–132, 1943.

SPECIFIC LANGUAGE DISABILITY TEST (SLDT) (GRADES SIX, SEVEN, AND EIGHT)

Neva Malcomesius

Educators Publishing Service, 1967

Cost   12 test booklets, $4.00; cards and charts, $3.00; manual, $.70; specimen set (one manual, one booklet), $1.00

Manual, 13 pages; test booklet, 10 pages, 10 subtests

Time   1 hour 15 minutes to 2 hours, administration; 10–25 minutes, scoring

Linda Swisher   *University of Arizona*

Purpose   The manual states that the Specific Language Disability Test was designed to identify the eight out of every 100 students with a degree of dyslexia that requires special training. In addition, in materials provided it is claimed that the results can be used in the design of remedial programs. The materials are described as usable for both individual and group testing. The manual states that "before the tests are given, each student's eyes, ears, and IQ should be checked."

Administration, scoring, and interpretation   Subtests I–V evaluate visual discrimination, visual memory, and visual-to-motor coordination. Tests VI–X evaluate perception in auditory discrimination, auditory-to-visual coordination, auditory-to-motor coordination, and comprehension. All tests involve the ability to follow the spoken instructions. The same tests are considered appropriate for the three grades (six, seven, and eight) for which the test was developed.

The manual gives brief instructions as to how each test is to be administered and evaluated. For example the evaluation section for Test 1 has four sentences of which the first is, "Note the handwriting; if it is biased, the student probably has some motor incoordination."

Evaluation of test adequacy   No data concerning test construction, reliability, or validity are provided. No rationale for the selection of test categories or items is provided.

Summary   Because it has no descriptive data or underlying rationale for its construction, this test cannot be recommended.

TEST OF LISTENING ACCURACY IN CHILDREN (TLAC)

Merlin J. Mecham, J. Lorin Jex, and J. Dean Jones

Communication Research Associates, Inc., 1968, 1973

Cost $35.00

Six-page individual and seven-page group testing examiner's manuals; one pad of group test score sheets, 25 individual test score sheets, one reel-to-reel tape, one cassette tape, one film strip

Time 15–20 minutes, administration; 2–4 minutes, scoring

Kathleen Pendergast *Seattle (Washington) Public Schools*

Purpose As its title indicates, and according to an article written by one of the authors, the Test of Listening Accuracy in Children measures verbal listening accuracy in children. The purpose is not further clarified in the manual.

Administration, scoring, and interpretation The TLAC may be administered to a group or to individual children. In group testing, the children see three pictures projected from a film strip onto a screen, they hear a series of three words played from a reel-to-reel tape recorder, and they mark an individual score sheet (A–B–C) indicating the position of the one correctly pronounced word. These score sheets are corrected by using an acetate key. In individual testing, the child looks at three pictures in a test booklet, listens to three words from a cassette tape recorder, and points to the one picture that is correctly pronounced. The examiner marks the individual test score sheet with a plus for correct and a minus for incorrect responses. For both individual and group testing, correct responses are totaled. The total score may be converted into a percentile score rated from "very poor" to "superior" according to grade level. No age score is derived to identify the amount of deficit.

The results of the normative data led the authors to conclude that "listening accuracy, as measured by the present test, seems to be a developmental phenomenon which plateaus rapidly between the 4th and 6th grades" (Mecham 1971).

Evaluation of test adequacy The TLAC used accepted practices for test construction in its design. Normative data were collected appropriately, and the internal consistency of the test was analyzed by use of the Kuder–Richardson analysis of variance technique. This method yielded a high reliability for each grade level tested.

The words in the test are presented with some background noise which may require a slightly different listening skill than most auditory discrimination tests. The test may identify a deficit not apparent on the other tests.

The sequence of three words is presented fairly rapidly and each sequence is presented with barely enough time to mark the score sheet. In individual testing this requires a degree of manual dexterity and practice on the part of the examiner. The test has 86 items that require maximum attention for 15 to 20 minutes. Some examiners feel this is too long for young or distractible children. Older children tend to become bored toward the end of the test. Scores from the individual and group test do not appear to be comparable at second grade level, and there are no percentile rankings above second grade for individual test administration.

The strengths of this test are that the presentation is controlled by the taped instructions, the recording and scoring system for the individual test are simple, the illustrations are good, and the test package is well constructed and fairly durable. The weaknesses of the test are that it is too long and becomes boring; the instructions are too difficult and inadequate for young children; norms on individual test administration do not go above second grade; norms are presented according to grade, not age, which can cause some inequities; some children have difficulty marking the group recording sheets; and there is no discussion relating the skills tested to communication skills or remediation of identified deficits. The authors present no rationale for creating the test nor do they discuss the skill it measures. Therefore, the examiner is limited in the implications to be drawn from either a high or low score.

Summary   The TLAC is an attractive test of no stated purpose. It is limited in its potential clinical usefulness by excessive length, difficult instructions for young subjects, and truncated normative data. In its present form, it might be more useful as a research tool than as a clinical tool. Further research may reveal implications for clinical use but at present its value is limited.

Reference

Mecham, M. J.   Measurement of verbal listening accuracy in children. *J. Learning Dis.* 4: 257–259, 1971.

A TEST OF SOUND DISCRIMINATION

Orvis C. Irwin

Published in Orvis C. Irwin, *Communication Variables of Cerebral Palsied and Mentally Retarded Children.* Springfield, Ill.: Charles C Thomas, 1972
Two equivalent forms, A and B

Cost $20.75
Manual and test forms are not available except as a part of the book

Ruth M. Lencione *University of California at Los Angeles*

Purpose A Test of Sound Discrimination was one of a series of research studies conducted by Irwin that culminated in a standardized test for children with either cerebral palsy or mental retardation. It was designed to be used with children between the ages of six and 16 years.

Administration, scoring, and interpretation Forms A and B contain 30 pairs of words, five of which are foils, with the target sound in the initial, medial, and final positions of words. Only those children who have had a prior hearing test and have adequate hearing for speech are to be given the test. The test procedure includes having the examiner speak each pair of words slowly and clearly at a conversational level, taking care to separate the two words of the pair by a slight pause. The child is asked to indicate whether the words are same or different. A check on how well the child is attending is afforded by the five foils; responses to the foils are not included in the final score.

Evaluation of test adequacy Test construction was accomplished by assembling a pool of 135 paired words from a variety of sources. This pool was reduced to 100 pairs after consultation with a speech–language pathologist familiar with the speech problems of cerebral-palsied children. These items were then divided into two groups of 50 for the purpose of developing equivalent forms. As a preliminary tryout, one 50-item test was administered to 86 cerebral-palsied children in six rehabilitation centers; the other 50 items were administered to 129 cerebral-palsied children.

The results from these tryouts were subjected to item analysis based on the criteria of discriminating power of the item, uniqueness, and difficulty. Each test was reduced to 25 items and then standardized on two samples of cerebral-palsied children drawn from widely different geographic areas. Form A was standardized on 153 children six to 16 years old ($M = 9$-6 years) from southwestern and eastern states, while Form B was standardized on 260 children six to 17 years old ($M = 10$-9 years) from northcentral and northwestern states.

Reliability of the forms was determined by the internal consistency of the tests and a comparison of the means for boys and girls in the two geographic areas. Results were similar for both forms. Based on a Kuder–Richardson formula, r was .87 for Form A, and .88 for Form B. In each case, the means for boys and girls either within or between the two geographic areas did not differ significantly. The correlation between forms was .90.

Validity was based on the relation of the scores to chronological age, mental age, and ratings of general language ability. Using the method of extreme groups, the results indicated a significant chronological and mental age progression in the scores, as well as a significant difference between mean scores of children rated good and poor in general language ability.

Additional data are provided about the effect of spasticity and athetosis, the effect of the degree of severity of cerebral palsy, and the effect of position of the target sound in the initial and final position of words. The means of scores of spastics and athetoids were alike; and the means of scores of children medically diagnosed as mildly, moderately, and severely involved were alike. On Form A, the difference for the mean scores for sounds in the initial and final positions indicated that the final position was significantly more difficult than the initial position. Results from Form B did not confirm this finding, as the differences between means for sounds in the three positions were nonsignificant. A replication with Form A with a sample of 260 children indicated no difference between scores for sounds in initial and final positions.

A similar procedure was followed to study the reliability and validity of Form A for use with retarded children. The standardization group consisted of 76 retarded children from six to 17 years old ($M = 12-5$ years) from Hawaii and northwestern states.

Examination of internal consistency resulted in an r of .81, compared with .87 for the cerebral-palsied group. Neither sex nor geographic differences were obtained.

Vocabulary, abstraction, and mental classification were used as validating criteria. The method of extreme groups produced significant differences in the expected direction for each comparison.

Norms, as such, are not provided. The means and standard deviations reported as well as the relative difficulty of the items are derived from groups with an age span of 10 to 11 years. Thus, the data are not reported in a manner that allows for a comparison of a particular child's sound-discrimination abilities with that of others of similar age or physical or mental condition.

Summary   At the time A Test of Sound Discrimination was developed, it provided an additional adjunct in the battery of quantitative tests developed by Irwin designed to investigate the speech–sound status of cerebral-palsied and retarded children. This test, used in conjunction with the Integrated Articulation Test (qv) (Irwin 1972) provided speech–language pathologists with a valid index of communication abilities and disabilities and provided objective data for use in planning speech therapy.

With the advent of alternate methods of communication such as communication aids and, when possible, total communication, the need for discrete tests of sound discrimination is no longer as critical as it was a decade ago. Irwin's work served as a springboard for innovative management procedures with groups of communicatively handicapped children.

Reference

Irwin, O. C. *Communication Variables of Cerebral Palsied and Mentally Retarded Children.* Springfield, III.: Charles C Thomas, 1972.

THE VISUAL AURAL DIGIT SPAN TEST (VADS)

Elizabeth M. Koppitz

Grune and Stratton, 1977

Manual (monograph), 200 pages, $15.50; test cards and scoring sheets (ordered separately), $6.75

Time 15–20 minutes, administration and scoring

William S. Rosenthal *California State University, Hayward*

Purpose The Visual Aural Digit Span Test, also known as the VADS Test, provides a standardized measure of short-term memory and what the author describes as intersensory integration. According to Koppitz the test is meant to be used as a diagnostic tool in assessing learning disabilities in school-age children. Based on her own research (Koppitz 1971), the author has found that learning-disabled children who require long-term special education have serious difficulty in integration and recall. Thus by evaluating these two functions, this test is not only diagnostic but intended to be predictive of educational outcome as well.

Administration, scoring, and interpretation The VADS Test consists of four subtests, each of which requires the child to reproduce a series of two-digit to seven-digit numbers under different conditions. The number sequences are presented on a set of 26 VADS Test stimulus cards. The Aural–Oral subtest involves the aural presentation of the digit series and their oral recall. The Visual–Oral subtest involves the visual presentation of digits and their oral recall. The third and fourth subtests, Aural–Written and Visual–Written, are similar to the first two subtests except that the responses are written instead of spoken. In the aurally presented portions of the test, digits are presented by the examiner at the rate of one per second. Visually presented portions are shown to the child for ten seconds.

A child receives credit when either one of two trials is reproduced correctly for a given digit series length. Testing begins at different digit series lengths depending on the subtest, the child's age, and the child's presumed capability. Each subtest is ended when the child misses both trials of a given sequence of digits.

Scores for each of the four subtests are easily arrived at. They are simply the number of digits in the longest series correctly reproduced. These four subtest scores are then used to calculate six additional combination scores. Combination scores are the additive value of any two subtest scores. Thus the scores on the Aural–Oral and Aural–Written subtests can be combined to yield what is called the Aural Input score. Similarly, combination scores called Visual Input, Oral Expression, and Written Expression may be calculated. The combined scores of the Aural–Oral and Visual–Written subtests result in what is called the Intrasensory score. Combined scores of the Visual–Oral and Aural–Written subtests yield the Intersensory Score. Finally, the added values of all four subtests result in the Total VADS Test Score. There are, in all, 11 measures that can be calculated from a single test administration.

Test results may be interpreted in two ways, by using normative data or by qualitative analysis of the child's test performance. The VADS Test normative data permit the comparison of each of the 11 obtained and derived scores for a given child with the means, standard deviations, and percentile scores of the child's age-mates (5.5 to 12) or grade-mates (kindergarten to sixth grade). A separate section of the test manual guides the examiner through an analysis of the child's qualitative performance that includes the formation, size, and arrangement of digits on the written response subtests.

Evaluation of test adequacy   The reliability of the VADS Test was established by a test–retest procedure conducted by the author. The procedure is weak in several respects. Only one examiner administered the test. The test–retest interval was highly variable, ranging from one day to 15 weeks. Only children with learning and behavior problems were tested. With these limitations noted, reliability coefficients ranged from a low of .72 to a high of .92.

The normative data for the VADS Test are statistically sound. They are obtained from 810 children divided into ten age groups (5–6 to 12–11), all of approximately the same size. Both sex and ethnic distributions approximate the rates in the general population. Geographical distribution of the normative sample is heavily skewed to the Northeast (New York State) and to medium-sized urban areas, but includes children from the Midwest, West, and South.

The test manual treats the issue of test validity in meticulous detail. Separate chapters relate VADS Test performance to school achievement, learning difficulty, and IQ. In each instance consistent, statistically significant, though not always strong relationships are demonstrated between these variables and VADS Test scores for both normal and LD children. Since the test is intended to be diagnostic, the pattern or profile of subtest scores is considered significant. In a separate chapter, various test profiles are evaluated both statistically and through the presentation of detailed case history examples.

The fact that the test manual departs in form and format from what is usually expected of test manuals may confound the casual user. The manual is, in fact, a 200-page monograph. The huge amount of tabular and descriptive data presented may confuse some users and result in unreliable and invalid interpretations of test results.

The VADS Test is of little use in the evaluation of children with language disorders. It is not a test of language function, nor is it claimed to be. In fact, nowhere in the manual is any attempt made to relate performance on this test with language ability. In the first place, the test is intended for children beginning at age 5.5. By that age language is well established in normal children. If a language disorder exists at that age, a test such as this is not needed to detect it. Furthermore, use of the test would not aid in evaluating the nature of such a disorder should it be present.

In a similar vein one can question the need for this test in detecting other kinds of cognitively based problems such as reading, writing, and learning disorders since such disorders are also obvious when they are present. A claim might be made that the VADS Test can uncover the root cause of such disorders. However, that premise is based on the belief that cognitive functions represented by language behavior, reading, writing, and the learning of academic material are composed of a set of discrete but integrated perceptual skills. Memory, recall, sequencing, and sensory integration are among the skills presumed to underlie such functions. However, an increasing body of research argues against this premise. For example, Rourke (1975), who has studied extensively children with reading disorders as well as other learning disabilities, has found that so-called perceptual disorders are not specific to sensory modalities such as vision and audition. Rather, they are central in nature due to fundamental attentional deficits.

A decision to use or not to use this test will depend to a great extent on what theoretical construct the tester adheres to. Even so, the examiner who is persuaded by the "perceptual skills" approach might better consider using a test which measures more directly linguistic behavior, such as the Illinois Test of Psycholinguistic Abilities (qv). At best the VADS Test is a screening device and adds little to the information obtainable by the use of larger test batteries.

Summary The Visual Aural Digit Span Test (VADS Test) is an easily administered test that can be quickly scored and interpreted by use of well researched normative data. The test is intended to measure memory, recall, and sensory integration in children from 5.5 to 12 years of age. It is offered as a diagnostic test for children with learning disabilities. However, its diagnostic utility is contingent on a theoretical construct that is controversial and increasingly under question. It may be used as part of a screening battery but ought not to be used as a major source of decisions about the child's performance or placement.

References

Koppitz, E. M. *Children with Learning Disabilities: A Five-Year Follow-Up Study.* New York: Grune and Stratton, 1971.

Rourke, B. P. Brain-behavior relationships in children with learning disabilities: a research program. *Amer. Psychol.* **30**: 911–920, 1975.

WASHINGTON SPEECH SOUND DISCRIMINATION TEST (WSSD TEST)

Elizabeth M. Prather, Adah Miner, Margaret Anne Addicott, and Linda Sunderland

Interstate Printers and Publishers, Inc., 1971

Instruction booklet, 7 picture cards, pad of 64 test forms, and plastic folder, $7.95

Time 15–20 minutes, administration; 2 minutes, scoring

John H. Saxman *Syracuse University*

Purpose The purpose of the Washington Speech Sound Discrimination Test is to provide a quick evaluation of speech–sound discrimination ability in children ranging from three years of age to kindergarten level. The authors state in the preface to the manual that it is not considered to be a sophisticated diagnostic instrument. They state further, however, that critical analysis of the test results can indicate the existence of a sound discrimination deficiency and delimit the type(s) of error(s) present. The test is suggested for use in assessing and programing for children with speech-sound discrimination problems. In addition to clinical uses, the authors suggest that the test has application as a research instrument.

Administration, scoring, and interpretation The test is composed of five subtests, each consisting of a key word and a variable number of foils designed to represent incorrect productions of the key word. The five key words, each depicted on picture cards, are cup, fish, sun, cracker, and toothbrush. Foils for subtests 1 (cup) and 2 (fish) were derived by changing one or two articulatory production features of one phoneme in the key word, in a manner based on Koenigsknecht and Lee (1968) procedures. The remaining three subtests use foils derived by changing the test phonemes /s/, /r/, /ð/ and /ө/ to commonly substituted phonemes based on substitution frequencies presented by Van Riper and Irwin (1958). All five subtests include foils derived by omitting one sound from the key word, e.g., kʌ for kʌp.

Administration of the WSSD Test is basically a three-step procedure. The first two steps are referred to as the preliminary teaching–testing procedure in which (1) receptive vocabulary for the five key words is tested and (2) the task involved in the main test is demonstrated and trained. Following successful demonstration that all five key words are in the subject's receptive vocabulary and that the subject understands and can perform the listening task, the test is administered.

The format for administration is as follows: The picture for the first subtest (cup) is placed on a table before the subject. The examiner then says: "Here is the cup. When I say cup, point to the cup. (Pause.) Cup." The subject responds, the correct response being a point to the picture, or several acceptable variations such as covering or touching the picture card and giving a verbal or gestured form of a yes-no response. The examiner continues: "Good. Now listen carefully. Point only when you hear cup. (Pause.) Cup." Several repetitions of the key word are given to reinforce the pointing response. Then the 15 items on the test form in subtest 1 are spoken. Each of the remaining subjects is presented in the same manner as described for the first. The subtests are administered sequentially. A reinforcement phrase "Good listening" is used throughout the test. The phrase is cued by an asterisk on the form next to test items on which it is to be used. The reinforcement schedule is a random distribution.

Correct responses (e.g., pointing, covering, etc., when the key word is said, *not* pointing when a foil is spoken) are indicated on the WSSD Test form by the symbol (+). Incorrect responses are indicated on the form by the symbol (−). An incorrect response would be pointing, etc., when a foil is spoken or *not* pointing when the key word is said by the examiner. The total right and the total wrong are computed for each subtest by summing the pluses and minuses. The score on the WSSD Test is the total correct for all subtests. The WSSD Test has a total of 53 items.

A scoring table is given on the test form that contains four age levels, 3.5, 4.0, 4.5, and kindergarten, with means and standard deviations of correct responses for each age. The means are 35, 40, 46, and 50 with associated standard deviations of 8, 7, 3, and 3, respectively. The examiner is instructed to ". . . locate the age level or levels which most closely approximate the score obtained and report the age level of func-tioning to the nearest half year." Scores below 27 (one standard deviation below the 3.5 year mean) are reported only as a raw score. The examiner is cautioned to recog-nize the large variability for the two younger age groups and to ". . . allow scores at these young ages to range substantially above and below the means."

Evaluation of test adequacy The WSSD Test has several positive features relative to other speech sound discrimination tests. The test uses only five words, each of which is pretested to ensure that it is within the receptive vocabulary of the subject. The picture cards, though small (approximately 2" x 3"), are easily recognized as repre-senting the objects depicted. The test form is simple and the scoring procedure is straightforward.

The test does not require a verbal response, a feature which is attractive for use with nonverbal children. In addition, the child is not required to make a same–different discrimination that seems to affect performances on some other sound discrimination tasks (Weiner 1967). Perhaps the strongest feature of the test is that provision is made for demonstration and training on the task involved in the test prior to test administration.

There are several limitations of the WSSD Test that require comment. A first limitation concerns the nature of the task itself. It is questionable whether the task assesses speech-sound discrimination. It is more likely that the task is an identification task in that no contrastive or discriminative response is required. Perhaps the test should be renamed the Washington Speech-Sound Identification Test.

Unfortunately, the details of test construction and the rationale underlying the selection of stimulus items are not easily available to the reader. The manual does not contain information of this nature, and the only references that might assist the reader in evaluating the rationale are unpublished manuscripts.

Major reservations about this test must be stated because neither the validity nor reliability of the instrument has been established. The origin of the WSSD Test was a 66-item test reported by Addicott and Sunderland (1969) in an unpublished master's thesis. The manual does not report sufficient information to assess construct validity. There is no indication of criterion-related validity. The only reliability information re-ported is intertester reliability (100 percent agreement) and a correlation coefficient of .9847 for the relationship between the original 66-item test and the 53-item WSSD

Test. Without either validity or reliability measures, questions concerning item selection criteria, basic test rationale, and the use of no response as a response become debatable.

One final serious limitation concerns the interpretation of the test scores from the scoring table. The standardization sample is extremely small for the 3.5, 4.0, and 4.5 age groups ($N = 20, 23,$ and 21, respectively). Considering the small N and the large variability, the Discrimination Age derived from the table has no credibility.

Summary   The test proposes an interesting approach to the problem of assessing speech sound recognition abilities in children. Unfortunately, publication of this test seems premature because the standardization norms are inadequate and there are no validity or reliability data available with which to evaluate the test. Its use cannot be recommended until appropriate standardization, validation, and reliability procedures are reported.

References

Addicott, M. A. and L. Sunderland   *Speech Sound Discrimination Skills of Preschool Children.* Master's Thesis, University of Washington, 1969.

Koenigsknecht, R. and L. Lee   Distinctive feature analysis of speech sound discrimination in three-year-old children. Paper presented at the American Speech and Hearing Association Convention, Denver, November, 1968.

Van Riper, C. and J. V. Irwin   *Voice and Articulation.* Englewood Cliffs, N.J.: Prentice-Hall, 1958.

Weiner, P. S.   Auditory discrimination and articulation. *J. Speech Hearing Dis.* **32**: 19–28, 1967.

Part IV
Appraisal of Aphasia

Introduction

Fourteen test instruments designed for the assessment of acquired language dysfunction are reviewed in the following section. These tests, some identified as tests of aphasia, others represented as tests of communicative functions, represent a fairly wide range of points of view concerning the dissolution of language and how it should be appraised.

To assess a patient's ability to process language, we must determine how efficiently the patient recognizes, retains, and comprehends various kinds of input—auditory, visual, gestural, tactile; how well he or she integrates and interprets this input and formulates a response to it; and how well he or she produces various types of output—oral, graphic, and gestural—both imitatively and spontaneously. The spectrum of possible stimuli and responses is huge with several possible levels of complexity to be represented; test responses are multifaceted requiring interpretation with regard to completeness, promptness, accuracy, and efficiency. Comprehensive evaluation of every conceivable type of language content and structure with every possible mode of input coupled with every possible mode of output would tax one's ingenuity and result in a test battery of impractical length. A sampling procedure is necessary. The tests here reviewed reflect varying opinions about how the sampling should be done, how the responses should be scored, how patterns of test responses should be interpreted, and what conclusions should be gleaned from the whole process.

Since theoretical and clinical interest in aphasia began to flourish about a hundred years ago, investigators have used a variety of techniques of their own creation or borrowings from their professional colleagues to answer questions that intrigued them about the disorder. Early in this century Pierre Marie insisted that patients be examined systematically with tests of increasing difficulty so that even mild language dysfunction could be detected. Probably Sir Henry Head (1926) was the first to introduce discipline into the area of aphasia assessment. In his two-volume *Aphasia and Kindred Disorders* he devoted a chapter to "Methods of Examination." He stated (Vol. 1, p. 145):

An inconstant response is one of the most striking results produced by a lesion of the cerebral cortex. . . . It is not a sufficient test to hold up some object, and ask the patient to name it; at one time he may be able to do so, at another he fails completely. No conclusion can be drawn from one or two questions put in this way; his power of responding must be tested by a series of observations in which the same task recurs on two or more occasions. . . . Not only is it necessary to arrange the tests in sequence, but each set must be placed before the patient in several different ways. . . . The order in which each single test follows another in the series remains the same throughout the various methods of examination; this alone makes it possible to draw any conclusion from the inconstant responses which are so disconcerting. . . . It is also important to graduate the severity of the task before concluding to what extent the patient can speak, read or write.

For purposes of studying 26 patients in detail, Head developed a battery of tests strongly suggestive of today's tests: tests for naming and recognition of common objects and colors; reading and writing simple phrases; clock setting; following oral and written instructions; using gestures in imitation and on command; repeating the alphabet, days, and months; reading and telling about a paragraph; telling and writing about a picture; performing arithmetic problems; naming and using coins; drawing; finding one's way around; and playing games.

In their "clinical and psychological study" of aphasia, Weisenburg and McBride (1935) emphasized the importance of standardized examination procedures. In practically the same breath they added (p. 132):

But, however great the effort for standardization, examinations for aphasia can never be routine procedures, for not only must particular tests be added to analyze specific disturbances, but the standard tests must sometimes be altered to throw more light on unusual difficulties.

They also cautioned (p. 133) that

tests must be arranged to differentiate between the quality of the comprehension and the quality of the response. In other words, studies of expression in speech or writing must be independent of the extent to which the patient has understood, and studies of comprehension must involve responses such as checking a word or drawing a line which are as little as possible influenced by the patient's expressive defects.

To accomplish their purposes Weisenburg and McBride used some of the same kinds of tests Head had designed (automatic word series; saying the alphabet; naming objects, colors, and pictures; repeating words, phrases, and sentences; writing to dictation); in addition they recorded the spontaneous speech and reactive responses of patients and also built into their procedure many existing standardized tests of achievement in reading, writing, spelling, and arithmetic. They administered these tests, largely designed for children, to groups of normal adults and developed norms against which to compare adult aphasic responses. For some patients testing time consumed 94 hours. An average of 19 hours was spent in testing each individual patient. In the appendix to their book they listed two "short batteries" for use with severe and "slighter" disorders, both requiring from two to three hours of administration time.

Over the years neurologists, psychologists, and speech–language pathologists involved in clinical assessment of aphasic patients have developed tests designed for their needs, most involving relatively brief samples of language behavior, mostly unstandardized, often without explicitly described procedures or scoring criteria, often based on no clear conceptualization of language and its disturbances. Some of these screening instruments were published and used in the United States including those of Chesher (1937), Wells and Ruesch (1945), and Halstead and Wepman (1949).

Such instruments did not suffice. As Schuell et al. wrote (1946, p. 60):

> While an examiner might have been satisfied with a simple screening test 20 or 30 years ago, concern has now passed to fine-grained description that will afford sufficient detail to make possible differential diagnosis, determination of prognosis, and evaluation of progress in therapy.

The purposes of aphasia testing today are summarized by Goodglass and Kaplan (1972, p. 1) thus:

> The examination for aphasia may be geared to any one of three general aims: (1) diagnosis of presence and type of aphasic syndrome, leading to inferences concerning cerebral localization; (2) measurement of the level of performance over a wide range, for both initial determination and detection of change over time; (3) comprehensive assessment of the assets and liabilities of the patient in all language areas as a guide to therapy.

The tests available to aphasiologists today approach these goals with different degrees of completeness and success. A scrutiny of the tests reveals that developments in the assessment of aphasia have moved in a positive direction in several respects:

1   Without reaching for the limits illustrated by Weisenburg and McBride, many test instruments represent an admirably comprehensive coverage of language processes, allowing ready identification of significant and even negligible deficits in many aspects of communicative behavior. For example, the Minnesota Test for Differential Diagnosis of Aphasia (MTDDA) is composed of 47 subtests for detailed testing in five major areas of possible disturbance. The Boston Diagnostic Aphasia Examination (BDAE) is comprised of 31 subtests and an evaluation of conversational speech, plus supplementary groups of 13 language and 14 nonlanguage tests. The reviews of the tests that follow indicate that most of the tests yield an estimate of the patient's ability to perform in all modalities—listening, reading, speaking, and writing. And many of the subtests comprising these tests contain a sufficient number of items to foster satisfactory test reliability.

2   These tests evidence progress in building objectivity and quantification into aphasia assessment. Several tests contain well detailed specifications concerning how they are to be administered, scored, and interpreted, and most provide for some degree of quantification of the results, building into the test construction the kind of orderliness and quantification which Kaplan (1959) had in mind in developing her "Descriptive Continuum of Language Responses in Aphasia," a quantification scheme which can be applied to any test results. For example, the MTDDA provides a clinical rating scale to quantify the patients's performance in each area. The Functional Communication Profile (FCP) yields ratings on a nine-point scale and a percentage score indicating a patient's general language ability. The Porch Index of Communicative Ability (PICA) represents the ultimate in quantification, each of a patients's 180 responses being rated on a 16-point multidimensional scale, yielding finally an overall test score as well as separate scores on verbal, gestural, and graphic subtests. The BDAE provides for a conversion of raw scores into

z-scores for intertest comparison and comparison of patients with a standardizing group. Several tests involve translation of results into profiles.

3 Some tests now provide some basis for prediction of a patient's recovery from aphasia. By following her patients through a course of therapy until dismissal from hospital, Schuell (1964) was able to show that placement in one of her five major groups of aphasic patients on the basis of initial testing with the MTDDA was a reasonable predictor of outcome. So she concluded (1965, p. 7), "The overall pattern of aphasic impairment is a better predictor than age, educational, or occupational level, extent of neurological involvement, or initial severity of aphasia." Predictions with the MTDDA are based upon administration of the test when the patient is neurologically stable, at approximately three months post onset. Porch has shown that the PICA administered at one month post onset predicts test score at six months post onset, using either of two prediction methods. It has been shown that higher intake scores on the FCP predict higher outcome scores and that prognosis for recovery is more guarded as intake scores decrease on this measure.

Regrettably, the various tests here reviewed have not moved as far as we might hope in demonstration of various types of validity. The tests vary widely with regard to content validity, sampling as they do in quite different ways the universe of language behaviors that aphasia involves. The record is somewhat better with regard to construct validity, but no test during its construction and standardization was subjected to an adequate test of its concurrent validity. Except for the Functional Communication Profile, which "attempted to quantify the communication behaviors which a patient actually uses in the course of interaction with others" (Sarno, p. 1), test makers have not dealt with the matter of how test scores relate to one's functional communication in real-life situations. Only lately has work begun to clarify this relationship. Holland (1977), supported by a grant from the National Institute for Neurological and Communicative Disorders and Stroke, has developed a measure of functional communication adequacy entitled Communication Assessment for Daily Living (CADL) and has begun to use it in study of the concurrent validity of the FCP, BDAE, and the PICA. Preliminary data indicate that correlations are high, patients tending to perform similarly on the various measures.

Another curious failure in aphasia test development relates to the general absence of built-in ways of distinguishing aphasic patients from patients with language disorders that might be confused with aphasia. Although the title of the MTDDA suggests that this instrument might have been designed for the purpose, the only groups other than aphasic patients to whom the test was administered during the standardization process were normal subjects. The term "differential" in this case refers to the placement of patients within five different subgroups of aphasia characterized by different overall patterns of performance and different prognoses of recovery. The PICA yields profiles which are suggestive of two nonaphasic syndromes—namely, apraxia of speech (Wertz and Rosenbek 1971) and "bilateral involvement" (Johnson and Porch 1968; Porch 1971). It has also demonstrated accurate differentiation between persons "simulating" aphasia or malingering and real aphasic patients (Porch and Porec 1977; Porec and Porch 1977). Test makers have not demonstrated that aphasia can be differentiated from syndromes of confusion, dementia, or psychosis through the use of their tests. Using an adaptation of the MTDDA, Halpern, Darley, and Brown (1973) delineated the patterns of language performance characteristic of patients diagnosed as aphasic, apraxic in speech, confused, and demented, and DiSimoni, Darley, and Aronson (1977) used a similar test battery to derive a profile of language performance of chronic schizophrenic patients. It is to be hoped that future test development will provide instruments which with increasing precision can differentiate language-impaired patients whose performance may superficially resemble that of aphasic patients but in whom the neurologic or psychiatric basis for the disorder is importantly different.

Frederic L. Darley

References

Chesher, E. C. Technique for clinical examination in aphasia. *Bulletin of the Neurological Institute of New York* 6: 134–144, 1937.

DiSimoni, F. G., F. L. Darley, and A. E. Aronson Patterns of dysfunction in schizophrenic patients on an aphasia test battery. *J. Speech Hearing Dis.* 42: 498–513, 1977.

Goodglass, H. and E. Kaplan *The Assessment of Aphasia and Related Disorders.* Philadelphia: Lea and Febiger, 1972.

Halpern, H., F. L. Darley, and J. R. Brown Differential language and neurologic characteristics in cerebral involvement. *J. Speech Hearing Dis.* 38: 162–173, 1973.

Halstead, W. C. and J. M. Wepman The Halstead–Wepman aphasia screening test. *J. Speech Hearing Dis.* 14: 9–15, 1949.

Head, H. *Aphasia and Kindred Disorders.* New York: Macmillan, 1926. Reprinted by Hofner, New York, 1963.

Holland, A. L. Developing a measure of functional communication adequacy: communication assessment for daily living. Project Report for the National Institute for Neurological and Communicative Disorders and Stroke, 1977.

Johnson, M. G. and B. E. Porch The differential effects of unilateral versus bilateral cerebral lesions on performances involving comparable visual and auditory tasks. Paper presented at the Annual Convention of the American Speech and Hearing Association, Chicago, 1968.

Kaplan, L. T. A descriptive continuum of language responses in aphasia. *J. Speech Hearing Dis.* 24: 410–412, 1959.

Porch, B. E. A comparison of unilateral and bilateral PICA profiles on brain-damaged adults. Paper presented at the Annual Convention of the American Speech and Hearing Association, Chicago, 1971.

——— and J. P. Porec Medical-legal applications of PICA results. In R. H. Brookshire (ed.), *1977 Clinical Aphasiology Conference Proceedings.* Minneapolis: BRK Publishers, 1977, pp. 302–309.

Porec, J. P. and B. E. Porch The behavioral characteristics of "simulated" aphasia. In R. H. Brookshire (ed.), *1977 Clinical Aphasiology Conference Proceedings.* Minneapolis: BRK Publishers, 1977, pp. 299–301.

Sarno, M. T. *The Functional Communication Profile: Manual of Directions.* New York: New York University Medical Center Institute of Rehabilitation Medicine, 1969.

Schuell, H. *Differential Diagnosis of Aphasia with the Minnesota Test.* Minneapolis: University of Minnesota Press, 1965.

———, J. J. Jenkins, and E. Jiménez-Pabón *Aphasia in Adults: Diagnosis, Prognosis, and Treatment.* New York: Hoeber, 1964.

Weisenburg, T. and K. E. McBride *Aphasia: A Clinical and Psychological Study.* New York: Commonwealth Fund, 1935.

Wells, F. L. and J. Ruesch In *Mental Examiners Handbook* (2nd ed.). New York: Psychological Corporation, 1945, pp. 48–50.

Wertz, R. T. and J. C. Rosenbek Appraising apraxia of speech. *J. Colo. Speech Hearing Assn.* 5: 18–36, 1971.

APHASIA LANGUAGE PERFORMANCE SCALES (ALPS)

Joseph S. Keenan and Esther G. Brassell

Pinnacle Press, 1975

Cost $23.10

Manual, 110 pages; reading scale cards; score sheet, 2 pages; cumulative record, 1 page

Time 20–30 minutes, administration; 10–15 minutes, scoring

E. Gene Ritter *Indiana University*

Purpose Believing that all tests of aphasia available in 1970 had objectionable features, the authors of the Aphasia Language Performance Scales wished to design an instrument that (1) would require a minimum of time to administer and analyze, (2) could be used in any physical setting and without "considerable paraphernalia," (3) would provide the clinician helpful information for planning therapy, and (4) would not be so formal as to "break down . . . rapport." They also wanted their scales to measure the language performance of all aphasic patients regardless of type of aphasia or severity of the language deficit.

Administration, scoring, and interpretation The patient may earn a maximum of 10 points in each of the four scales—Listening, Talking, Reading, and Writing, which are given in that order. The examiner assigns one point for each patient response that might be expected of a normal subject. Self-corrections are given full credit. Each examiner is expected to determine what constitutes an error or a reasonable response delay that would necessitate the use of a prompt. If after the prompt the patient responds well, the examiner awards one-half a point.

In the Talking Scale there are only eight test items, but the patient may still earn the maximum of 10 points. If the patient names more than the required minimum number of items or repeats more than the minimum number of phrases, bonus points are awarded.

In each scale items are given in order of increasing difficulty. Not all the easier items need be given since the examiner, in pretest conversation with the patient, determines the appropriate beginning level for each scale. Testing in each scale is terminated when the patient has reached his or her ceiling, usually defined as two consecutive failures following prompts.

To administer the scales, in addition to the manual one needs an ALPS score sheet, the ring-bound reading scale cards, a stopwatch, some coins and keys, a tablet, a pencil, and a pen. The ALPS can usually be administered in 20 to 30 minutes and requires an additional 10 to 15 minutes to score and analyze the responses. Although administration of the ALPS does not require a "technical expert," the authors insist that the scales do require a "clinician" for proper presentation and scoring. They state in the test manual (p. 32) that a clinician is one who will focus on the patient's behavior rather than upon the test and will

> stand alone and declare what he thinks and what he proposes. He cannot stop with the test results, but must add his own considered judgment. We believe that clinical work demands this personalized approach, with a risk of error and a potential for excellence.

The authors have arbitrarily related scores from each of the scales to degrees of language impairment. They provide the following guide: profound, 0 to 1.0; severe, 1.5 to 3.0; moderate–severe, 3.5 to 5.0; mild–moderate, 5.5 to 7.0; mild, 7.5 to 9.0; and insignificant, 9.5 to 10.0.

Evaluation of test adequacy   The ALPS underwent nine revisions, some of which lasted only as long as 11 days and others surviving 18 months. The present form, in use since October 1972, was published in 1975.

In the ALPS manual the authors mention several prepublication studies related to the reliability and validity of the Scales. Although the information is far from overwhelming, the results are generally adequate. One study indicated that in the hands of an experienced ALPS examiner, the scales had satisfactory test–retest reliability over a three-to-five-week period with 22 aphasic patients. The authors, in studying the extent to which the scales are truly arranged in order of increasing difficulty, reported data within the .005 confidence level when using the Richardson–Kuder Formula 20 for internal reliability (p. 22).

Two studies are reported in which overall and modality mean scores of aphasic patients on the Porch Index of Communicative Ability (PICA) were compared with ALPS modality results. A study by Flugrath and Zyski used 12 aphasic patients while another by Basili and Diener studied 50 patients (Basili et al. 1974). In both studies high correlations were found indicating that, in general, the ALPS and the PICA both did well in measuring the language usage of aphasic patients. Ability to equate the two tests for excellence, however, is not implied. In any sampling of language behavior, the clinician obtains just that—a sample. When the sample is too long and exhaustive, the patient's true ability is masked by fatigue and analysis is too time consuming to be considered practical. However, when the sample is too brief, its value is compromised in that not enough information is available to help the clinician discern the patient's language problem or to provide help in planning therapy. The ALPS tends to be too brief for a comprehensive view of the patient's language ability.

Summary   The ALPS is a good screening instrument. It can be administered with a fair degree of informality although the authors provide specific statements which must be "spoken verbatim to the patient" (p. 36). Thus the authors have succeeded in designing an instrument to meet half of their objections to other tests of aphasia. Instead of having an instrument that can be given in "any" location, Keenan and Brassell concede that the scales should be administered in a quiet room and that the clinician and patient should face each other over the corner of a table where test objects may be placed. In reference to the original four goals, the most important deficit relates to the provision of helpful information for planning therapy. In this respect, the ALPS does no better than most other tests of aphasia and less well than the Minnesota Test for Differential Diagnosis of Aphasia (qv) and the Porch Index of Communicative Ability (qv).

Reference

Basili, A. G., S. Diener, J. M. Flugrath, G. H. Horsfall, and B. J. Zyski   Comparisons between the Aphasia Language Performance Scales and two established tests of aphasic impairment. Paper presented at annual convention, American Speech and Hearing Association, Las Vegas, November 7, 1974. Abstract: *Asha* 16: 552, 1974.

APPRAISAL OF LANGUAGE DISTURBANCE (ALD)

Lon Emerick

Northern Michigan University Press, 1971

Cost $27.00

Manual, 8 pages; test booklet, 6 pages

Time One to two hours administration and scoring

Audrey L. Holland   *University of Pittsburgh*

Purpose   The purpose of the Appraisal of Language Disturbance, according to its author, is "to provide a systematic approach for the evaluation of linguistic impairment in adult aphasic patients." It permits the clinician "to perform a comprehensive inventory of the patient's communicative abilities with respect to the various modalities of input and output and central integrating processes."

Administration, scoring, and interpretation   The test, which is reported to take from one to two hours to administer, is given individually to aphasic patients. The testing kit contains stimulus cards for visual and reading assessment, color shapes for testing visual agnosia and for sorting and arranging tasks, and a hand puzzle for an object assembly task. All auditory comprehension and speech items are presented in the test protocol booklet, which includes instructions for each of the 51 hierarchically arranged subtests designed to explore the following aspects of language: (1) auditory stimuli for spoken, matching, gestural, and written responses; (2) gestural stimuli for matching to pictures and objects; (3) visual stimuli for gestural responses; (4) visual stimuli for oral and written responding; (5) some aspects of "central language comprehension" involving matching, assembling, sorting, categorizing, and manding; and (6) some aspects of abilities "peripheral to symbolic language" (sic) including tactile recognition, arithmetic ability, and motility of the oral mechanism. In addition, the tester is also required to administer the Peabody Picture Vocabulary Test.

The tester is instructed to record the accuracy of each response as well as the manner of each error, although no provisions are made in the test booklet for such systematic recording. Test scores are then to be recorded on a summary form in the booklet that requires translation of each major modality subsection's correct raw score into a five-point rating scale. This rating scale uses "1" to indicate "all or almost all responses correct," and so on to 5, "all or almost all responses incorrect." Results scaled in this manner are said to produce a profile of each aphasic patient's particular language deficit in terms of the input and output factors previously mentioned.

Evaluation of test adequacy   Potential ALD items were initially assigned to the various subcategories of the test, as well as arrayed on a continuum of "simple-to-difficult," by normal adult speakers. The items were then presented to a second set of normal language users to ferret out confusing items and further refine the hierarchical placement within subtests. No data resulting from these procedures are presented in the manual.

Test–retest reliability was computed using 39 neurologically stable aphasic patients, with a resulting *r* of .81. Interrater reliability was estimated at .86 for the 39 patients each tested by two clinicians. Time interval between tests was not specified.

No measures of construct, content, or criterion-related validity were obtained for the ALD.

In view of the somewhat unimpressive stability data and the frank lack of validity data, the ALD has substantial limitations in terms of its usefulness with aphasic adults. The conceptual model (Wepman) on which the test is based is solid enough. However, if or how this test relates to the Wepman model has not been experimentally examined, nor have many of its basic assumptions. For example, no data are presented to substantiate that subtest items are representative of equal-appearing intervals or that they even represent values of a single stimulus dimension. Also unexamined is the assumption that each subtest represents an equally important aspect of the language act, even though all contribute equally to the development of an individual's profile. This assumption is particularly problematical since the items leading to entries on this form vary in number from 1 to 30.

Throughout the manual and test booklet definitions are fuzzy. For example, transforming the numerical data to the rating scale depends on the tester's own decision as to what values constitute "almost all correct," etc. The instructions are also inexact. For example, some items require multiple responses (as in saying the letters of the alphabet) and no indication is given the tester as to what constitutes "passing" such items.

ALD does present some fresh areas for consideration in inventorying aphasic language performance. For example, one subtest requests the patient to identify errors in verbally presented material; another requests the patient to furnish antonyms for a set of stimulus words. Such tasks represent provocative leads for further study or rehabilitation tasks. Unfortunately the author himself has not followed these leads and provided normative data.

Summary   The ALD is long and probably somewhat arduous to take. These problems, as well as its lack of substantiating data, make it of questionable value to the aphasia tester for the traditional uses of description and prognosis.

BOSTON DIAGNOSTIC APHASIA EXAMINATION (BDAE)

Harold Goodglass and Edith Kaplan

Lea and Febiger, 1972

Cost $11.50

Manual, 80 pages (in book entitled *The Assessment of Aphasia and Related Disorders*); test stimulus cards; examination booklet, 32 pages

Time One to four hours, administration; 30 minutes, scoring

Joseph R. Duffy *University of Massachusetts*

Purpose The authors state in the manual (p. 1) that the Boston Diagnostic Aphasia Examination was designed to meet three general aims: "(1) diagnosis of presence and type of aphasic syndrome, leading to inferences concerning cerebral localization; (2) measurement of the level of performance over a wide range, for both initial determination and detection of change over time; (3) comprehensive assessment of the assets and liabilities of the patient in all areas as a guide to therapy."

Administration, scoring, and interpretation The test is organized into five major sections. The first, Conversational and Expository Speech (nine items), assesses speech responses during conversation and a free narrative response. Scoring involves the rating of six speech characteristics (melodic line, phrase length, articulatory agility, grammatical form, paraphasia, and word finding) on a seven-point, equal-interval scale and assignment of a severity rating on a six-point scale of oral communication. The profiles derived from these scales are crucial to diagnosis of the "type" of aphasia. The severity rating and some of the speech characteristic ratings are plotted on a z-score profile, which is also used in classifying patients.

The Auditory Comprehension section (four subtests) requires simple pointing, yes–no responses, or the carrying out of commands in response to verbal stimuli of varying length and complexity. Some subtests are organized so that responses to different semantic word categories, body parts, and right–left discrimination can be examined separately. Scoring is largely plus–minus, although points awarded on some subtests vary according to response latency and the amount of information required to elicit an accurate response.

The Oral Expression section (11 subtests) includes measures of verbal and nonverbal diadochokinesis; automatic overlearned sequences; manual rhythm repetition; repetition of words and phrases; word and sentence reading; naming to picture, body part, and verbal stimuli; and a word fluency test. Scoring is primarily plus–minus, although point awards may vary according to speed of repetition, latency, number of responses, or articulatory adequacy. A tally of the number and type of articulatory and paraphasic errors is also kept, with the pattern of paraphasic breakdown contributing importantly to the determination of diagnostic classification.

The Understanding Written Language section of the test (four subtests) requires pointing responses on tasks involving visual matching of words and letters across different writing styles, and identification of written words to verbal stimuli. Abilities to identify spelled words orally, comprehend written words by picture-pointing, and complete (comprehend) written sentences and short paragraphs by selecting appropriate written choices are also assessed. All scoring is plus–minus.

The last section of the test, Writing (four subtests), examines the motor aspects of writing, the ability to recall isolated written letter and number symbols, the ability to write dictated words and sentences, and the ability to write the names of pictured objects and a narrative about a pictured situation. Rating scales and plus–minus scoring are used to score responses.

Interpretation of test results is based upon analysis of the severity rating scale, the rating scale profile of speech characteristics, and the pattern of performance across subtests and modalities after raw scores have been converted to z-scores. (The z-score profile makes subtests comparable and shows the patient's pattern of breakdown relative to the large sample of patients on whom the test was standardized.) Test interpretation is primarily geared toward placing patients into diagnostic categories based on the "classical" anatomical typologies of aphasia. The major dichotomy between fluent (posterior lesion) and nonfluent (anterior lesion) aphasia is based on the profile exhibited on the speech characteristics rating scale, while finer distinctions among the fluent aphasias are based on the z-score profile as well as the profile of speech characteristics. The test manual coherently discusses the presumed anatomical substrate and psychological nature of the communicative breakdown; it illustrates and discusses the test profiles characteristic of Broca's, Wernicke's, anomic, and conduction aphasia, transcortical sensory and transcortical motor aphasia, and alexia with agraphia. Also discussed are several so-called pure aphasias and callosal disconnection syndromes, but their associated profiles are not specifically described.

Several supplementary language and nonlanguage tests are also presented in the test manual. They include subtests that explore psycholinguistic factors in auditory comprehension and verbal expression, repetition disorders, tests for disconnection syndromes, a "parietal lobe" battery, and tests for nonverbal apraxia. With the exception of the parietal lobe battery, these supplementary tests lack statistical norms. While they increase the comprehensiveness of the test and are certainly of interest to speech–language pathologists, they will not be further evaluated because they are not part of the standardized aphasia battery.

Evaluation of test adequacy Standardization was conducted on an acceptably large sample of 207 patients. The z-score conversions for the various test measures are based on data from varying numbers of these patients. It is important for the test user to realize that the standardization sample was chosen to include a greater proportion of patients with relatively isolated symptoms and small lesions than would have been the case if all available patients had been selected. This biased sampling can be justified from the standpoint that it was suited to illustrating differences among patients for the purpose of highlighting the localization and different underlying psychological components of aphasia. However, the clinical speech–language pathologist is cautioned that the characteristics of the standardization sample may not accurately reflect the characteristics of the aphasic population found in most clinical settings in which severe aphasia and large lesions occur with relatively great frequency. The development of local norms may be necessary to adjust for these differences in severity and selectivity of impairment if z-scores are to be considered valid.

The degree of reliability of the BDAE varies according to the criteria used. The authors present data which indicate good internal consistency for all test measures containing a series of scorable items. Interjudge reliability coefficients for the rating scale of speech characteristics based on ratings of 99 patients are, on the average, acceptable, although two of the six scales showed relatively low reliability ($r = .78$ and .79). While not presented in the test manual, good interjudge reliability for the severity rating scale, the rating scales of speech characteristics, and assignments to some of the aphasia classifications has been demonstrated elsewhere (Goodglass, Quadfasel, and Timberlake 1964). Unfortunately, interjudge reliability for the remainder of the test is not reported, although the demonstrated acceptable reliability of some of the more difficult-to-score portions of the test suggests that other portions may also be reliable. On the other hand, intra- and interjudge reliability may be somewhat compromised by a lack of clear, specific directions for administration and scoring on some subtests.

As a test of language ability, the BDAE is valid in the sense that it requires language performance on verbal and written comprehension and expression measures at different levels of complexity without excessive contamination by irrelevant modalities, education, intelligence, or experience. It may have greater content validity, in terms of completeness, than other aphasia tests because of its unique inclusion of measures of the qualitative characteristics of speech, which the authors defend as being among the most prominent features of aphasic speech.

The test was not designed to have predictive validity as a measure of prognosis for language recovery, and no prognostic capabilities are claimed for it. To the extent that results may yield profiles which roughly correspond to various classical forms of aphasia, the test can be said to "predict" type of aphasia, at least for the type of patient in the standardization sample. The test's capacity for determining site of lesion (anterior vs. posterior) has received indirect support from several studies that have compared localization data with performance on scales similar or identical to the test's rating scales of speech characteristics (Goodglass, Quadfasel, and Timberlake 1964; Kerschensteiner, Poeck, and Brunner 1972; Benson 1967). However, with the exception of a small number of case illustrations, the test manual presents no localization data for its standardization sample and no information about the accuracy of or confidence which may be placed in predictions regarding locus of lesion. This is a significant shortcoming for a test designed to allow inferences about localization.

The test monograph contains correlational data and results from factor analysis that support the validity of the belief that breakdowns in different psychological components underlying language are associated with different behavioral syndromes. The authors indicate, for example, that the five principal factors (reading and writing, spatial-quantitative-somatognosic, fluency, auditory comprehension, and paraphasia) derived from factor analysis of test results are sufficient to separate all of the major aphasic syndromes, with the possible exception of anomic aphasia. Whether the test's differentiation among various types of aphasia should be considered as due to differences in language impairment, severity, or the presence or absence of associated but nonaphasic deficits, remains an unresolved matter of debate. (Darley [1977], for example, has suggested that the difference between fluent and nonfluent aphasia is a reflection of the presence or absence of apraxia of speech in association with aphasia.) However, the existence of this debate (which raises questions about the construct validity of any aphasia test that classifies patients) does not compromise the validity of the BDAE as a measure of different forms of breakdown in the communication process.

Several clinical strengths can be ascribed to the BDAE. First, its more than 270 items rank it among the most comprehensive of aphasia batteries. It may also contain the most systematic sampling of various input and output modality combinations of any standardized aphasia test (Brookshire 1973). Second, the ability to convert raw scores to z-scores allows the clinician validly to determine the patient's relative strengths and weaknesses and chart changes in these profiles in objective fashion. Third, the unique inclusion of the rating scale of speech characteristics provides the clinician with a useful tool for describing the primary features of speech output. This rating scale is also among the test's measures used to identify patients most likely to benefit from melodic intonation therapy (Sparks, Helm, and Albert 1974). Finally, because it highlights differences among patients and allows inferences about localization, neurologists may take a special interest in test results. The skillful speech–language pathologist may use it as a tool for bridging the gap between the gross evaluative subjectivity used by many physicians who employ classical terminology and the clinician's possible desire to employ a classification system that utilizes the same terms but with objective, descriptive, operational definitions.

The test also has several weaknesses that may negate its usefulness in some clinical settings. Some of these weaknesses are related to the test's purposes and design and may even be an outgrowth of the strengths listed above. First, the amount of useful information provided by the test may not warrant the amount of time required to obtain it. An accurate diagnosis of aphasia, acquisition of sufficient baseline data, and treatment planning can, in most instances, be obtained in less than the four hours it may take to give the BDAE. Second, the test offers no prognostic information, a serious limitation for any clinician desiring objective data for counseling and decisions about treatment. Third, the test does not directly generate any information about the planning of treatment programs, a clinical limitation not unique to the BDAE. Finally, clinicians in settings in which severe aphasia and large lesions occur with high frequency may find the test norms to be inappropriate or of limited usefulness.

Summary   The BDAE is a comprehensive test instrument that deserves special praise for operationally defining and standardizing the diagnosis of previously loosely defined and assessed classical, anatomical forms of aphasia. The test's clinical strong points include comprehensiveness, use of standardized data, the ability to distinguish among different patterns of performance, its unique inclusion of scales for measuring qualitative aspects of speech output, and its possible appeal to neurologists. Its clinical weaknesses include lengthy administration time, lack of prognostic and treatment planning information, and possible limited usefulness of its norms in settings where severe aphasia is frequently encountered. Clinical questions which remain unanswered about the test relate to the current lack of information on test–retest and interjudge reliability for all parts of the test, and the absence of information on the accuracy of inferences that may be drawn about locus of lesion.

While the BDAE has been listed as one of the most worthy aphasia tests to be developed in the past 25 years (Darley 1977), decisions regarding its use must be based on the clinician's beliefs about aphasia and his or her purposes in testing. The BDAE is recommended for use by clinicians with an interest in classical orientations to aphasia who wish to discover differences (and their possible explanations) in performance within and between patients, and who wish to speculate about the localization of lesions. Those clinicians who are more interested in aphasia as a unidimensional disorder and whose purpose for testing is to evaluate severity of communicative impairment, make prognostic statements, and plan treatment programs, may find other tests (Porch Index of Communicative Ability (qv), Minnesota Test for Differential Diagnosis of Aphasia (qv)) better suited to their needs.

References

Benson, D. F.   Fluency in aphasia: correlation with radioactive scan localization. *Cortex* 3: 373–394, 1967.

Brookshire, R. H.   *An Introduction to Aphasia.* Minneapolis: BRK Publishers, 1973.

Darley, F. L.   A retrospective view: aphasia. *J. Speech and Hearing Dis.* 42: 161–169, 1977.

Goodglass, H., F. A. Quadfasel, and W. H. Timberlake   Phrase length and the type and severity of aphasia. *Cortex* 1: 133–153, 1964.

Kerschensteiner, M., K. Poeck, and E. Brunner   The fluency–nonfluency dimension in the classification of aphasic speech. *Cortex* 8: 233–247, 1972.

Sparks, R., N. Helm, and M. Albert   Aphasia rehabilitation resulting from melodic intonation therapy. *Cortex* 10: 303–316, 1974.

EXAMINING FOR APHASIA

Jon Eisenson

The Psychological Corporation, (rev. ed.) 1954

Cost $9.00 (Manual and 25 record forms)
Manual, 73 pages; record form, 12 pages

Time 30 minutes to two hours, administration and scoring

Gerald J. Canter *Northwestern University*

Purpose Examining for Aphasia, one of the first commercially available aphasia test batteries, was designed to provide the clinician with a guided approach for evaluating aphasic language disturbances. Although the author indicated that the easier test materials can be used in assessing "congenitally aphasic" children, we will focus here on the use of the test with the population for which it was primarily intended—adult aphasic patients. In the manual, Eisenson states that results of the examination "enable the clinician to obtain an overall view of the patient's strengths and weaknesses" as well as determine the "level of ability within a given area of language function." Changes in test performance are taken as indicators of improvement and are considered of value in planning therapy.

Administration, scoring, and interpretation The test is dichotomized into primarily receptive and primarily expressive portions. Within each of these sections, a further division is made between subtests designed to test subsymbolic or low symbolic levels (agnosias, apraxias, automaticities, etc.) and those tapping higher symbolic levels (aphasias). This organization provided a model which was followed, with modifications, by many later constructors of aphasia tests.

Test administration is extremely flexible. The examiner is given the choice of administering either the receptive or the expressive portion first; the examiner may also choose to administer all the low-level tests (receptive and expressive) before the higher-level tests. More importantly, a variety of stimulus presentations are acceptable. For example, on the very first subtest, which is intended to reveal visual agnosia for common objects, the patient is instructed to do one of the following: name the object, point to the object named by the examiner, select the correct name from the choices given by the examiner, or demonstrate the use of the object. Success in utilizing any of these response modes would indicate that common object recognition through vision is intact. Failure in certain response modes but not in others would indicate a non-agnosic problem. Scoring of items is on a pass/fail basis, and the examiner is instructed to indicate the nature of the response on the record form.

Evaluation of test adequacy Examining for Aphasia is not a standardized test. The author states: "Aphasic patients are characteristically too inconsistent in their responses to permit formal scoring standards to be developed meaningfully." In addition to a lack of quantitative scoring, no information is provided to indicate how well normal individuals might perform, although the author points out that some of the subtests—particularly those involving reading and writing—cover a wide range of mental ability and educational experience. Meaningful interpretation of a patient's performance thus requires considerable clinical judgment with respect to degree of impairment. Similarly, the interpretation of patterns of impairment demands clinical judgment and is in no way "automatized" by the organization of the test results on the record form.

It is evident that Eisenson's test does not provide the clinician with any ready-made interpretation as to degree of impairment, clinical type of aphasia, or prognosis. The absence of standardization data further limits the clinician in using this instrument as a measure of progress, since we have no information on the temporal stability of aphasic patients' performance on the test. (The author's statement, cited above, that aphasic patients are too inconsistent to allow for standardized scoring has been amply shown to be incorrect by the successful standardization of several aphasia tests since the publication of Examining for Aphasia.)

Summary   Despite the total lack of psychometric merit, these test materials have a place in the diagnostic armamentarium of the clinical aphasiologist. The stimulus materials themselves (pictures, colors, printed words and letters, etc., which are included in the spiral-bound manual) are excellently printed and are superior to parallel materials included in some other tests—materials that sometimes appear to provide undesirable difficulties of visual perception that may confound the results. In the hands of an experienced examiner, these materials can provide the basis for a thorough, systematic assessment of the aphasic patient. But it must be emphasized that without intelligent test administration and sound clinical judgment based on experience with aphasic patients, Examining for Aphasia will not provide diagnostic information as useful as the more recent standardized tests do. Some clinicians may not be satisfied with those tests because they consider that a highly structured procedure is not appropriate or sufficient to explore the extraordinarily diverse speech and language alterations that occur in the aphasic population. For them, a set of materials such as those provided in Examining for Aphasia can be used flexibly as they seek to understand the nature of aphasic patients' problems.

FUNCTIONAL COMMUNICATION PROFILE (FCP)

Martha T. Sarno

Institute of Rehabilitation Medicine, New York University Medical Center, 1969

Cost $5.00

Manual, 32 pages, $4.00; conversion chart, 1 page; form sheet, 1 page; pack of 25 form sheets and 2 copies of conversion chart, $1.00

Time 10–20 minutes, administration; 2 minutes, scoring

Linda Swisher *University of Arizona*

Purpose The Functional Communication Profile (FCP) was designed to describe the language performance of an aphasic patient in an informal setting (Taylor 1965). The manual states that it is an attempt to "quantify the communication behaviors which a patient actually uses in the course of interaction with others." Unlike the " 'clinical performance' elicited in formal language tests that often sample artificial behaviors," it measures "functional performance . . . the unforced, voluntary, and habitual utterances which characterize normal spoken language" (Sarno 1969, pp. 1–2).

Administration, scoring, and interpretation Forty-five specific communication behaviors are rated on a nine-point scale after conversation between an experienced speech–language pathologist and a patient. These communication behaviors are divided into five categories: movement, speaking, understanding, reading, and a miscellaneous category that includes writing and calculation. After summing the ratings in each category, the examiner uses a conversion chart to derive a weighted score and ultimately an overall percentage score indicating the patient's effectiveness in everyday communication. The interview takes between 10 and 20 minutes, with two minutes for scoring.

In addition to being a nontask-oriented procedure, the FCP differs from the usual aphasia test in that "normal" on the rating scale refers to the clinician's judgment of the patient's premorbid abilities. No normative data are considered appropriate. For example, an overall score of 50 indicates that the patient was judged to be functioning with 50 percent of estimated premorbid proficiency. The patient's age, educational level, and employment are all considered by the clinician in arriving at an estimation of premorbid level.

The clinician also takes into account the patient's compensatory behavior. For example, lacking useful oral production, the patient may indicate the numbers of the hospital floor to the elevator operator by holding up the appropriate number of fingers. While this was not normal behavior premorbidly, the patient might be rated fair to good on this item because of an ability to compensate for verbal impairment. Other nonlinguistic variables such as speed, accuracy, and consistency of performance are considered in arriving at ratings. For example, a patient may be accurate in all behaviors but may perform so slowly that a normal rating cannot be assigned.

By way of illustration, the Understanding category is reproduced in Fig. 1. The behaviors to be rated represent a continuum of increasing difficulty, with a range from "awareness of gross environmental sounds" to "understanding of rapid complex conversation." A guide to the meaning of normal, good, fair, and poor judgments on the rating scale is: all normal, 100 percent; all good, 75 percent; all fair, 50 percent; and all poor, 25 percent. For example, if a patient responds affirmatively to the calling of his or her name, a rating of normal or 100 percent on the item "Understanding of own name" might be assigned. If, on the other hand, the patient was asked during the interview to "Pick up the pen and give it to me" and picked up the pen but did not carry out the complete instruction, the patient might be rated fair, or 50 percent, for "Understanding verbal instructions."

	Normal		Good		Fair		Poor		0	
									Awareness of gross environmental sounds
									Awareness of emotional voice tone
									Understanding of own name
									Awareness of speech
									Recognition of family names
									Recognition of names of familiar objects
									Understanding action verbs
									Understanding gestured directions
									Understanding verbal directions
									Understanding simple conversation with one person
									Understanding television
									Understanding conversation with more than two people
									Understanding movies
									Understanding complicated verbal directions
									Understanding rapid complex conversation

(Left margin label: Understanding)

Fig. 1 Understanding section of the Functional Communication Profile.

Evaluation of test adequacy Studies reported in the manual indicate high interrater and intrarater reliability of both overall and individual category FCP scores, ranging from .87 to .95. Similarly high interrater reliability and test–retest reliability have been reported by Anderson, Boureston, and Greenberg (1971).

With regard to validity, Anderson, Boureston, and Greenberg (1971) found a systematic relationship between performance by aphasic patients on the FCP and the Minnesota Test for Differential Diagnosis of Aphasia (qv). They indicated that the FCP is useful because it is reliable and brief and results can be explained in nontechnical language. Further, the possible effects of learning resulting from repeated use of more formal tests are minimized.

Needham and Swisher (1972) reported that the FCP Understanding category covers a wider range of difficulty than the Token Test for adults with aphasia. The latter was found to be quite difficult for many patients. An unexpected finding was that Understanding ratings on the FCP appear to be lowered by the presence of verbal apraxia or dysarthria in patients. As in previous studies (e.g., Anderson, Boureston, and Greenberg 1971) a relationship was found between performance on supposedly nontask-oriented items (FCP) and task-oriented scores (Token Test; in-house Aphasia test) when patients with obvious expressive speech problems were excluded.

Overall FCP scores have been found to correlate significantly with measures of functional communication in the home (Holland 1978). The FCP has demonstrated value as a predicter of recovery from aphasia. Sands, Sarno, and Shankweiler (1969) reported that a higher overall FCP intake (premanagement) score predicts a higher outcome score and that prognosis for recovery must be more guarded as intake scores decrease.

The manual expressly states that the FCP is "not intended as a single measure of language performance . . . nor as a substitute for comprehensive and systematic linguistic analysis of aphasic behavior." It "is not concerned with the etiology, pathology, or reasons for a patient's impairment . . . . It is hypothetically possible that an individual in an acute depression might achieve a low FCP speaking score if he produces little speech" (pp. 1, 15). The FCP Profile likewise "does not suggest a rationale or directions for treatment" but is primarily "of descriptive value, that is, the ratings suggest patterns of verbal behavior for the individual patient" (p. 2).

Summary The FCP can be rapidly administered and the results are easily understood by persons without a background in speech–language pathology. FCP scores correlate highly with measures of aphasia that require much more time to obtain, including measures of functional communication in the home. Little information for planning intervention is provided by this measure. No other evaluation tool permits as rapid an overall assessment of a patient's general pattern of impairment in an informal setting. It admirably fulfills the purpose for which it was intended.

References

Anderson, T., N. Boureston, and F. Greenberg   Rehabilitation predictors in completed stroke. Final report to the U. S. Soc. Rehab. Service. Minneapolis: Sister Kenny Rehabilitation Institute, American Rehabilitation Foundation, 1971.

Holland, A.   Personal communication, 1978.

Needham, L. S. and L. P. Swisher   A comparison of three tests of auditory comprehension for adult aphasics. *J. Speech Hearing Dis.* 37: 123–131, 1972.

Sands, E., M. T. Sarno, and D. Shankweiler   Long-term assessment of language function in aphasia due to stroke. *Arch. Phys. Med. Rehab.* 50: 202–206, 222, 1969.

Taylor, M. L.   A measurement of functional communication in aphasia. *Arch. Phys. Med. Rehab.* 46: 101–107, 1965.

HALSTEAD APHASIA TEST, FORM M.

Ward C. Halstead, Joseph M. Wepman, Ralph M. Reitan, and Robert F. Heimburger

University of Chicago Industrial Relations Center, undated

Cost $12.00

Manual, 17 pages; bound test cards; record form, 1 page

Time 1 hour, administration; 30 minutes, scoring

Ronald S. Tikofsky *Florida International University*

Purpose This form of the original Halstead–Wepman Aphasia Screening Test (Halstead and Wepman 1949) was designed to meet the neurologist's need for a pocket-size aphasia screening examination that can be used while making rounds. The test items and sequence of presentation for Form M is the same as that for the original test, which is no longer in print. The essential difference between the two versions is in the use of a plastic stimulus booklet and small record form for Form M, as opposed to a large "test dial" and large record form on which to record patient responses used in the original test.

Administration, scoring, and interpretation Test stimuli are presented to the patient through a window in the test booklet. Instructions to the examiner appear on the back of a stimulus card behind the back cover of the booklet. The booklet must be rotated after item 22.

Specific instructions for administration are given in the manual which accompanies the test kit. These instructions include comments to aid the examiner in presenting stimuli and eliciting responses. The manual provides little guidance to the examiner for differential scoring of the patient's responses. Each item is scored separately on a right-or-wrong basis. Some general suggestions made in the manual with respect to evaluation of severity of impairment will not prove to be very helpful to the novice examiner. No detailed information in reference to scoring or interpretation of findings is offered. A sample "Diagnostic Code and Profile" is presented. This profile is a duplicate of the original Halstead–Wepman Aphasia Screening Test. The authors state that the items relate to categories of dysfunction such as agnosia, visual form agnosia, auditory agnosia, and verbal agnosia, and that a profile can be established by circling items missed by the patient. Four basic types of aphasia are suggested: Global, Expressive-Receptive, Expressive, and Receptive. The user is given no information about the criteria to be used in determining from the profile how a patient is to be classified.

Evaluation of test adequacy No data are presented in the manual nor have studies been published which deal with the validity or reliability of this instrument. Schotland (see Tikofsky 1966) in an unpublished master's thesis criticized the original Halstead–Wepman Aphasia Screening Test as an inadequate measuring instrument because it included no norms and presented no data concerning reliability and validity. Her criticisms of the original test hold for Form M since it is only a miniaturized version of the original. The authors attest to the clinical usefulness of the Halstead–Wepman Aphasia Screening Test on the basis of their experience and that of others who have used the test. Results of the patient's performance are not subject to quantification. Information relative to item selection and standardization procedures is not available to the potential user of this instrument. One gets the impression that test items were selected on the basis of clinical experience and intuition.

This test has only limited clinical utility given the range of aphasia tests currently available to speech–language pathologists. At best it can serve as a weak screening device for establishing which patients warrant or can tolerate full language evaluation. In comparison to Schuell's Short Examination for Aphasia (Schuell 1957), this test comes off a poor second. Form M, which is the only form of the test available, has for all practical purposes outlived its usefulness. It has not been revised since its original publication some time in the 1950s (no specific copyright date is given) and thus does not reflect contemporary concepts in the field of aphasia testing.

Summary This test has interesting historical value, but it is of only limited usefulness for present-day aphasia evaluation. In comparison to other available instruments, including screening tests, it would be ranked low, and it is probably not in wide use. The test should not be used by the inexperienced clinician since little guidance is provided for interpretation and classification.

References

Halstead, W. C. and J. M. Wepman The Halstead–Wepman Aphasia Screening Test. *J. Speech Hearing Dis.* 14: 9–15, 1949.

Schotland, H. L. An evaluative study of two tests for aphasia. Unpublished masters thesis, University of Iowa, 1953. (See R. S. Tikofsky, Language problems in adults. Chapter 11, pp. 261–284, in R. W. Rieber, and R. S. Brubaker (eds.), *Speech Pathology.* Amsterdam: North Holland Publishing Co., 1966.)

Schuell, H. M. A short examination for aphasia. *Neurology* 7: 625–634, 1957.

THE LANGUAGE MODALITIES TEST FOR APHASIA (LMTA)

Joseph M. Wepman and Lyle V. Jones

Education-Industry Service, 1961
Two equivalent forms: I and II

Cost   Complete Kit, $35.00
Instruction manual, 15 pages, $1.00; administration manual, 91 pages, $3.00; filmstrip, $7.00; subject response booklet, 27 pages, $0.75, package of 10, $4.50; examiner's record book, 21 pages, $0.75, package of 10, $4.50; scoring summary-history form, 4 pages, $0.25, package of 10, $1.75

Time   Two to five hours

Robert H. Brookshire   *Minneapolis Veterans Administration Hospital*

Purpose   According to the authors, the Language Modalities Test for Aphasia is designed "for both clinician and research use." It is "easy to use and interesting to the patient. From its results, the best approaches to therapy are easily determined. In addition, because of its standardization, it provides a research tool for both intra-individual changes and inter-individual comparisons." Two equivalent forms (Form I and Form II) of the LMTA are provided.

Administration, scoring, and interpretation   Test stimuli are presented from a 35mm film strip projected onto a screen. The test contains a screening section (the first 11 items), followed by two "cycles" of 23 stimulus items each. According to the authors, the "cycles" allow the examiner to administer the LMTA in two or three sessions without disrupting the patient's performance.

   Responses are scored right–wrong (screening and matching items) or according to a six-category system of error types (oral and graphic response items). The examiner is encouraged to supplement scores with longhand notation and to transcribe errors verbatim, where appropriate. Scoring examples for oral and graphic responses are included in appendices to the administration manual.

   General directions for summarization and interpretation of results are included in the manual. No standardized procedures by which the examiner might summarize and interpret patient performance are offered, although a Scoring Summary Sheet is provided as part of a four-page "Subject's Personal Medical History" form.

Evaluation of test adequacy   The original version of the test was administered to 168 aphasic patients. Of these 168, 130 exhibited right hemiparesis, five exhibited left hemiparesis, and three were bilaterally paralyzed. The remaining 30 evidently exhibited no paresis or paralysis.

   The high proportion of individuals in the sample with hemiparesis suggests that the sample used to validate the LMTA may have contained an inordinate number of individuals with anterior lesions. The presence of bilaterally hemiparetic patients indicates that at least some of the patients in the sample had bilateral brain damage. Such sampling bias may weaken the generality of the authors' statements concerning test validity and may compromise the results of their factor analyses and analyses of variance. In general, the procedures followed in selecting the normative sample and in evaluating the validity and reliability of the LMTA are incompletely described. Only age, educational level, and time post onset of aphasia are reported for the normative sample. No information is given about the composition of the sample in terms of etiology, site of lesion, or existence of complicating conditions.

Data regarding the equivalence of Forms I and II consist of tables indicating (1) that equivalent numbers of stimulus-response type combinations are included in the two forms, (2) generally high correlations (above .80) between the number correct on Forms I and II, and (3) equivalent mean proportions of correct responses, by stimulus and response types, for Forms I and II.

A table of interscorer reliabilities is presented, based upon 6000 responses, scored independently by different judges. The reliabilities reported are generally high (.878 and above), but the description of the procedures by which these measures were obtained is so ambiguous that the dependability of these results cannot be estimated.

The authors cite the results of a factor analysis as evidence for the validity of the LMTA. According to the authors, the results of "several factor analyses" generated the following factors: (1) oral responses to visual stimuli, (2) oral responses to auditory stimuli, (3) written responses to auditory stimuli, (4) written responses to visual stimuli, (5) matching auditory or visual stimuli to pictures. No details of the factor analyses are given. Therefore, no confident conclusions can be drawn regarding the validity of the LMTA from these analyses. No information is provided regarding the relationships of LMTA scores to other measures of language abilities. Thus the user of the LMTA is provided little information on which to make a confident decision about the test's validity.

The filmstrip format for stimulus presentation can be cumbersome and awkward. The user may find it helpful to cut the filmstrip into separate frames and mount the frames in $2'' \times 2''$ slide mounts, so that a standard slide projector can be used to present test stimuli.

Because of limited information about the reliability and validity of the LMTA, it would probably best be used as a screening test, unless the user cared to take the time necessary to establish local norms. The LMTA might also be useful as a within-patient test of general progress in treatment, although the lack of clear data concerning test–retest reliability might compromise its usefulness in this respect.

Summary   Lack of normative information and deficiencies in information about the reliability and validity of the LMTA appear to preclude its use as a primary tool for assessing the aphasic individual's language abilities. At its current stage of development, the LMTA appears to be more suitable as a screening test, or as an auxiliary test, administered as an adjunct to a more extensive and better-standardized language examination.

THE MINNESOTA TEST FOR DIFFERENTIAL DIAGNOSIS OF APHASIA (MTDDA)

Hildred Schuell

University of Minnesota Press, Revised edition, 1972

Cost $24.00
Manual, 23 pages, $2.00; Monograph *Differential Diagnosis of Aphasia with the Minnesota Test,* 108 pages, $6.00; two packs of stimulus cards, $10.00; test booklet, 7 pages, pack of 25 for $6.00

Time 1½ to 2½ hours, administration and scoring

Ann Zubrick and Aaron Smith *University of Michigan Medical School*

Purpose and development of test Beginning with the first version (Form I 1948), Schuell's construction and continuing refinements of the Minnesota Test for Differential Diagnosis of Aphasia marked a major advance in the development of standardized, objective, and comprehensive measures of language functions in adult aphasic patients. The underlying rationale in her development of the MTDDA derived from her accumulating data in intensive and extensive diagnostic studies of 155 successive aphasic adults admitted to the Minneapolis Veterans Administration Hospital between 1955 and 1958, and of a second group of selected cases admitted between 1965 and 1970.

Thus her continuing revisions of the MTDDA were based on empirical evidence and increasingly emphasized the importance of differentiating the nature and degree of impairments of the basic "higher" or mental functions that underlie the processing of symbols in all four language modalities from impairments of the sensory and motor functions involved in each specific language modality. For example, Schuell (1950) observed that paraphasia was not simply a uniform speech disorder resulting from destruction of a circumscribed area within the left "dominant" hemisphere but might reflect disruptions of mechanisms that must be organized in preparation for speech. The various degrees and possible forms of paraphasia and other language disorders might therefore be due to various pathological alterations in the sensory and motor mechanisms involved in integrative as well as expressive and receptive language functions. Similarly she differentiated (1) perseverative errors in speech indicative of sensory deficits in patients who are unaware of their errors from (2) errors indicative of motor deficits in patients who recognize and try to correct perseverative speech errors.

The MTDDA was thus an increasingly refined distillation of an initially wide number of language and nonlanguage tests routinely administered to the Minneapolis VA Hospital aphasic population. Unlike Marie and Head, in addition to testing 50 normal adults as controls, Schuell took into account the various changes in the form and severity of language disorders in the different language modalities as a function of "spontaneous recovery" shortly after onset of aphasia as well as a function of therapy in test–retest comparisons of patients with persisting aphasia.

The successive revisions of the MTDDA from 1948 to 1972 ultimately resulted in the elimination of certain nonlanguage tests. When factor analysis revealed clustering around five major factors underlying aphasic language disturbances, some language tests were discarded. The results of the analysis led Schuell to conclude that despite apparent differences in the degrees of impairment of the four language modalities, aphasia was a unitary disorder. Thus, like Hughlings Jackson, Finkelnburg, Kussmaul, Marie, and others, Schuell's continuing refinements of the MTDDA reflected an increasing focus on the complex nature of normal language functions and the role of sensory and motor deficits as determinants of the nature and degree of aphasic disturbances.

Accordingly, Schuell classified her heterogeneous aphasic populations on the basis of descriptive and prognostic criteria into five major and two minor groups. In contrast to earlier models, the divisions were not contingent on the specific site, type, or extent of lesion, age, education, and other variables. Instead the groups were differentiated according to functional language capacity (mild to severe) and the specific effects of associated visual, auditory, or sensorimotor impairment.

Tests of the 50 normal subjects showed occasional random errors indicating care- lessness or limited education. This was not the case for aphasic patients. Their indi- vidual and collective error scores and marked intratest scatter demonstrated that Schuell's test selections were appropriate as an index of functional language and that the items were sufficiently discriminating, reliable, and valid to identify significant changes in the various language modalities from admission to discharge following language rehabilitation.

In addition to the test manual, Schuell (1965) wrote a separate monograph, *Dif- ferential Diagnosis of Aphasia with the Minnesota Test*. The term "differential diag- nosis" usually applies to diagnostic studies designed to establish the etiology or identify specific disorders in patients with equivocal or diverse overlapping signs and symptoms of unknown etiology. However, *"The Minnesota Test for Differential Diagnosis of Aphasia* was designed to permit the examiner to observe the level at which language performance breaks down in each of the principal language modalities, since this is essentially what there is to observe in aphasia" (Schuell 1965, p. 3). Thus, the MTDDA was designed first to differentiate subjects with normal language and patients with other disorders but intact language functions from patients with aphasia. While the MTDDA provides an effective tool for such dichotomous differentiations, the only kind of real "differential diagnosis" it provides in routine studies of normal or diverse clinical populations is definition of the presence or absence of aphasia.

As the term was used by Schuell, "Differential diagnosis is the basis of both de- scription and prediction in aphasia" (Schuell 1965, p. 5). In this context, the term therefore refers to the ability of the MTDDA to differentiate specific subgroups within the generic category of aphasia. Thus Schuell described seven presumably discrete aphasic syndromes according to the severity of language disorders based on MTDDA performances and the presence or absence of various associated nonlanguage disorders. The MTDDA, however, was not designed for differentiation of patients with loose associational thought processes, dementia, confusion, severe hearing loss, memory loss, or other nonaphasic disorders which variously manifest in language disturbances dif- ferent from the specific categories of aphasia described by Schuell. Although this is an important and not infrequent problem in differential diagnostic studies, there are as yet no data or guidelines indicating the usefulness or limitations of the MTDDA in such clinical applications.

Administration, scoring, and interpretation   The MTDDA consists of 57 subtests com- posed of varying numbers of items. The subtests are categorized into five groups repre- senting primary areas of language/symbolic disturbance (auditory, visual and reading, speech and language, visuomotor and writing disturbances, and disturbances of numerical relations and arithmetic processes). Most items are scored correct or incorrect. In general the scoring is unambiguous. Speech and language subtests require some clinical judgments to be made, but the bases for making them are well covered in the manual. However, the dichotomous correct or incorrect scoring criteria make no provision for quantitative differences within the correct–incorrect categories.

The relative difficulty of items in the subtests and possible weighting of one with another might also benefit from further refinements. It is assumed that there is a graduated, linear increase in difficulty of the items within each group of subtests. By and large, this is the case, but there are exceptions. In the examination of auditory disturbances, the subtests increase in difficulty from recognition of common words to understanding a paragraph. Results on the last two subtests (digit and sentence repetition) may be confounded by speech impairment in some aphasic patients, rather than reflecting reduced auditory retention.

Objective results are supplemented by a clinical rating (0–6, representing the range from no observable impairment to no functional capacity) and a diagnostic scale (0–4, representing the range from no impairment to no performance on relevant tests). The clinical rating represents easily determined and well specified criteria obtainable from clinical observation interviews of family or observation from other sources. The diagnostic scale summarizes overall clinical performances from the various sections into headings representing functional performance categories.

The test results may be reported as numerical indices of severity of language impairment that can then be used in test–retest comparisons. Schuell made no claims for the test outside of the criteria she selected to assign patients to a broad-based category of disorder and severity. For each of her five major groups she detailed a prognostic outcome based on clinical findings of the therapy given at the Minneapolis VA Hospital. Since she documented the clinical population she used, her results should allow for population comparisons. However, comparison of individual aphasic patients with Schuell's groups should be made cautiously. Smith's study (1972) of chronic aphasic patients suggested that while the percentage errors on the MTDDA were correlated with overall language gains (the fewer the errors, the greater the long-term language gains), other significant predictors of language recovery from aphasia included the status of the whole brain relative to preservation of nonlanguage functions, somatosensory functions, age, and especially motivation.

Evaluation of test adequacy The MTDDA consists of an administrative manual, two spiral-bound books of test plates, and a standard recording booklet. The examiner must furnish a box of specified common objects, a stopwatch, flashlight, pencils, and writing paper. Initially developed as a research tool, a research edition was published in 1955. The standard form appeared in 1965 and was revised in 1972. Statistical analysis using factor analysis (Varimax and Oblimin Factor matrices) with correlations between the sections revealed continued validity as the population N increased and also showed stability in test–retest conditions.

A short form of the test was described (Schuell 1957) for medical personnel. This is not a standardized form and is not meant to substitute for the longer form. Rather, it provides a means by which a physician may systematically approach diagnostic testing in aphasia. However, just as the continuing refinements of the long form derived from empirical findings in systematic reevaluations of the MTDDA, Schuell's critical assessments of its efficacy and limitations finally prompted her to disclaim the short form as a useful clinical instrument (Schuell 1966). Instead, she continued her efforts to improve the validity and sensitivity of the MTDDA based on systematic reviews of the results obtained in initial diagnostic studies and on follow-up studies of treated and untreated aphasic patients.

Users of the long form, while requiring no special training, require some background knowledge of testing procedure and language defects. Distribution of the test is primarily to speech–language pathologists and psychologists.

Schuell cautioned against definitive interpretation of the test results when the patient is "neurologically unstable." She suggested that the examiner extend the testing over more than one session when fatigue or illness make this advisable and stated that the patient should be able to sit for a period of two hours when formal testing is instituted. Since variability of performance, fatigue, and the effects of spontaneous remission are all well documented facets of acute neurological impairment, her caution is well heeded. She did not report how many of her subjects may have had results that were open to interpretation for these reasons. Pooling large numbers of patients tested variously post-ictus may tend to hide individual variation in test scores; aphasia testing done three to six months post-ictus (the period usually defined as "spontaneous remission") should therefore be interpreted conservatively for prognostic purposes.

Schuell's population, while heterogeneous, was not vastly discrepant from that seen in any large neurological service. Aged, diffusely damaged, and ill patients were excluded from the study. Those retested (75 out of 155) who had undergone therapy were possibly a more select population than those who did not receive therapy, and a larger pooling of subjects would possibly have yielded different proportions in each of the diagnostic categories. Such problems, arising out of difficulties inherent in such studies, should not detract from a general acceptance of findings, carefully accrued.

Smith (1971, 1972) has shown the usefulness of the MTDDA as a standardized instrument in the systematic examination of aphasic patients. His results obtained from 126 chronically impaired aphasic patients supported Schuell's finding of aphasia as a unitary disorder. He did not investigate the validity of Schuell's subgroups for prognostic purposes. Standard administration and scoring procedures were used except that in items requiring dichotomous (yes–no) responses, error scores were doubled to allow for chance. However, as noted earlier, "Certain subtests designed as measures of a single language component may be confounded by involvement of other language components. For example, responses to A-9 (designed to assess auditory disturbances) must be made in speech" (Smith 1971, p. 179).

In the manual for their Boston Diagnostic Aphasia Examination (BDAE) (qv) also based on studies of aphasic patients in a VA Hospital (Boston), Goodglass and Kaplan noted the marked discrepancy between Schuell's findings of "impairment in general ability" and their own claims of confirmation of the variously modified Broca's "motor," Wernicke's "sensory," "conduction," and other presumably discrete anatomically based aphasic syndromes. They attribute the increasing reports of a unitary "deficit" and quantitative findings in Schuell's and other studies of aphasia to "cases in which large lesions are the rule, implicating, simultaneously, functionally diverse areas. Small lesions producing isolated disorders occur less frequently and therefore have a smaller effect in any study which groups all cases together" (Goodglass and Kaplan 1972, pp. 2–3). Thus they imply that the nature of the aphasic population is a critical factor in the standardization of aphasia tests. They indicate that their approximately 200 aphasic subjects were highly selected cases with "small lesions." However, unlike Schuell's carefully detailed descriptions of the nature of aphasiogenic lesions, age, education, sex, and other variables, Goodglass and Kaplan do not report comparable data for their standardization sample, including the selection criteria. Nonetheless, although their arguments cannot be readily dismissed, it is intriguing to note that both Broca's and Wernicke's initial claims of dichotomous syndromes of motor vs. sensory aphasia were also based on preconceived hypotheses and studies of a small number of old stroke patients who were much more like Schuell's than the highly selected Boston VA aphasic population.

Summary No single test for aphasia is adequate for evaluation of all aphasic patients. The MTDDA is no exception. However, it is recommended as a thoroughly researched and increasingly refined tool. While it is not sensitive to very mild aphasia, its value is enhanced when combined with other tests as described below. Its values for prediction and prognosis in acute aphasia need further study. In our experience, clinicians and students learn to administer it rapidly and accurately.

The MTDDA provides no measures of nonlanguage sensory and motor functions for assessing the presence of associated visual, constructional, spatial, memory, and other nonlanguage deficits, the functional status of the right hemisphere, and of the brain as a whole. However, when complemented with a neuropsychological test battery, the MTDDA and overall findings provide a comprehensive and detailed clinical picture of the nature and degree of language and associated nonlanguage and of residual intact functions that have potentially significant prognostic implications. The overall findings also provide bases for assessing the individual aphasic patient's capacities to benefit from language therapy. In our experience, regardless of the nature or severity of aphasic disorders, patients with normal nonverbal visual-ideational reasoning and the absence of left-sided manual motor or somatosensory deficits indicating intact right hemisphere functions have demonstrated significantly greater improvement after language therapy than do aphasic patients with evidence of bilateral cerebral involvement.

There is also a need for MTDDA studies of other aphasic populations, especially those with "small" lesions, to evaluate the validity of the argument by Goodglass and Kaplan and also concurrent studies with the BDAE to assess the strengths and weaknesses of both tests. We also hope that despite Schuell's death her colleagues will continue the work she did so ably and assiduously to provide the field with a further refined edition of the MTDDA.

References

Goodglass, H. and E. Kaplan *The Assessment of Aphasia and Related Disorders.* Philadelphia: Lea and Febiger, 1972.

Jenkins, J. J., E. Jiménez-Pabón, R. E. Shaw, and J. W. Sefer *Schuell's Aphasia in Adults: Diagnosis, Prognosis, and Treatment.* (2nd ed.). New York: Harper & Row, 1975.

Schuell, H. Paraphasia and paralexia. *J. Speech Hearing Dis.* 15: 291–306, 1950.

——— A short examination for aphasia. *Neurology* 7: 625–634, 1957.

—— *Differential Diagnosis of Aphasia with the Minnesota Test.* Minneapolis: University of Minnesota Press, 1965.

—— A re-evaluation of the short examination for aphasia. *J. Speech Hearing Dis.* **31**: 137–147, 1966.

Smith, A. Objective indices of severity of chronic aphasia in stroke patients. *J. Speech Hearing Dis.* **36**: 167–207, 1971.

——, R. Campoux, J. Leri, R. London, and A. Muraski *Diagnosis, Intelligence, and Rehabilitation of Chronic Aphasics: Final Report.* SRS Grant 14-p-55198/5-01. Ann Arbor: University of Michigan Department of Physical Medicine and Rehabilitation, 1972.

NEUROSENSORY CENTER COMPREHENSIVE EXAMINATION FOR APHASIA (NCCEA)

Otfried Spreen and Arthur L. Benton

University of Victoria Neuropsychology Laboratory, 1969.

Cost $35.50
Manual, 49 pages; monograph, 75 pages; answer booklet, 22 pages, pack of 20; Profiles A, B, and C, packs of 20 each; recorded tape; set of plastic tokens; reading cards; photographs of four trays with objects. Additional manuals, $3.00; additional packets of 20 answer booklets and Profiles A, B, and C, $12.00 per packet

Time 60 minutes, administration; 20 minutes scoring: control tests require additional 20 minutes, administration; and 10 minutes, scoring

Frederick R. Greenberg *Glenrose Hospital, Edmonton, Alberta, Canada*

Purpose The implicit purpose of Neurosensory Center Comprehensive Examination for Aphasia is the comprehensive examination of the language skills of patients suspected of being dysphasic. The authors (Spreen and Benton 1977, p. 1) write, "[The examination helps to] assess understanding and production of language, retention of verbal material, reading and writing."

Administration, scoring, and interpretation The examination consists of 20 "language" tests and four "control" tests. Thirty-two different objects arranged in four trays of eight objects each are utilized in the administration of eight of the language tests and three of the control tests. Duplicate sets of objects are required for the three control tests. The 20 language subtests are identified as follows:

1. Visual Naming
2. Description of Use
3. Tactile Naming, Right Hand
4. Tactile Naming, Left Hand
5. Sentence Repetition
6. Repetition of Digits
7. Reversal of Digits
8. Word Fluency (qv)
9. Sentence Construction
10. Identification by Name
11. Identification by Sentence (Token Test, qv)
12. Oral Reading (Names)
13. Oral Reading (Sentences)
14. Reading Names for Meaning (Pointing)
15. Reading Sentences for Meaning (Pointing)
16. Visual-Graphic Naming
17. Writing of Names
18. Writing to Dictation
19. Writing (Copying)
20. Articulation

Subtests 1–9, 12, 13, and 20 require oral responses. Subtests 10, 11, 14, and 15 require gestural responses. Subtests 16, 17, 18, and 19 require graphic responses.

The four control tests are identified as follows: C-1. Tactile Visual Matching, Right Hand; C-2. Tactile Visual Matching, Left Hand; C-3. Visual Visual Matching; and

C-4. Form Perception. C-1 is administered if errors occur on Language Test 3; C-2 is administered if errors occur on Language Test 4; C-3 is administered if errors occur on Language Tests 1 or Control Tests 1 or 2; C-4 is administered if errors occur on Language Tests 12, 13, 14, or 15.

After scores are calculated for each subtest and, where appropriate, corrections made for age and education, the scores are plotted on one of three profile sheets. Profile A plots scores according to percentile ranks for normal adults, Profile B plots scores according to percentile ranks for aphasic patients, and Profile C plots scores according to percentile ranks for brain-damaged nonaphasic patients.

Interpretation of the resulting profiles is, for the most part, left to the examiner. The authors state merely that with Profile A (normal adults) a percentile rank of 40 or above can be expected for subjects without language disturbance. "Ranks in the 30 to 40 range indicate minimal difficulties in performance; ranks in the 20 to 30 range indicate mild impairment; ranks below 20 indicate more severe dysfunction" (Spreen and Benton 1977, p. 12).

Evaluation of test adequacy   The test manual, record forms, and accompanying material fall short in assisting the user to interpret the test results. Although not specified in the test manual, it is apparent that only experienced examiners will be able to use the examination and interpret the results. Within the test manual itself minimal information is provided regarding the construction of the test and the sample groups from which normative data (percentile ranks) were derived. Notably lacking is information regarding content validity, criterion-related validity, construct validity, and reliability. Those subjects are mentioned by reference to previously published and unpublished material, but the user is obliged to review those references rather than having information available in the manual as might be expected. Some of the references (Lawriw 1976; Ludlow 1977; Wertz 1977) were not available to the reviewer.

Benton (1967) has described the manner in which the NCCEA was constructed and how norms for adult aphasic patients were established. Not explained, however, is how "... the appropriate corrections for the influence of age and educational level were made and the corrected scores were converted into percentile rank scores. ..." Sample profiles are provided for patients whose referral diagnoses were "expressive aphasia," "anomia," "jargon aphasia," "Gerstman's syndrome," and "global aphasia." The normative data are derived from a group of "normal" subjects and "adult aphasics," with the number of individuals in each group not specified.

In a study by Kenin and Swisher (1972) the NCCEA was administered to 15 patients and results were compared with the overall score from Sarno's (1969) Functional Communication Profile (FCP) (qv). This study showed that the NCCEA demonstrated changes in patients' language function when FCP overall scores were used as an outside criterion measure. The authors note that the NCCEA did not sample an adequate range of behavior except in the auditory comprehension area.

Crockett (1976) compared results of the NCCEA for 57 aphasic patients with their scores on the Verbal Rating Scale (VRS), a 17-item scale used to rate recorded samples of the speech of the aphasic patient. The 17 dimensions of communication rated were rate of speech, prosody, pronunciation, hesitation, phrase length, effort, pauses, press of speech, perseveration, word choice, paraphasia, communication, naming, grammar, interstitial connectives, use of inflections, tense and gender, and understanding of spoken language. The high correlation coefficients between the 17 mean scores and similar NCCEA subtests can be interpreted as indicative of NCCEA subtest validity. In a later report Crockett (1977) demonstrated that scores on the NCCEA differentiated four groups of patients statistically derived from scores on the VRS, thus providing further evidence of test validity.

Of interest but little use is the inclusion with the test package of a monograph, The Spreen–Benton Aphasia Tests, Normative Data as a Measure of Normal Language Development (Gaddes and Crockett 1973). The monograph describes a research project designed to determine the usefulness of the NCCEA for examining children's language and to that purpose presents data for normal children. Far more useful to the potential user would be a more detailed discussion of the validity and reliability of the test and information regarding the interpretation of results obtained on adult subjects.

The clinical usefulness of this test will vary as a function of examiner skill and the severity of patients' language impairment. For patients with mild impairments or subtle linguistic deficits, the test is not sufficiently discriminating, i.e., there is insufficient "top." For severely impaired patients, the relative simplicity of many of the subtests will yield useful information regarding language dysfunction that would be missed in other tests with too little "bottom."

The test is not convenient to administer. The manipulation of four trays of objects for the language tests and eight trays for the control tests is awkward and time consuming. The presentation of some auditory-oral tasks via recorded tape is also awkward and time consuming, particularly if a recorded subtest is discontinued prior to its end because of repeated patient failure. When that occurs, the examiner must advance the tape to the beginning of the next recorded subtest, and there are no editing cues available to facilitate this forward movement of the reel.

The potential user of the test should understand that in addition to the materials that come with the test it will be necessary to purchase two sets of objects (1978 cost about $25.00). Also required will be a reel-to-reel tape recorder, stopwatch, and the construction of a box for presenting the tactile subtests.

Summary   This is a useful test for severely impaired brain-injured communication-impaired adults if administered by a skilled and experienced examiner. The paucity of information in the test manual regarding test construction and interpretation of results influences this reviewer to rank the test low in comparison with other available examinations for aphasia, e.g., Porch Index of Communicative Ability (qv), and Minnesota Test for Differential Diagnosis of Aphasia (qv). On the other hand, the relatively low cost of the test may be justification for having it available in those instances where it would be useful.

References

Benton, A. L.   Problems of test construction in the field of aphasia. *Cortex* 3: 32–58, 1967.

Crocket, D. J.   Multivariate comparison of Howes' and Weisenburg and McBride's models of aphasia on the Neurosensory Center Comprehensive Examination. *Perceptual and Motor Skills* 43: 795–806, 1976.

——— A comparison of empirically derived groups of aphasic patients on the Neurosensory Center Comprehensive Examination for Aphasia. *Journal of Clinical Psychology* 33: 194–198, 1977.

Gaddes, W. H. and D. J. Crockett   *The Spreen–Benton Aphasia Tests, Normative Data as a Measure of Normal Language Development,* Research Monograph No. 25. Victoria: Neuropsychology Laboratory, University of Victoria, 1973.

Kenin, M. and L. P. Swisher A study of patterns of recovery in aphasia, *Cortex* **8**: 56–68, 1972.

Lawriw, I. A test of the predictive validity and a cross-validation of the Neurosensory Center Comprehensive Examination for Aphasia. Doctoral dissertation, University of Victoria, 1976.

Ludlow, C. L. Recovery from aphasia: a foundation for treatment. In M. Sullivan and M. S. Kommers (eds.), *Rationale for Adult Aphasia Therapy.* Omaha: University of Nebraska Medical Center, 1977.

Sarno, M. T. *The Functional Communication Profile. Manual of Directions.* New York: New York University Medical Center, Institute of Rehabilitation Medicine, 1969.

Spreen, O. and A. L. Benton *Neurosensory Center Comprehensive Examination for Aphasia.* 1977 Revision. Victoria, B. C.: Neuropsychology Laboratory, Department of Psychology, University of Victoria, 1977.

Wertz, R. T. Appraisal and diagnosis in aphasia: evaluating the effects of treatment. In M. Sullivan and M. S. Kommers (eds.), *Rationale for Adult Aphasia Therapy.* Omaha: University of Nebraska Medical Center, 1977.

ORZECK APHASIA EVALUATION (OAE)

Arthur Z. Orzeck

Western Psychological Services, 1964

Cost $1.50

Examiner's manual, 4 pages; protocol booklet, 4 pages

Time 30–40 minutes

Elisabeth H. Wiig *Boston University*

Purpose The author states that he designed the Orzeck Aphasia Evaluation to (1) provide a scale suitable for effective screening for suspected brain damage, (2) supplement other psychological, neurological, and medical examination, (3) provide a clinical-rating type of quantification of organicity, and (4) offer a practical frame of reference for structuring therapy.

Administration, scoring, and interpretation The OAE is presented as a clinical interview in which biographical and medical information is obtained initially. Subsequently, the 26 test items are presented to screen for (1) apraxias of speech, writing, design, and calculation; (2) visual, auditory, design, finger, and left–right agnosia; and (3) visual, tactile, and auditory suppression. The responses are rated for degree of pathology on a four-point scale from severe to no pathology. Judgments for the rating of responses are to be made "on the basis of . . . clinical experience." The author proposes that "the presence of *any one* sign suggests some brain damage" and discusses possible relationships between various problems, dominance, and the location of the organic damage.

Evaluation of test adequacy The OAE manual does not present information concerning the validity of the test. The user is told nothing about the content, construct, or criterion-related validity of the test. Similarly there is no evidence presented in the manual that the interexaminer or test–retest reliability of the test has been considered.

Summary The limitations in the construction of this overly brief test reported above limit the clinical use of the OAE severely. In comparison with competing tests of aphasia, the OAE would be ranked lowest. This reviewer does not recommend the use of the OAE by speech–language pathologists.

PORCH INDEX OF COMMUNICATIVE ABILITY (PICA)

Bruce E. Porch

Consulting Psychologists Press, Inc., 1967.
Manual, Volume II, revised 1971

Cost $70.00, kit in attaché case; $60.00 in cardboard container
Manual, Volume I, 57 pages, $5.00; Volume II, 116 pages, $7.50; Manuals $11.50 if bought together. Two sets of 10 test objects; test format

booklet, 24 pages, $4.50; set of cards for each reading subtest, $6.00; set of cards for visual matching subtest, $6.00; packs of 50 score sheets, ranked response summaries, modality response summaries, aphasia recovery curve profile sheets, predictive data summary sheets, and rating of communicative deficits sheets, $2.50 each

Time 1 hour average (range 22 to 143 minutes) for aphasic patients, administration; 20 minutes (range 13 to 49 minutes) for normal subjects (Duffy et al. 1976); 30 minutes, scoring

Malcolm R. McNeil *University of Colorado*

Purpose The expressed purpose of the Porch Index of Communicative Ability is twofold: the PICA was designed psychometrically to provide a stable means of evaluating patient change, and it was designed as a tool for communicating with other professionals, in quantitative terms, about a patient or a population of patients.

Administration, scoring, and interpretation The PICA has set a model in aphasia testing for standardization in both administration and the scoring of patient behaviors. The testing environment, the patient and tester seating, test object alignment, stimulus presentation, stimulus repeat and cue presentation, subtest ceiling (three consecutive item rejections), and the overall speed and tempo of test administration are strictly specified.

Four verbal, two auditory, two reading, two gestural, and two visual matching subtests are presented in a hierarchical manner progressing from least to most information relative to what the test requires and how the tasks are to be performed. Six graphic subtests follow, arranged under the same hierarchical constraints.

A 40-hour workshop followed by supervised experience in administering the test to ten aphasic patients and scoring it is generally considered adequate for learning to administer, score, and interpret the PICA. In addition, the following reliability standards have been established for PICA scoring: *Advanced competence,* 90–100 percent score agreement; *General competence,* 80–89 percent score agreement; *Basic competence,* 70–79 percent score agreement; *Training level,* 60–69 percent score agreement (needs practice scoring under competent supervisor or needs to retake a basic workshop); *Pre-Workshop scoring level,* below 60 percent score agreement.

A 16-point binary choice, multidimensional category scoring system is used to evaluate patient performance. The five dimensions of accuracy, responsiveness, completeness, promptness, and efficiency describe multidimensionally several processes involved in the reception, perception, association, integration, conceptualization, formulation, and expression of information.

Multidimensional scoring is an attempt to combine the advantages of plus–minus scoring (ease) with the advantages of descriptive note taking (more information captured). It also attempts to overcome the weaknesses and limitations of both scoring systems. As Porch (1971b) suggests, it would be impractical to learn a scoring system that would encompass all possible permutations of the five dimensions listed. By combining those dimensions found by others to describe aphasic behavior best, and by eliminating what he considered to be less important combinations of dimensions, Porch constructed a 16-point scoring system which captures considerable information about the adequacy of the response as well as some information about mediational strategies used to arrive at the response.

The dimension of *accuracy* is defined as the degree of correctness or rightness of a given response and encompasses the scores 8 through 16 in the scoring system; different degrees of incorrectness are represented by scores 1 through 7. *Responsiveness* relates to the ease with which an appropriate response is elicited, or the amount of information needed by the patient in order to give a correct response. (Correctness is operationally defined in the PICA as a behavior which can be scored as an 8 (cued) or above.) This dimension is represented primarily by the scoring categories of 8, 9, and 10. *Completeness* is defined as the extent to which the task is carried out in its entirety and refers to such variables as grammatic, syntactic, or semantic qualities of the act. The scoring categories of 11, 12, and 15 represent this dimension. The dimension of *promptness* relates to the degree of immediateness with which a response is completed. The scoring categories of 11 and 13 describe deficits in this dimension. *Efficiency* is defined as the proficiency of the response and relates exclusively to the motoric aspects of the behavior. It is represented by the scoring category of 14.

The binary choice aspect of the scoring system refers to the process of arriving at a particular score from the 16 categories. This process necessitates the scorer's asking a series of questions about the response under consideration: Did the patient attempt to do the task? Was the response correct or incorrect? If correct, was it completed without extra information from the examiner? Each positively answered question leads to a higher score, and each negatively answered question necessitates the consideration of a lower score. Thus each yes–no answer leads to another question which leads to another yes–no answer until the appropriate score is deduced.

The PICA is based on a cybernetic model of information processing. As such, the five dimensions listed above must describe some aspects of the central nervous system's underlying mechanism. There is at least logical reason to believe that the underlying mechanism would be similar, if not the same, for motor behavior as for receptive–integrative behavior. Completely independent of Porch, neurophysiologists such as Evarts arrived at essentially the same dimensions to describe motor behavior, a fact that offers concurrent validity for the dimensions of behavior evaluated by the PICA.

Each response on each ten-item subtest receives a score from the 16-point scale. All ten scores are then averaged to express a mean overall measure of severity for the subtest. In order for mean scores to be used validly, to judge severity of performance on a given subtest, the scoring system must have at least an ordinal, if not interval, ranking (Labovitz 1970). Ordinality of a scoring system implies that a score of 6 is better than a score of 3, though not necessarily twice as good. Intervality, on the other hand, implies that a score of 6 is twice as good as a score of 3, or that 12 is twice as good as 6. If the ordinality of the PICA scoring system were not established, mean scores could not be interpreted (Van Demark 1974) and commonly used statistical treatment of PICA data would be invalid (Prescott and McNeil 1973).

Porch (1967) attempted to evaluate the hierarchical relationship of the 16 categories. He suggested that the rank ordering of his categories seemed to correspond to case history descriptions of patients during recovery. He also described a clear correlation between his categories and those arranged hierarchically by Kaplan (1959) and Wepman and Jones (1961) in their scoring systems. Porch also commissioned 12 speech pathologists, naive to the PICA, to arrange the 16 categories into a "clinically logical order." High positive correlations with his rank ordering offered an operative rationale for its use.

McNeil, Prescott, and Chang (1975) have questioned the PICA ordinality on other grounds. They suggested that there may be two different and independent types of ordinality for the PICA: one type refers to the judging of behaviors as to the severity of brain damage and aphasia either with loss of function with insult or return of function after insult; the other type refers to the perceived acceptability of performance, or an ordinality for "functional communication." Acceptability ratings from videotaped behaviors by 26 speech pathology graduate students, also naive to the PICA, revealed discrepancies between hierarchies arranged by Porch and those judged for acceptability of communicative style from watching behaviors. Twenty-seven percent of all combinations evaluated were judged to be questionably ordinal, and 3 percent of the total combinations were found to be unordinal. Generally repeats (score of 9) and self-corrections (10) were judged to be more acceptable than incomplete (12) and incomplete delayed (11) responses.

Duffy and Dale (1977) further evaluated the ordinality issue, having subjects rank-order written descriptions of the 16 categories as Porch did originally. A different hierarchy was reached from that found by Porch. Generally the dimensions of completeness and responsiveness were interchanged, as McNeil et al. (1975) had found. Next they correlated their rank ordering of the categories with the PICA rank ordering. Positive correlations exceed .90. Finally they asked, "Does the difference between the two scales make a difference as far as the clinical, statistical uses to which the PICA scale is generally put?" To determine this, they compared the two category hierarchies on the results of 50 aphasic patients randomly selected from a large population of completed tests. The correlations between the two scoring scales exceeded .99 for each individual subtest, as well as for gestural, verbal, graphic, and overall means. Given this level of predictability, the authors concluded that "PICA summary score results obtained with the PICA scoring scale can be considered equivalent to those which would be obtained using an interval level scale." Thus mean scores appear to represent levels of severity of aphasic behavior, and parametric statistical treatment of these means is appropriate.

As questioned by Silverman (1974) and explained by Porch (1974) and Van Demark (1974), mean scores on the PICA do not represent a specific category of behavior. In other words a mean of 12 on a subtest does not represent a mean behavior of incompleteness. Indeed, as Silverman (1974) noted, a 12 may not even have appeared in that subtest. However, as Porch (1974) commented, mean scores, whether subtest, modality, or overall, are never to be interpreted thus. Results of Duffy and Dale's (1977) study suggest that mean scores can be interpreted validly as measures of severity of aphasic deficits.

Evaluation of test adequacy   The structure of the PICA is based, like that of most other published tests of aphasia, on the concept that modalities can be affected to different degrees and that language usage is disturbed rather than the competence of the rules underlying language usage. The PICA is also based on the premise that aphasic deficits are primarily convergent in nature (the patient is asked to give a specific function of an object) as opposed to divergent (where the patient would be asked to give as many functions as possible of a specific object). With these facts in mind, the PICA would not be interpreted as a measure of a patient's ability to manipulate or generate specific linguistic constructions. Likewise, it would not be interpreted as a measure of divergent thinking. The following psychometric principles of test construction incorporated in the PICA's construction, validation, and standardization make it a useful test for constructing patient treatment programs (particularly the programmed stimulation type as outlined by LaPointe 1977) as well as a sensitive measure of patient change for research and clinical accountability.

The demonstration of a test's *construct validity* requires both an empirical and logical attack. As suggested above, the dimensions of behavior that the PICA assesses have logical and concurrent support. The behaviors assessed by the 16-point scoring system have been noted in the scientific literature as important behaviors associated with brain damage and aphasia. The scoring system appears to be valid and ordinal for describing severity of aphasia. Concurrent validity for the PICA model exists; the concepts of testing different levels of the major input and output modalities are representative of nearly all testing models for aphasia. Likewise, most models recognize levels of processing such as reception, perception, association, integration, conceptualization, formulation, and expression represented by Porch's (1967) model.

Concurrent validity of the PICA has only recently been established. Holland (1977) used Pearson product–moment correlations from a group of 80 patients with aphasia to establish the relationship of performance on her yet unpublished aphasia test (Communication Assessment for Daily Living—CADL) with the Functional Communication Profile (Taylor 1965), the Boston Diagnostic Aphasia Examination (Goodglass and Kaplan 1972), and the PICA. She also ran correlation coefficients on the PICA and the other two tests. The FCP correlated .86, the BDAE correlated .88, and the CADL (a test designed to elicit behavior that is more interpretable in terms of functional communication than in other existing tests for aphasia) correlated .93 with the PICA. These data suggest that patients tend to perform similarly on these measures. They also suggest high concurrent validity for the PICA.

Porch suggests that the PICA has good *predictive validity* relative to predicting the overall severity of the individual's test score at six months post onset when the initial test is administered at one month post onset. This prediction is based on the observation that the average of the nine highest subjects that is found to correspond, in percentile, to the patient's overall score at one month post onset, best represents the patient's six-month mean overall severity level. Six-month predictions can also be made by another method if the patient is beyond one month post onset at the time of the initial test, following a premade set of prediction curves (the high overall prediction or HOAP Slope). Clinical observations by many aphasiologists as well as data provided by Porch, Wertz, and Collins (1973, 1974) support the predictive validity of the PICA.

The *content validity* of the PICA, the degree to which the test content is representative of the class of situations or subject matter about which conclusions are to be drawn, must be evaluated on several dimensions. The PICA surveys 18 different tasks from the almost endless continuum of possible tasks. It appears to assess an adequate range of subtest difficulty for talking, reading, pantomiming (gesturing), visual matching, and writing. However, only two subtests directly assess the auditory modality, the modality of primary deficit in aphasia according to some aphasiologists (Schuell,

Jenkins, and Jiménez-Pabón 1969). Criticism offered by Boone (1972, pp. 1354–1355) summarizes this weakness.

> There is no way in using the PICA to determine where auditory verbal abilities break down specific for such parameters as length of instruction, complexity of linguistic instruction, auditory memory length, auditory sequencing complexity, etc.

(Berry [1976] has proposed several additional subtests to assess the auditory modality in greater depth using the same PICA test objects and scoring system. This addition may eliminate this major weakness in the PICA.) Overall, however, the PICA possesses a range of task difficulties with which to describe the mildly to severely impaired aphasic patient. This severity range is narrow in the auditory modality. Porch (1971) suggested that a test of aphasia have a relatively large number of homogeneous subtest items per subtest because brain-damaged persons are often inconsistent in their processing and responding. The PICA has 10 homogeneous items per subtest, an apparently adequate number for describing patterns of disturbed processing such as "tuning in" and "fading out" behaviors in aphasic patients (DiSimoni, Keith, Holt, and Darley 1978). It therefore appears adequate in this dimension of aphasia test construction.

Four factors of stimulus selection have been controlled in the construction of the PICA:

1 *Intrasubtest homogeneity* refers to all aspects of the stimulus, i.e., the materials used and the manner in which they are presented. If held constant within a subtest, control of the patient's input and output modalities can be maintained. The same modalities for the input of the instruction and the input for the stimuli and output responses are maintained within each PICA subtest. Porch (1967) conducted a split-half reliability study using odd–even items of each subtest. He also used an analysis of variance combining the results of 30 patients and three scorers. Results demonstrated good internal consistency for each subtest and that the ten PICA items are relatively homogeneous.

2 The homogeneity of items across subtests *(intersubtest homogeneity)* increases the validity of interpretation of performance differences between and among subtests. If changes in performance occur between two subtests, the change can be judged reliably to be the result of a change in modality or the linguistic complexity of the task. This factor is controlled in the PICA and is a potent factor in making the PICA a clinically interpretable test.

3 The stimuli and the tasks to be performed should be as culture-free *(cultural loading)* as possible. Inspection of the ten objects used in all subtests suggests that they are relatively culture-free and free from ambiguity. One possible exception to this is use of the cigarette, which frequently evokes a strong emotional reaction from a patient, either positive or negative. Porch suggests scoring a rejection of that item as an acceptable attempt at doing the task.

4 *Linguistic, educational,* and *IQ loading:* consistent with the cybernetic model on which the PICA is based, the test construction requirements offered by DeRenzi and Vignolo (1962) set another psychometric requirement for judging the adequacy of the PICA. The authors suggest that a test for auditory comprehension (also applicable to the assessment of other modalities) in aphasia should be free

from educational biases and unusual lexical items or syntactic structures since they depend primarily on the experience of the individual. They also suggest that the test should be free from intellectual factors. Duffy, Keith, Shane, and Podraza (1976) found, in their standardization of the PICA on normal subjects, that education was a significant factor for overall and modality scores. The subject education level was specified in the population on which the test was standardized (Porch 1967). It is currently indeterminable whether either of these results is due to the stimulus items or the tasks required, since individual item performance has not been correlated with educational level. There is, however, little reason to suspect that performance on any of the ten items would be affected by educational or intellectual factors. All ten PICA nouns are high and relatively equal in frequency of occurrence in the English language.

The tasks involved in the 18 PICA subtests do not differ markedly from those assessed by most other aphasia test batteries (Schuell 1965; Wepman and Jones 1961; Eisenson 1954; Emerick 1971). All these tests assess the basic language usage tasks of reading, writing, listening, talking, and gesturing. All assess more than one level of difficulty for each of these areas, and all assess different levels of complexity of talking such as naming and sentence usage.

Three subfactors of task selection might be considered in the judgment of the validity and interpretability of the tasks in a test for aphasia:

1   *Intrasubtest homogeneity* refers to the maintenance of the same input modalities for the stimuli and the task instructions, as well as the maintenance of the same task and the same output modality (as well as the same amount of output within that modality) within any given subtest. This homogeneity of tasks, modalities, and amounts of response required allows for intersubtest comparisons to be made, based only on the change of tasks. The PICA has managed to control this factor well. Other tests such as the Language Modalities Test for Aphasia (Wepman and Jones 1961) (qv) and the Minnesota Test for Differential Diagnosis of Aphasia (Schuell 1965) (qv) are deficient in one or more of these intrasubtest homogeneity considerations.

2   *Cultural loading,* as with the stimulus selection considerations, refers to the biasing on a cultural or subcultural level of the test results, due in this instance to the tasks being performed. The PICA appears to be as culture-free as possible and is generally applicable across at least English-speaking American subcultures. The test has been successfully used in England, Australia, and several other countries.

3   If a test for aphasia is free from *linguistic, education,* and *IQ loading,* it is implied that the instructions and the response requested do not include unusual linguistic structures or content, are within range of intellectual normality, and are not influenced by educational factors. The PICA appears to be free of linguistic and intellectual factors. The educational factor was specified in the original 150 patients in the standardization data provided by Porch (1967). In addition, the educational level of these patients was correlated with PICA scores. Nonsignificant and low correlation coefficients were obtained for the mean overall score (.12), mean gestural score (.11), and mean verbal score (−.11). A positive and statistically significant but substantively insignificant correlation of .32 was found for mean graphic scores.

The inconsistency of findings between Duffy et al. (1976) and Porch (1967) relative to the influence of educational level on performance on the PICA might be explained in several ways. Biographical factors such as educational level may be important differential factors for normal performance on the PICA and be inconsequential once the patient becomes aphasic as long as he or she is not illiterate. Further research will have to answer this question; however, the tentative conclusion that the PICA is not biased by educational factors for the aphasic patients seems warranted. Holtzapple (1972) has discussed the influence of total illiteracy on PICA profiles as well as its influence on the validity of PICA predictions. The influence of illiteracy must be considered.

Standardization   The biographical characteristics were specified for each individual in the original 150-subject pool (Porch 1967). The factors of age, race, sex, educational level, occupational status, native language, handedness, etiology, and weeks post onset, as well as the overall time taken to complete the test, were specified. In 1971 the administration, scoring, and interpretation manual was revised and normative data for an additional 130 left hemisphere-damaged patients (total = 280) and 100 bilateral hemisphere-damaged patients were provided. Biographical characteristics of the additional subjects were not described in the revised manual, however.

The task and item instructions are well specified for the administration of the PICA. Deviancy from the standardized manner calls for specification of a nonstandard administration for that test. This type of administration standardization enhances the validity of interpretation of the test results when two different testers administer the test or when the same tester administers it on two separate occasions.

Stimulus presentation has been controlled in PICA administration. Although the arrangement of the stimuli are slightly altered between the first 12 subtests and the final six graphic subtests, the left to right ordering is preserved in both arrangements. This is the usual order that patients follow for the unspecified presentation order in subtests I, II, IV, A, and B.

Normative data are provided in several ways. Volume II (1971) provides for the conversion of gestural, verbal, and graphic modality mean scores into percentile scores. Subtest mean scores are provided at five decile steps. The average of the nine highest and nine lowest subtests and overall mean scores can also be converted to percentile scores. All data were derived from a heterogeneous sample of 280 left hemisphere-damaged aphasic patients. Percentile scores for bilateral hemisphere-damaged aphasic patients are provided at five decile steps for the mean overall, gestural, verbal, and graphic scores as well as for each subtest. These data were derived from a heterogeneous sample of 100 bilateral hemisphere-damaged aphasic patients.

At least three types of reliability should be discussed with the other standardization criteria for any test. *Test–retest reliability:* The test–retest reliability of the PICA, averaged for 40 subjects with two weeks or less elapsed time between tests, was high. Stability coefficients were: overall, .98; gestural, .96; verbal, .99; graphic, .96. Changes that occurred between the first and second tests averaged .38 points and were all in the positive direction, indicating either a small learning effect or the effects of physiological recovery.

Interjudge Reliability   Responses from 30 patients were scored for the entire PICA battery by three trained scorers. Porch (1967) approached the stability of scores in several different ways. First, he found a significant difference between scorers on subtests III, C, and E, using analysis of variance. Scorers also differed significantly on the overall and gestural response levels. Estimates of reliability derived from the analysis of variance data were .93 or above for all individual subtests and .97 or above for overall, gestural, verbal, and graphic response means. It can be concluded that high interjudge reliability can be achieved after 40 hours of training in using the multidimensional scoring system of the PICA.

Intrajudge Reliability This refers to the stability of the scorer, scoring the same behaviors twice on two separate occasions. This necessitates videotaping the test administration and scoring it at two different times. If the test is scored first while administering the test and at a later time from the videotape, the additional variable of *live-versus-video* scoring must be considered unless multiple replays of the tape are prohibited. Neither of these types of scorer reliability has been addressed with the PICA. However, intrajudge reliability can be assumed to be high since test–retest reliability was found to be high.

DiSimoni, Keith, Holt, and Darley (1975) have reported on two shortened forms of the PICA that correlated highly with the overall PICA score. Using stepwise regression analyses on 222 completed PICA's, they found that results from one subtest (I) could predict the overall score about 77 percent of the time ($R = .88$). Results from two subtests (I, VII) predicted the overall about 88 percent of the time ($R = .94$). Three subtests (I, VII, and D) predicted about 94 percent ($R = .97$); four subtests (I, VII, D, VI) predicted about 96 percent ($R = .98$); seven subtests (the above four plus F, II, IV) predicted 98 percent; and ten subtests (the above seven plus B, XII, VIII) predicted the overall 100 percent of the time.

In addition to looking at subtests as a means of shortening the PICA, DiSimoni et al. (1975) evaluated individual PICA items for their power of predictability. Although the ten items are of relatively equal difficulty, the pencil was found to be the most highly predictive ($R = .98$), 96 percent of the time correctly predicting the overall score. The pencil and knife together raised the prediction to 98 percent ($R = .99$). Five items (pencil, knife, comb, cigarette, and quarter) correctly predicted the overall score at a 100 percent level ($R = 1.00$).

These findings strongly suggest that the PICA is redundant for predictability purposes, both across subtests and items within subtests. Item redundancy would be expected since the test was designed for its homogeneity of items. DiSimoni et al. (1975, p. 497) summarize the implications of their findings:

This is not to say that we believe that one can now begin to give only four complete subtests or one or two items across the board and use the formulae to predict overall mean scores. However, it is our belief that a short form of the test can be developed which will predict overall score without significant error. We, of course, can say nothing about the reliability of such a shorter instrument nor about its prognostic value or its usefulness in detecting patterns of patient behavior as these aspects of the test were not explored in this study. . . . What remains is to devise several shortened forms of the PICA, using protocols suggested by the data, and to administer the complete form and shortened forms to aphasic patients. In this way the actual effectiveness of some plausible combinations of subtests can be tested.

In addition to these qualifications of their results, DiSimoni et al. (1975) as well as Porch (1970) suggest that there may be other reasons for maintaining the long form of the PICA. Aphasic patients have been reported to show what Porch (1970) called "tuning in" and "fading out" behaviors during a single subtest. Shortening the PICA to five or fewer items might not allow for those clinically significant patterns to emerge. DiSimoni, Keith, Holt, and Darley (1978) verified that these patterns occur on 11 of the ordered PICA subtests when all ten items are administered. Other patterns of processing deficiency have been described by Brookshire (1972) that might be lost if the number of items was reduced from ten.

Therefore, shortened forms of the PICA are possible to create, standardize, and validate. However, their uses may be more restricted than those of the current test.

Strengths of the Test   The PICA has proven to be a valuable tool for clinical, research, medical–legal, and professional accountability purposes. In its clinical use, it has proven valuable for differentially diagnosing normal subjects from aphasic patients with about 92 percent accuracy (Duffy et al. 1976). Using a discriminant function statistical analysis, Porch, Friden, and Porec (1977) found about a 98 percent accurate differential performance on the PICA between persons "simulating" aphasia or malingering, and real aphasic patients. Porec and Porch (1977) also described unquantified behaviors elicited by the PICA that further differentiated malingerers from aphasic patients.

As a measure of aphasia, the PICA stands alone in its objectivity in helping make treatment decisions. Because of its prognostic power, psychometric construction, and internal consistency, accurate and valid judgments can be made relative to who demonstrates potential for recovery (and therefore who can benefit from treatment) and who does not.

Because of its rigor in holding to psychometric principles of test design, including a highly standardized administration procedure as well as high reliability, the PICA has been used extensively as a dependent measure in research with aphasia. It is currently probably the most widely used research instrument.

Forensic aphasiology, the medical–legal aspects of expert testimony in cases involving aphasia, may well be the responsibility of the speech pathologist, as Rada, Porch, and Kellner (1975) have suggested. The stability of test results, the quantitative nature of the test, and the predictive power offered by the PICA have caused it to be accepted as evidence in court. Information relative to the overall competence of the aphasic patient may be provided by analysis of PICA results, as was demonstrated by Rada et al. (1975). In addition, the PICA's ability to discriminate between malingerers and aphasic patients makes it a tool that appears useful and acceptable as evidence for the expert medical witness.

Decisions regarding third-party payment for speech pathology services require documentation of the positive effects of treatment. The quantified and reliable nature of PICA results has made it an accepted tool for this purpose. As with treatment decisions, the PICA offers valuable guidelines for deciding when further treatment is not beneficial.

Unlike the Boston Diagnostic Aphasia Examination (Goodglass and Kaplan 1972) (qv), little research has been conducted with the PICA relative to describing patterns of behavior for purposes of classifying patients, describing specific aphasic syndromes, or localizing site of lesions. Barnes (1975) has, however, provided some data supporting its usefulness for localizing site of lesion. Wertz, Rosenbek, and Collins (1972) demonstrated that the verbal behavior elicited by the four verbal subtests of the PICA, when used in combination with a battery of verbal tasks designed to elicit apraxia of speech (Wertz and Rosenbek 1971), was sufficient for correct identification of nearly 100 percent of their apraxic population. Johnson and Porch (1968) and Porch (1971a) have described patterns of PICA performance that differentiate left hemisphere-damaged aphasic patients from those with bilateral hemisphere damage. The crucial feature was differential performance on comparable visual and auditory tasks.

The structure of the PICA has provided a basis for plotting and investigating recovery patterns in the aphasic patient. The influence of such factors as illiteracy (Holtzapple 1972) and etiology of aphasia (McNeil 1972) on the recovery patterns has been discussed.

Cautions in PICA Interpretation   Martin (1977) has written a critical essay on the PICA. This reviewer believes that his criticisms (most of which are valid) might better be translated as cautions in interpretation of PICA results, rather than taken as evidence for the PICA's invalidity. The following six interpretation cautions are based upon Martin's (1977) essay:

1   When a task is performed incorrectly or not performed at all, the question should be asked as to whether the patient understands what he or she is being asked to do. Stimulus repetition alone does not ensure understanding. Although the PICA standardization does not allow for practice items, practice on particular items or subtests for familiarization purposes can always be done when the test has been completed. Even the inclusion of sample or practice items on a test does not absolve the tester from responsibility for a thorough evaluation of test performance.

2   While the PICA offers considerable information about structuring therapy for the individual aphasic patient, it does not quantify or even specify all of the important behaviors necessary for treating the patient with aphasia (Porec and Porch 1977). Even if the basic PICA categories were all described in a given response, the terminal PICA score would not always reflect all of the important behaviors of the patient. The experienced PICA tester usually writes down the entire process the patient goes through to arrive at a terminal response. The process is recognized as being equally as important as the product for differential diagnosis, planning therapy, and describing the nature of the deficit.

3   The PICA attempts to assess some of the underlying reasons for communication breakdown through specific modalities. It does not evaluate either unstructured conversational speech or situations in which different modalities are combined for added communicative effectiveness. PICA results projected to these situations must be made with caution.

4   The lack of social intervention by the tester while administering the PICA "may provide less control of the comprehension variable than some tests which allow for intervention" (Martin 1977). However, the ordering of the subtests from least to most information about how to perform the task nearly always eliminates the potential problem of frustration. It should also be noted that explanation of why failure has occurred on a particular response has proven unfruitful (Holland and Sonderman 1974).

5   It is improper to use the mean scores from subtests II, III, V, VI, VII, VIII, X, and XI as a measure of patient's gestural ability. Since these subtests assess pantomime,

reading, auditory comprehension, and picture and object matching, they are obviously not homogeneous as strictly gestural tasks. The gestural modality score may be used only as a mean score against which to measure change; it should not be thought of as representative of a patient's actual gestural abilities.

6 Many different types of behavior and even different processing strategies are subsumed under each category of the scoring system. This occurs because those behaviors are assumed to be at about the same level on the severity continuum. However, as Martin (1977) has noted, this remains an assumption since it has never been addressed either experimentally or on a logical basis.

Summary The PICA is a highly standardized, psychometrically designed test for aphasia. It is based on a model that places the emphasis on processing rather than on linguistic deficits. Its 16-point multidimensional scoring system appears to approximate an equal-appearing interval scale and can therefore be used to quantify aphasic deficits. It has good construct, concurrent, and predictive validity as well as test–retest, interjudge, and intrajudge reliability.

The PICA has proven valuable as a clinical, research, medical–legal, and professional accountability tool. Its purpose of providing a valid, stable means of evaluating patient change and providing a tool for communicating with other professionals about a patient or population of patients has been largely fulfilled. It has been used successfully for differential diagnosis among normal subjects, apraxic patients, and left hemisphere-damaged and bilateral hemisphere-damaged aphasic patients. Its major uses have been for the structure of therapy, plotting and predicting patient recovery, and as a dependent variable in aphasia research.

Although the PICA has good concurrent validity, the degree to which it measures "functional communication" is unresolved. Because of the quantifiable nature of the PICA it is highly susceptible to misuse and misinterpretation. It requires extended training and extreme (possibly more than for other aphasia tests) caution with regard to interpretation of results. An extremely narrow range of subtest difficulty for assessing the auditory modality is a weakness of the test battery, warranting supplementation by additional auditory tests.

References

Barnes, J. E. The PICA as a diagnostic tool in the localization of cerebral function in patients with tumors of the brain. Unpublished Ph.D. Dissertation, Ohio State University, 1975.

Berry, W. R. Testing auditory comprehension in aphasia: a clinical alternative to the Token Test. In R. H. Brookshire (ed.), *Clinical Aphasiology Proceedings*. Minneapolis: BRK Publishers, 1976, pp. 43–63.

Boone, D. R. Porch Index of Communicative Ability. In O. K. Buros, (ed.), *The Seventh Mental Measurements Yearbook. Vol. II.* Highland Park, N. Y.: Gryphon Press, 1972, pp. 1354–1355.

Brookshire, R. H. The role of auditory functions in rehabilitation of aphasic individuals. In T. E. Wertz and M. J. Collins (eds.), *Clinical Aphasiology Conference Proceedings*. Madison: Veterans Administration, 1972, pp. 66–72.

DeRenzi, E. and L. A. Vignolo The Token Test: a sensitive test to detect receptive disturbances in aphasics. *Brain* 85: 556–678, 1972.

DiSimoni, F. G., R. L. Keith, D. L. Holt, and F. L. Darley Practicality of shortening the Porch Index of Communicative Ability. *J. Speech and Hearing Res.* 18: 491–497, 1975.

——— "Tuning in" and "fading out": performance of aphasic patients on ordered PICA subtests. In preparation, 1978.

Duffy, J. R. and B. J. Dale   The PICA scoring scale: Do its statistical shortcomings cause clinical problems? In R. H. Brookshire (ed.), *Clinical Aphasiology Conference Proceedings.* Minneapolis: BRK Publishers, 1977.

Duffy, J. R., R. L. Keith, H. Shane, and B. L. Podraza   Performance of normal (non-brain-injured) adults on the Porch Index of Communicative Ability. In R. H. Brookshire (ed.), *Clinical Aphasiology Conference Proceedings.* Minneapolis: BRK Publishers, 1976, pp. 32–43.

Eisenson, J.   *Examining for Aphasia.* New York: Psychological Corporation, 1954.

Emerick, L. L.   *Appraisal of Language Disturbance.* Marquette: Northern Michigan University Press, 1971.

Goodglass, H. and E. Kaplan   *The Assessment of Aphasia and Related Disorders.* Philadelphia: Lea and Febiger, 1972.

Holland, A. L.   Developing a measure of functional communication adequacy: communication assessment for daily living. Project Report for the National Institute for Neurological and Communicative Disorders and Stroke, 1977.

Holland, A. L. and J. C. Sonderman   Effects of a program based on the Token Test for teaching comprehension skills to aphasics. *J. Speech Hearing Res.* 17: 589–598, 1974.

Holtzapple, P.   The influence of illiteracy on predicting recovery from aphasia. In T. E. Wertz and M. J. Collins, (eds.), *Clinical Aphasiology Conference Proceedings.* Madison: Veterans Administration, 1972, pp. 48–54.

Johnson, M. G. and B. E. Porch   The differential effects of unilateral versus bilateral cerebral lesions on performances involving comparable visual and auditory tasks. Paper presented at the Annual Convention of the American Speech and Hearing Association, Chicago, 1968.

Kaplan, L. T.   A descriptive continuum of language responses in aphasia. *J. Speech Hearing Dis.* 24: 410–412, 1959.

Labovitz, S.   The assignment of numbers to rank order categories. *American Sociological Review* 35: 515–524, 1970.

LaPointe, L. L.   Base 10 programmed stimulation: task specification, scoring, and plotting performance in aphasia therapy. *J. Speech Hearing Dis.* 42: 90–105, 1977.

McNeil, M. R.   Recovery from aphasia resulting from arteriovenous malformation: a report of three cases. In T. E. Wertz and M. J. Collins (eds.), *Clinical Aphasiology Conference Proceedings.* Madison: Veterans Administration, 1972, pp. 113–127.

———, and E. C. Chang   A measure of PICA ordinality. In R. H. Brookshire (ed.), *Clinical Aphasiology Conference Proceedings.* Minneapolis: BRK Publishers, 1975, pp. 113–124.

——— and T. E. Prescott   Assessment of auditory disorders associated with aphasia: The Revised Token Test. Paper presented at the Conference on Clinical Aphasiology, Albuquerque, 1973.

Martin, A. D.   Aphasia testing: a second look at the Porch Index of Communicative Ability. *J. Speech Hearing Dis.* 42: 547–562, 1977.

Porch, B. E.   *Porch Index of Communicative Ability. Volume 1: Theory and Development.* Palo Alto, Calif.: Consulting Psychologists Press, 1967.

———   PICA Brain Teaser. *PICA Talk* 2: 2, 1970.

———   A comparison of unilateral and bilateral PICA profiles on brain-damaged adults. Paper presented at the Annual Convention of the American Speech and Hearing Association, Chicago, 1971a.

———   *Porch Index of Communicative Ability. Volume 2: Administration, Scoring, and Interpretation* (Rev. ed.). Palo Alto, California: Consulting Psychologists Press, 1971b.

———   The use of homogeneous subtest items in assessing aphasia. Paper presented at the Annual Convention of the American Speech and Hearing Association, Chicago, 1971c.

———   Comments on Silverman's "Psychometric Problem." *J. Speech Hearing Dis.* 39: 226–227, 1974.

———, T. Friden, and J. Porec   Objective differentiation of aphasic versus nonorganic patients. Paper presented to the International Neuropsychology Society, Santa Fe, New Mexico, 1977.

Porch, B. E., T. E. Wertz, and M. J. Collins   Recovery of communicative ability: patterns and predictions. Paper presented to the 11th Annual Meeting of the Academy of Aphasia, Albuquerque, 1973.

—— A statistical procedure for predicting recovery from aphasia. In B. E. Porch (ed.), *Clinical Aphasiology Conference Proceedings*. New Orleans: Veterans Administration, 1974, pp. 27–37.

Porec, J. and B. E. Porch   The behavioral characteristics of "simulated" aphasia. In R. H. Brookshire (ed.), *Clinical Aphasiology Conference Proceedings*. Minneapolis: BRK Publishers, 1977, pp. 297–301.

Prescott, T. E. and M. R. McNeil   Measuring the effects of treatment of aphasia. Paper presented at the Conference on Clinical Aphasiology. Albuquerque, 1973.

Rada, R., B. E. Porch, and R. Kellner   Aphasia and the expert medical witness. *Bulletin of American Academy of Psychiatry and the Law* 3: 231–237, 1975.

Schuell, H. M.   *Minnesota Test for Differential Diagnosis of Aphasia*. Minneapolis: University of Minnesota Press, 1965.

Silverman, F. H.   The Porch Index of Communicative Ability (PICA): a psychometric problem and its solution. *J. Speech Hearing Dis.* 39: 225–226, 1974.

Taylor, M. L.   A measure of functional communication in aphasia. *Archives of Physical Medicine and Rehabilitation* 46: 101–107, 1965.

Van Demark, A. A.   Comment on PICA interpretation. *J. Speech Hearing Dis.* 39: 510–511, 1974.

Wepman, J. M. and L. V. Jones   *Studies in Aphasia: An Approach to Testing*. Chicago: Education—Industry Service, 1961.

Wertz, R. T. and J. C. Rosenbek   Appraising apraxia of speech. *J. Col. Speech and Hearing Assoc.* 5: 18–36, 1971.

Wertz, R. T., J. C. Rosenbek, and M. J. Collins   Identification of apraxia of speech from PICA verbal tests and selected oral-verbal apraxia tests. In R. T. Wertz and M. J. Collins (eds.), *Clinical Aphasiology Conference Proceedings*. Madison: Veterans Administration, 1972, pp. 175–190.

SKLAR APHASIA SCALE (SAS)

Maurice Sklar

Western Psychological Services, 1966

Cost $16.50 per complete kit
Manual 23 pages, $3.50; test materials, $8.50;
record booklet, 4 pages, pack of 25 for $3.50

Time 30 to 60 minutes

Harvey Halpern *Queens College of the City University of New York*

Purpose The purpose of the Sklar Aphasia Scale (SAS) is to evaluate objectively speech and language problems caused by brain damage. This is done by examining skills in auditory verbal comprehension, reading comprehension, oral expression, and graphic production.

Administration, scoring, and interpretation The SAS consists of a series of four subtests representing the four language areas listed, each subtest containing 25 items. As an illustration, oral expression is tested by having the patient do the following: name five objects; repeat five single words and sentences; evoke five functional speech responses (name, address, etc.); evoke five sentences after looking at a picture; and evoke five sentences after reading a paragraph.

Scoring is done by rating the patient's response to each test item, either a 0, correct response with no assistance; 1, correct response with assistance; or 2, no response or incorrect response. The scores for each of the 25 items are summed and the total is multiplied by 2, the resultant grand total representing the percentage of impairment for that subtest. For example, if a patient received a 2 on each of the 25 items in a subtest, the total would be 50, multiplied by 2, yielding a score of 100 which represents 100 percent impairment for that subtest. A total language impairment score is obtained by adding the four subtest impairment scores and dividing by 4. The total impairment score is then interpreted as follows: 0-10 percent = no impairment; 11-30 percent = mild impairment; 31-60 percent = moderate impairment; 61-90 percent = severe impairment; 91-100 percent = total or global aphasia. The author claims that on the basis of the total impairment score, a prognosis for recovery can be made: the lower the total impairment score, the better the prognosis.

Evaluation of test adequacy The test manual reports some validity studies (Sklar 1963). One compared the scores of 12 adult aphasic patients on the SAS with scores on three other aphasia tests. Correlations were .92 with Eisenson's Examining for Aphasia (qv); .85 with The Halstead-Wepman Aphasia Screening Test; and .97 with Schuell's Short Examination for Aphasia. These correlations indicate that the SAS is tapping language activity similar to that measured by the other aphasia tests.

Other validity studies (Sklar 1963) discussed in the manual showed that the SAS correlated positively with general intelligence (Wechsler-Bellevue Intelligence Scale), visuomotor perception (Bender Visual Motor Gestalt Test), and the ability to assume the "abstract attitude" (Goldstein–Scheerer Cube Test). Results showed that as language deteriorated, so did general intelligence, visuomotor performance, and ability to abstract. Another study showed that results of the SAS correlated positively with severity of brain damage in the speech areas. An early standardization study involved giving the SAS to 20 adults with no known history of cerebrovascular accidents. Results showed that the SAS pointed to pathology in less than 6 percent of the subjects, indicating that its "language items were within the ability of average adults with eighth grade education or higher."

A study done by Cohen et al. (1977) using a German version of the SAS showed that the test can discriminate between aphasic and normal subjects, aphasic and brain-damaged patients without aphasia, and aphasic patients and chronic schizophrenic patients. However, the SAS did not discriminate between fluent and nonfluent aphasic patients.

The SAS is a highly portable test, easy to administer. Testing time ranges from 30 to 60 minutes, a valuable feature since the test can yield a good deal of information in a relatively short period of time, thus reducing patient fatigue. The simple scoring procedures and the resultant ability to rank patients quantitatively according to degree of impairment at onset of therapy has advantages especially regarding prognosis for rehabilitation.

A limitation of the SAS is that it does not reflect quantitatively what sort of error the patient made, only that the patient was incorrect. For example, it does not differentiate a morphologic-syntactic error (as when the patient says "keys" for "key") from a semantic error (as when the patient says "lock" for "key") in naming objects on the oral expression subtest. This apparent limitation was suggested in the study by Cohen et al. (1977) in which the SAS failed to discriminate between fluent and nonfluent aphasic patients.

Another limitation is found in the section of the oral expression subtest in which the patient is required to repeat after the examiner. The author claims that this section should help diagnose dysarthria and apraxia of speech. Scoring is based upon intelligibility, with the least intelligible response getting the worst score. Intelligibility is an inadequate single basis for differentiating dysarthric patients (with more consistent patterns of articulatory error, no trouble starting, no difference between automatic and volitional speech, and primarily distortion misarticulations) and patients with apraxia of speech (with inconsistent articulatory errors, trouble starting, better production under automatic speech conditions, primarily substitution misarticulations, and intermittent ability to evoke a correct production after a number of faulty attempts).

Summary   The SAS is a valuable diagnostic tool because it is easy to administer, can yield a good deal of information in a relatively short period of time, is easy to score, and yields a quantitative overall impairment rating that may be used as a prognostic indicator for rehabilitation. Although it has limitations in not reporting quantitatively the type of error the patient made and in failing to assess dysarthria and apraxia of speech, the SAS compares quite favorably with the other tests used in aphasia evaluation.

References

Cohen, R., D. Engel, S. Kelter, G. List, and H. Strohner   Validity of the Sklar Aphasia Scale. *J. Speech Hearing Res.* **20**: 146–154, 1977.

Sklar, M.   Relation of psychological and language test scores and autopsy findings in aphasia. *J. Speech Hearing Res.* **6**: 84–90, 1963.

THE TOKEN TEST (TT)

Ennio DeRenzi and Luigi A. Vignolo

Unpublished. The Spreen–Benton form is a subtest in the Neurosensory Center Comprehensive Examination for Aphasia (qv). The Revised Token Test by Malcolm R. McNeil and Thomas E. Prescott is published by University Park Press.

Alternate forms include those of Orgass and Poeck (1966), Boller and Vignolo (1966), Spreen and Benton (1969), and Spellacy and Spreen (1969)

Time 61-item original form, approximately 15 minutes (range from nine to 34 minutes, VA Cooperative Study on Aphasia, 1977b), administration; 5 minutes, scoring

Robert T. Wertz *Veterans Administration Hospital, Martinez, California*

Purpose The Token Test is a measure of auditory comprehension designed to detect mild "receptive" disturbances in aphasic patients who demonstrate no apparent difficulty understanding auditory stimuli contained in traditional tests. Other uses include measuring recovery from and planning treatment for aphasia and assessing development of auditory comprehension in children.

Administration, scoring, and interpretation Berry (1973) estimates that there are at least six forms of the Token Test. All are modifications of the original test developed by DeRenzi and Vignolo (1972). All employ auditory commands requiring the subject to manipulate tokens varying along three dimensions—color, shape, and size.

DeRenzi and Vignolo (1962) developed a five-part Token Test employing 20 tokens. Parts I through IV were comprised of 40 auditory commands, ten in each part, and Part V consisted of 22 commands; however, one was omitted in the initial report. Tokens varied along three dimensions—color, (red, blue, green, yellow, white), shape (circles and rectangles), and size (large and small). Parts I through IV systematically increased the length of the auditory stimulus (e.g., "Pick up the red circle" in Part I was increased to "Pick up the small yellow circle and the large green rectangle" in Part IV). Part V manipulated the syntactic complexity of the auditory stimulus (e.g., "Put the red circle on the green rectangle."). Ten large tokens, five large circles and five large rectangles, were used in Parts I, III, and V. All 20 tokens—five large circles, five small circles, five large rectangles, and five small rectangles—were used in Parts II and IV. Responses, though not specified in the initial report, were scored pass/fail.

Orgass and Poeck (1966) modified the original Token Test slightly by specifying 61 items and the arrangement of the tokens and modifying the scoring system. Patient responses were scored according to each element in each command. For example, "Pick up the *red circle*" could receive a total of 2, 1 for red and 1 for circle, and "Pick up the *small yellow circle* and the *large green rectangle*" could receive a total score of 6. More than 250 errors could be made on the test.

Boller and Vignolo (1966) introduced a second modification. They specified that patients "touch" rather than "pick up" the tokens, scored each item pass/fail, scored items separately when the stimulus was repeated, and returned to the original 62 items.

Spreen and Benton (1969) include a modification of the Token Test in their Neurosensory Center Comprehensive Examination for Aphasia (qv) as a subtest for "Identification by Sentence." They substitute squares for rectangles, use "part" scoring developed by Orgass and Poeck (1966), and reduce the number of items to 39. Six parts are administered, A–F; however, there is no break between parts since all 20 tokens are present in all parts. Auditory stimuli have been changed to "Show me" on Parts A–C and "take" on Parts D and E. The total possible score is 163 points. Instructions are given for discontinuing the test after a specified number of items are failed and for prorating a score based on the number of items completed.

Spellacy and Spreen (1969) selected 16 items from the 39 used by Spreen and Benton to provide a Short Form of the Token Test. Seventy-eight points are possible, using "part" scoring. At least one item is taken from each of the five parts; however, most come from Part F.

Finally, McNeil and Prescott (1973, 1978) have developed a Revised Token Test comprised of ten parts with ten items each. A 15-point multidimensional scoring system similar to that used in the Porch Index of Communicative Ability (qv) is employed to obtain a mean score for each part. Token shape (circles and squares) are standardized as are token color, size, and placement. The length of the auditory commands is systematically manipulated across parts, and Part V of the original De Renzi and Vignolo version is expanded into four parts containing two types of sentences (one with prepositional phrases and one with adverbial clauses) of two different stimulus lengths.

Evaluation of test adequacy   Considerable effort has been exerted to investigate the psychometric properties of the Token Test. Unfortunately, no single version has received a complete psychometric evaluation.

All forms appear valid, since all are reasonably accurate in differentiating aphasic patients from the nonaphasic. Using critical cutoff scores, Orgass and Poeck (1966) differentiated 84 percent of their aphasic patients from normal subjects and nonaphasic brain-injured patients. Spellacy and Spreen (1969) report similar success—89 percent for the Spreen and Benton form and 82 percent for the Short Form. The test, in its various forms, correlates significantly with performance on other measures of aphasia. Swisher and Sarno (1969) found significant correlations between Token Test scores and performance on the Functional Communication Profile (qv). Faglioni, Spinnler, and Vignolo (1969) observed that Token Test performance correlated significantly with a test for identification of meaningful sounds in a group of aphasic patients but not in nonaphasic patients with right hemisphere lesions. And Wertz, Keith, and Custer (1971) report that performance on Part V of the Token Test is significantly correlated with Porch Index of Communicative Ability (qv) overall, gestural, and auditory subtest (VI and X) scores in aphasic patients.

Reliability, expressed by coefficient alpha for the Spreen and Benton version is .95 for "part" scoring and .92 for pass/fail scoring, and reliability on the Short Form is .92 for "part" scoring and .87 for pass/fail scoring (Spellacy and Spreen, 1969). Gallaher (1970) observed acceptable test–retest reliability. Aphasic patients tested three times within eight days produced test–retest correlations ranging from .91 to .98. Even patients in the early stages post onset (28 to 105 days) showed test–retest reliability at .90. Finally, interscorer agreement, reported in the Veterans Administration Cooperative Study (1977a), is .99 for the Boller and Vignolo adaptation.

Several sets of norms are available. Spreen and Benton (1969) provide percentiles for normal subjects and aphasic patients, and Gaddes and Crockett (1973) have collected descriptive data (means and standard deviations) for normal children aged six through 13 years on the 39-item Token Test. Noll (1970) and his colleagues (Noll and Berry 1969; Noll and Lass 1972) also report descriptive data for children. Wertz and Lemme (1974), using the Boller and Vignolo version, list percentiles for normal subjects, aged four through 89 years, and samples of patients with left hemisphere lesions and patients with right hemisphere lesions. And Wertz et al. (1971) provide descriptive data (means, ranges, and standard deviations) on Part V (21 items) of the DeRenzi and Vignolo original form for normal subjects, aged five through 89 years, and percentiles for aphasic patients.

Finally, there is disagreement regarding the relationship between Token Test performance and several variables. Wertz et al. (1971) report a significant correlation between age and Token Test errors in both normal subjects and aphasic patients. Orgass and Poeck (1966) believe age has little influence on Token Test performance in subjects above 15 years. And Swisher and Sarno (1969) observed no influence of age on performance. Some (Orgass and Poeck 1966; Boller and Vignolo 1966) report poorer Token Test performance in aphasic patients with less education. Wertz et al. (1971) found a significant correlation between education and Token Test errors in normal subjects but not in aphasic patients. Swisher and Sarno (1969) report no influence of education on Token Test scores. Sex differences do not appear to influence Token Test performance in adults (Orgass and Poeck 1966) or children (Gaddes and Crockett 1973).

The Token Test appears to do what it was designed to do. It is a sensitive measure for detecting auditory disturbance in aphasia. DeRenzi and Vignolo (1962) found that it identified mild receptive disturbances in patients who had passed other auditory tests. Boller and Vignolo (1966) report that it is more sensitive to mild comprehension deficits than Marie's Three Paper Test.

Several additional clinical advantages have been observed. Orgass and Poeck (1966) believe Token Test performance is a good indication of aphasic severity. However, they found that it did not differentiate among types of aphasia. Similarly Poeck, Kerschensteiner, and Hartje (1972) found that it did not differentiate between fluent and nonfluent aphasic patients. Boller and Vignolo (1966) suggest that scores are not influenced by general intellectual deficit. They found no significant correlations between Token Test performance and Progressive Matrices performance. Further, the Token Test is sensitive to recovery from aphasia. Patients receiving individual or group treatment showed significant linear improvement on the Token Test during the first year postonset (Veterans Administration Cooperative Study 1977b).

Disagreement exists regarding the test's sensitivity to right hemisphere lesions. Aten, Wertz, and Collins (1972) found that left hemisphere patients scored significantly lower on all five parts of the Token Test than right hemisphere patients and normal subjects. No significant differences were observed between the right hemisphere and normal groups. Conversely, Swisher and Sarno (1969) report that their patients with right hemisphere lesions obtained significantly lower overall, Part IV, and Part V scores than their normal group. McClellan, Wertz, and Collins (1973) observed similar results; however, their right hemisphere patients were significantly below normals on Parts III and IV and overall scores. Thus the Token Test may be sensitive to right hemisphere involvement.

S, T, P, and C version does not exist; however, standardized instructions and a · recording responses have been employed in the Veterans Administration Co- e Study on Aphasia (1973).

eral sets of norms exist. For the F, A, and S form, Spreen and Benton (1969) percentiles for normals and aphasic patients, and Gaddes and Crockett (1973) lected descriptive (means and standard deviations) data for normal males and aged six through 13 years. For the S, T, P, and C form, Wertz et al. (1971) orted means, ranges, standard deviations, and percentiles for normal subjects, e through 89 years, and for aphasic patients. Wertz and Lemme (1974) provide les for normal subjects, aged four through 89 years, and for samples of nor- ts, patients with left hemisphere lesions, and patients with right hemisphere

h forms of the test appear to be valid indications of brain injury. All investiga- rkowski et al. 1967; Bechtold, Benton, and Fogel 1962; Fogel 1962; Wertz et ; and Aten, Wertz, and Collins 1972) report poorer performance in brain- ubjects than in normals. Further, Wertz et al. (1971) report that Word Fluency ance by aphasic patients is significantly correlated with Overall and Verbal per- e on the Porch Index of Communicative Ability (qv) and performance on Part Token Test (qv).

t–retest reliability remains to be established. Borkowski et al. (1967) report bal Word Fluency performance by normals is significantly correlated with ke–Lorge norms and estimates derived from the dictionary of the number of the English language beginning with each letter tested. Further, they report tice or fatigue effects in their normal or brain-injured samples. One report ns Administration Cooperative Study on Aphasia 1977a) on interscorer agree- dicates acceptable reliability ($r = .98$).

ally, Word Fluency performance appears to be significantly related to several . Borkowski et al. (1967) report that difficult letters, J and U, are most dis- ing for patients of high intelligence, and, conversely, easy letters, F, S, P, and est for differentiating the brain-injured from normals when both have low in- e. Wertz et al. (1971) report significant correlations between Word Fluency nd years of education in both normal subjects and aphasic patients. Further, served a significant relationship between performance and age in normal sub- t not in aphasic patients.

primary application of the Word Fluency Measure has been to detect brain ll investigators (Borkowski et al. 1967; Aten et al. 1972; Wertz et al. 1971; tz and Lemme 1974) report poorer performance in brain-injured adults than in . Aten et al. (1972) suggest that Word Fluency ability will also differentiate patients with left and right hemisphere lesions. Fogel (1962) believes the ver- of the test is sensitive to parietal lobe involvement; however, Milner (1964), itten production, reported significantly poorer performance in patients with tal lesions than in groups who had sustained either left temporal or right esions. Thus the test may be employed to appraise the presence of brain in- may have use in inter- and intrahemispheric localization.

d Fluency performance improves during recovery from aphasia. Aphasic receiving either individual or group treatment displayed significant linear ment in Word Fluency scores during the first year post onset (Veterans Ad- tion Cooperative Study on Aphasia 1977b). Rosenbek, Wertz, Collins, Green,

West (1973) and Holland and Sonderman (1974) used the Token Test to plan pro- grammed instruction for treating aphasic patients and to measure the results of that treatment. Both observed significant improvement in mild to moderately severely aphasic patients following treatment; however, Holland and Sonderman observed no change in severely aphasic patients. Neither investigator noted dramatic generalization to other "direction-following" tasks.

Gaddes and Crockett (1973) suggest that the Token Test would be an effective measure for studying development of auditory comprehension in children below the age of ten. Noll (1970) and Noll and Berry (1969) have demonstrated that Token Test performance improves during the early elementary school years. And Noll and Lass (1972) have reported possible sociolinguistic applications for the Token Test.

Generally the clinical strengths of the Token Test are those envisioned by its de- velopers, DeRenzi and Vignolo (1962). It requires little time to administer, no elaborate apparatus is necessary, it is not influenced by intelligence, it measures a wide range of linguistic difficulty, and it lacks redundancy. The Token Test will uncover auditory comprehension problems undetected by other measures. Clinical reservations include the fact that its difficulty renders it useless with severely aphasic patients, some syn- tactic constructions in Part V create ambiguity in scoring responses, and there is no es- tablished relationship between performance on the Token Test and "functional" auditory comprehension.

Summary The Token Test is a sensitive measure for detecting minimal auditory com- prehension deficits in aphasia. As such, it provides "top" to an aphasia appraisal bat- tery. It does not replace other measures; it supplements them. No information is obtained concerning a patient's ability to read, speak, or write; the test is confined to evaluating auditory comprehension. Unfortunately, several forms of the Token Test exist. While all are probably valid, sufficient differences among types can create dif- ficulty in interpretation.

References

Aten, J. L., R. T. Wertz, and M. J. Collins The effects of interhemispheric lesions on nonverbal and verbal visual and auditory sequential behavior. Paper presented at the 10th Annual Meet- ing of the Academy of Aphasia, Rochester, October, 1972.

Berry, W. R. A psychometric reconsideration of the Token Test. Paper presented at the Third Annual Conference on Clinical Aphasiology, Albuquerque, March, 1973.

Boller, F. and L. A. Vignolo Latent sensory aphasia in hemisphere-damaged patients: an experi- mental study with the Token Test. *Brain* 89: 815–830, 1966.

DeRenzi, E. and L. A. Vignolo The Token Test: a sensitive test to detect receptive disturbances in aphasics. *Brain* 85: 665–678, 1962.

Faglioni, P., H. Spinnler, and L. A. Vignolo Contrasting behavior of right and left hemisphere- damaged patients on a discriminative and a semantic task of auditory recognition. *Cortex* 5: 366–389, 1969.

Gaddes, W. H. and D. J. Crockett The Spreen–Benton Aphasia Test, normative data as a measure of normal language development. Research Monograph No. 25, Neuropsychology Laboratory, University of Victoria, 1973.

Gallaher, A. J. Temporal reliability of aphasic performance on the Token Test. Masters Thesis, Minneapolis: University of Minnesota, March, 1970.

Holland, A. L. and J. C. Sonderman Effects of a program based on the Token Test for teaching comprehension skills to aphasics. *J. Speech Hearing Res.* 17: 589–598, 1974.

McClellan, M. E., R. T. Wertz, and M. J. Collins   The effects of interhemispheric lesions on central auditory behavior. A paper presented at the American Speech and Hearing Association Convention, Detroit, October, 1973.

McNeil, M. R. and T. E. Prescott   *Revised Token Test.* Baltimore: University Park Press, 1978.

—— Assessment of auditory deficits associated with aphasia: the Revised Token Test. A paper presented at the Third Conference on Clinical Aphasiology, Albuquerque, March, 1973.

Noll, J. D.   The use of the Token Test with children. A paper presented at the American Speech and Hearing Association Convention, New York, November, 1970.

—— and W. R. Berry   Some thoughts on the Token Test. *Journal of the Indiana Speech and Hearing Association* 27: 37–40, 1969.

—— and N. D. Lass   Use of the Token Test with children: two contrasting socioeconomic groups. A paper presented at the American Speech and Hearing Association Convention, San Francisco, November, 1972.

Orgass, B. and K. Poeck   Clinical validation of a new test for aphasia: an experimental study of the Token Test. *Cortex* 2: 222–243, 1966.

Poeck, K., M. Kerschensteiner, and W. Hartje   A quantitative study on language understanding in fluent and nonfluent aphasia. *Cortex* 8: 299–304, 1972.

Spellacy, F. J. and O. Spreen   A short form of the Token Test. *Cortex* 5: 390–397, 1969.

Spreen, O. and A. L. Benton   *Neurosensory Center Comprehensive Examination for Aphasia.* Victoria, B. C.: Neuropsychology Laboratory, Department of Psychology, University of Victoria, 1969.

Swisher, L. P. and M. T. Sarno   Token Test scores of three matched patient groups: left brain-damaged with aphasia; right brain-damaged without aphasia; nonbrain-damaged. *Cortex* 5: 264–273, 1969.

Veterans Administration Cooperative Study on Aphasia, *Progress Report,* May, 1977a.

—— *Progress Report,* September, 1977b.

Wertz, R. T., R. L. Keith, and D. D. Custer   Normal and aphasic behavior on a measure of auditory input and a measure of verbal output. A paper presented at the American Speech and Hearing Association Convention, Chicago, November, 1971.

Wertz, R. T. and M. L. Lemme   Input and output measures with aphasic adults. Research and Training Center 10, Final Report, Social Rehabilitation Services, Washington, D. C., 1974.

West, J. A.   Auditory comprehension in aphasic adults: improvement through training. *Arch. Phys. Med. Rehab.* 54: 78–86, 1973.

WORD FLUENCY MEASURE (WF)

John G. Borkowski, Arthur L. Benton, and Otfried Spreen

Unpublished. Incl[...]
Neurosensory Cen[...]
tion for Aphasia, [...]
Alternate forms i[...]
T, P, and C."

Time "F, A, and [...]
tration; five minu[...]
four minutes, ad[...]
scoring

Robert T. Wertz   *Veterans Administration Hospital, Martinez, Califo[...]*

Purpose   The Word Fluency Measure is a controlled associat[...] the subject to produce as many words as possible beginning v[...] the alphabet over a given period of time. It is used to apprais[...] injured adults, particularly aphasic patients. Other applicatio[...] of the development of verbal fluency in children and chartin[...] tivity in aphasia.

Administration, scoring, and interpretation   At least two vers[...] Measure exist. Spreen and Benton (1969) include Word Flue[...] Neurosensory Center Comprehensive Examination for Apha[...] instructed to say as many words as he or she can think of in [...] with a letter of the alphabet specified by the examiner. Prop[...] word with a different ending are not permitted. Three letters[...] The patient's score is the sum of all admissible words for the [...] education corrections are applied and a percentile is obtain[...] norms are provided for aphasic and normal performance.

A second version, developed at Mayo Clinic, utilizes the [...] letters (S, T, P, C) are used, and proper names are permitted.[...] sum of all admissible words for the four letters. No correctio[...] education. Wertz and Lemme (1974) and Wertz, Keith, and C[...] mative data for this version for samples of patients with left [...] tients with right hemisphere lesions and age norms (four thro[...] subjects.

A written form of the Word Fluency Measure, attributed[...] employed by Milner (1964). The subject is given five minute[...] as possible beginning with the letter S. Then four minutes are[...] words beginning with C. The score is the total number of wo[...] vides no norms.

Evaluation of test adequacy   There is a paucity of psychome[...] on the Word Fluency Measure, and few attempts have been n[...] or reliability. Patient instructions, a form for recording respo[...] ing, and percentile ranks for normal subjects and aphasic pati[...] Neurosensory Center Comprehensive Examination for Aphas[...] (Spreen and Benton 1969) for the F, A, and S form of the te[...]

for the[...]
form f[...]
operati[...]

Se[...]
provid[...]
have c[...]
female[...]
have re[...]
aged fi[...]
percen[...]
mal ad[...]
lesions[...]

Bo[...]
tors (B[...]
al. 197[...]
injured[...]
perforr[...]
formar[...]
V of th[...]

Te[...]
that ve[...]
Thorne[...]
words [...]
no pra[...]
(Vetera[...]
ment i[...]

Fi[...]
variabl[...]
crimina[...]
T, are [...]
telliger[...]
ability [...]
they ol[...]
jects b[...]

Th[...]
injury. [...]
and We[...]
norma[...]
betwee[...]
bal for[...]
using v[...]
left fro[...]
fronta[...]
jury ar[...]

W[...]
patien[...]
improv[...]
minist[...]

and Flynn (1977) observed improvement in Word Fluency in an aphasic patient receiving treatment to resolve anomia. The test, therefore, appears to have value in measuring recovery from aphasia.

Normative data collected on children (Gaddes and Crockett 1973; Wertz et al. 1971; and Wertz and Lemme 1974) show that Word Fluency ability improves from age four through age 13. The measure could be used, therefore, to determine acquisition of verbal skills in children. There are, however, no reports of this application.

A potential strength of the measure is its ability to assess mild aphasia. Since the patient is limited only by his or her ability and the temporal constraints of the test, mildly aphasic patients can demonstrate performance not permitted by many traditional aphasia tests. For example, mildly aphasic patients who are 100 percent correct on traditional tests may show Word Fluency performance that transcends moderate involvement but falls short of normal. Thus the Word Fluency Measure provides "top" to aphasia appraisal batteries. Unfortunately, however, the range of ability demonstrated by normal subjects (Wertz and Lemme 1974) limits this application.

A limitation of the test is its difficulty for many aphasic patients. For example, the norms provided by Spreen and Benton (1969) indicate that 90th percentile performance by aphasic patients is essentially similar to 18th and 20th percentile performance by normal subjects. Further, production of a single word places the patient between the 30th and 35th percentiles on the Wertz et al. (1971) norms. Thus it is not very useful with severely aphasic patients.

Summary The Word Fluency Measure, a test of verbal output requiring subjects to state all of the words they can think of in one minute beginning with a letter of the alphabet designated by the examiner, is a sensitive indication of brain injury. Performance is influenced by intelligence and education. It is useful as part of a battery of tests to evaluate aphasia. Performance is significantly related to scores obtained on other measures of aphasia. However, it provides a limited measure of verbal skills, and there is no evidence that what is being measured is essential in functional communication. Further, the reliability of scores obtained is yet to be demonstrated.

References

Aten, J. L., R. T. Wertz, and M. J. Collins   The effects of interhemispheric lesions on nonverbal and verbal visual and auditory sequential behavior. Paper presented at the 10th Annual Meeting of the Academy of Aphasia, Rochester, October, 1972.

Bechtoldt, H. P., A. L. Benton, and M. L. Fogel   An application of factor analysis in neuropsychology. *Psychol. Rec.* 12: 147–156, 1962.

Borkowski, J. G., A. L. Benton, and O. Spreen   Word fluency and brain damage. *Neuropsychologia* 5: 135–140, 1967.

Fogel, M. L.   The Gerstmann syndrome and the parietal symptom-complex. *Psychol. Rec.* 12: 85–99, 1962.

Gaddes, W. H. and D. J. Crockett   The Spreen–Benton Aphasia Test, normative data as a measure of normal language development. Research Monograph No. 25, Neuropsychology Laboratory, University of Victoria, 1973.

Milner, B.   Some effects of frontal lobectomy in man. In J. M. Warren and K. Akert (eds.), *The Frontal Granular Cortex and Behavior.* New York: McGraw-Hill, 1964, pp. 313–334.

Rosenbek, J. C., E. F. Green, M. Flynn, R. T. Wertz, and M. J. Collins   Anomia: a clinical experiment. In R. H. Brookshire (ed.), *Clinical Aphasiology Conference Proceedings.* Minneapolis: BRK Publishers, 1977, pp. 103–111.

Spreen, O. and A. L. Benton *Neurosensory Center Comprehensive Examination for Aphasia.* Victoria, B. C.: Neuropsychology Laboratory, Department of Psychology, University of Victoria, 1969.

Veterans Administration Cooperative Study on Aphasia, *Protocol Manual,* 1973.

——, *Progress Report,* May, 1977a.

——, *Progress Report,* September, 1977b.

Wertz, R. T., R. L. Keith, and D. D. Custer Normal and aphasic behavior on a measure of auditory input and a measure of verbal output. Paper presented at the American Speech and Hearing Association Convention, Chicago, November, 1971.

Wertz, R. T. and M. L. Lemme Input and output measures with aphasic adults. Research and Training Center 10, Final Report, Social Rehabilitation Services, Washington, D.C., 1974.

Part V
Other Appraisal
Instruments

Introduction

The tests covered in this Part are those pertaining to stuttering, voice disorders, and basic concepts. Included, also, are a coding test and a developmental scale.

Considering the voluminous literature, both research and speculative, that exists about stuttering, it is rather curious that the only standardized tests are two attitude scales, one not adequately standardized and the other in need of more work, as indicated by the reviewers. Even if adequately standardized, attitude scales about stuttering would find no more than a limited place in the assessment batteries of some speech–language pathologists and none at all in the repertoire of others. They are not addressed to the kinds of observable behaviors that are ordinarily the target of therapy, and their diagnostic significance or predictive value has not been demonstrated.

What has long been needed in the area of stuttering are predictive tests. The speech–language pathologist needs to be able to identify at an early age those children who are likely to continue to be disfluent. Spontaneous remission rates are known to be high, and it would be useful to be able to predict which school-age children can be expected to stop stuttering and to know with what degree of confidence such predictions can be made. In some respects, this neglect seems almost irresponsible. Two factors are probably responsible. As long as the diagnosogenic theory of the etiology of stuttering was the theory of currency, interest in parental attitude rather than the stuttering behavior of children per se was necessarily the focus of attention. Perhaps more importantly, the development of such predictive tests would require longitudinal studies, which are inefficient and expensive. Some considerable effort would be needed to find and follow a population of sufficient size to develop and standardize such instruments.

Recognizing that some theories about the nature of stuttering would rule out differential approaches to the diagnosis and treatment of stuttering, it seems surprising that more effort has not been directed to the exploration of differences observable at onset or subsequently and what these differences might imply for treatment. Specifically, Van Riper has described four tracks of stuttering from onset to final development. It seems possible that a standardized approach to the collection and verification of these as well as other observations and subsequent development of a test with known reliability and validity would contribute to differential diagnosis and thereafter to the development and evaluation of differential treatment.

In the area of voice disorders, the need for standardized tests seems less apparent. Typically, a fairly uniform format of observations to be made is followed for assessment purposes. Criteria have been established for breath control and natural optimum pitch. Clinics with well equipped laboratories have a variety of instruments, such as those for making spectrograms and analyzing fundamental frequency. Many voice problems have physiologic correlates that are diagnostically significant.

The Wilson system is not a standardized test in the usual sense, but rather a more exacting classification system than the descriptive nomenclature usually employed. The published material is addressed to remediation; thus a fuller description of the reliability and validity of the classification system is not readily available. The system does address a significant problem in that it provides a means of "calibrating" the ears of the clinician. As indicated by the reviewer, the amount of time required to become competent with the system is uncertain. Whether this question reflects an innate difficulty in developing the listening skills necessary to make the kinds of judgments required or whether the training materials need revision so the learner may progress from gross to increasingly refined discriminations only further study can reveal.

The two "language" tests included here represent a somewhat different approach to sampling certain aspects of language in that they deal with restricted sets. That is, in comparison with tests that attempt to determine the extent of an individual's vocabulary or whose items have been selected as representative of certain concepts from which one can infer an understanding of similar concepts (comparative forms, for example), these tests are limited to a set of items selected as those requisite for success in particular grades. They were derived from what amounts to a task analysis. The problem addressed is not one of determining the extent of a repertoire, but rather whether the individual can do specific things or has specific understandings.

This approach is consonant with the philosophy of criterion-referenced instruction. Within this frame of reference, a test would not necessarily need to be standardized. It would have a parochial quality, as it would be developed for a specific situation, and it follows that one teaches to the test. Englemann is avowedly of this point of view; at least he was at the time the Basic Concept Inventory was published. However, the test with its "Fends" and "bizzers" is not consistently representative of this genre of tests. In any event, the test appears to have been abandoned by its author. It remains in its field edition, and reliability data, promised for 1968, have not appeared.

Evidently Boehm's intent was of broader scope, but certainly the approach to the selection of test items for the Boehm Test of Basic Concepts was of the task-analysis type. The approach has merit in that this type of test clearly identifies specific concepts within a specified set that have not yet been mastered. Whether it is appropriate to teach directly to the test items, as one would when using a criterion test, is open to question, as the reviewer points out in her discussion.

Coding or substitution tests are generally regarded as measuring one of a number of aspects of intelligence. Nonetheless, a symbol–digit test has been included (The Symbol Digit Modalities Test). Its purported usefulness as a large group screening test for minimal brain damage and learning disabilities as well as the claim for its application in cases of aphasia and other language and speech disorders warrants evaluation.

Finally, among the several published developmental scales, only one was included for review. The Denver Developmental Screening Test has brevity and ease of administration in its favor. It provides insights into other aspects of development of young children, though the speech–language pathologist probably will not be entirely satisfied with the language section according to the reviewer. With new mandates to provide service to very young, developmentally disabled children, the demand for developmental scales is likely to increase. Whether the speech–language pathologist will be called on to administer them or simply use the information from them supplied by professionals in other disciplines remains to be seen. Certainly, speech–language pathologists need a working knowledge of scales of this sort.

Maryjane Rees

BASIC CONCEPT INVENTORY (BCI)

Siegfried Englemann

Follett Educational Corporation, Field research edition, 1967

Cost $36.00

Manual, 48 pages, $3.60; picture cards, set of 9 for $3.60; test booklet, 7 pages, pack of 15 for $5.22

Time 20 minutes, administration; less than a minute, scoring

Katharine G. Butler *San Jose State University*

Purpose The author states that the purpose of the Basic Concept Inventory is to provide "a broad checklist of basic concepts that are involved in new learning situations in the first grade" (Manual, p. 1). In addition, he notes that the inventory has two functions: (1) to evaluate the instruction in certain beginning academically related concepts in terms of group instruction, and (2) to evaluate the instruction given to an individual child. Parenthetically, he indicates that a third function might be to group children based on BCI scores. Finally, the author states that the test is designed to be used for special groups of children (the culturally disadvantaged, slow learners, emotionally disturbed, and mentally retarded).

Administration, scoring, and interpretation According to the author, the BCI may be administered either by a trained examiner or a classroom teacher. If the test results are to be used diagnostically or for special placement of an individual child, it is recommended that a trained examiner administer it. If, on the other hand, the purpose is remedial instruction, a teacher will "probably gain a great deal of insight" (Manual, p. 5). It is not clear from the teacher's manual (which serves as the test manual) what the qualifications of the trained examiner might be. A review of the actual items indicates that the BCI might be appropriately used and interpreted by a speech–language pathologist or a psychologist. However, most of the manual is directed toward teaching young children certain linguistic forms. As the author notes, a more complete discussion of the content of instruction is contained in *Teaching Disadvantaged Children in the Preschool* by Bereiter and Englemann (1966).

The BCI is composed of three parts and 21 major items with several subitems for a total of 90 possible responses. It must be individually administered, and the author states that the typical administration time is 20 minutes. Part One requires the child to respond by pointing to pictures and by giving verbal responses to such questions as "Do you know which boy is the tallest?" The first 35 items require the child to point to an object or a person or to several objects or persons. The examiner asks, "Find the ones that cannot see," "Find the balls that are not white," or "Find the one that does not talk and does not bark." The final items in Part One require the child to hold up a hand, to hold up both hands, to touch an ear, and to touch both ears. Fifty-one of the 90 responses are within Part One of the test. The author indicates that the rationale behind the tasks in Part One is that the child should be able to follow basic instructions and should understand the content words utilized in those instructions. The concepts tested relate to plurals, the *not* concept, full statements as criteria for selection, and those stimuli that do not provide enough information to identify a particular object.

Part Two evaluates the child's ability to repeat statements and to answer the questions that are implied by those statements. The possible number of responses is 24, and the statements and questions include: "Listen: The bread is under the oven. Where is the bread? The bread is under the oven. Is the oven under the bread?" or "Listen: His present will be a dog or a bike. Say it. His present will be a dog or a bike. What do you think will happen? Will he get a dog? Will he get a bike?" The final two items in the section utilize such concepts as "Fends cannot crump. Say it. Fends cannot crump. Can fends crump? What can't fends do?" and "Only granders have bizzers. How could you tell a grander if you saw one? Only granders have bizzers. What's the only thing that has bizzers?" The author notes that the rationale for these items is that "statements that are used in everyday language and in the classroom should be familiar to the child," and views this section as a sentence repetition and comprehension task. Part Three (15 items) labeled "Pattern Awareness" requires the child to slap the table and clap, to repeat numbers such as 2-2, 8-8, 5-5, and to blend three words (flow—er, m—ilk, ta—ble).

The scoring of the 90 items is such that a low score indicates a high performance level; that is, no points are scored if a child successfully repeats a statement on the first trial, one point is given for success on the second trial, and so on. The examiner is required to make a judgment about the presence or absence of negative elements (*not* concept) or proper inflection ("*Fend* cannot crump" and "*Fends* cannot crump" are both considered correct).

Interpretation of the results is largely qualitative, although the author states that a child who misses 40 or more of the 90 items will probably have difficulty in new learning situations. The manual also notes that the type of analysis required to interpret performance contraindicates computing the subscores for the three areas. Six cases are presented, indicating how the performance on the three areas evaluated might be utilized.

Evaluation of test adequacy An evaluation of the appropriateness of this test is limited by the fact that it is an experimental edition and, as the author notes on page 44 of the manual, "BCI is published without sufficient validity and reliability data, and without age norms." The author declares that age norms are really inappropriate and are in reality "achievement norms." He also notes on page 45 that adequate data on reliability "will probably be available in 1968." Finally, he reports that predictive validity and construct validity for the BCI have not been established. Criterion-related validity is not reported in any statistical form, and it is difficult for the reader to determine what confidence can be placed in judgments or predictions regarding the individual child tested.

The BCI may be more useful to the classroom teacher, who utilizes the teaching methods advocated in the Bereiter and Englemann text, than to the speech–language pathologist attempting to analyze a child's language performance. This instrument was utilized to some extent during the early 1970s but with the advent of language sampling techniques, preschool language assessment strategies, and the requirements of nondiscriminatory evaluation of handicapped children, its clinical usefulness in linguistic analyses has decreased.

Over the past decade there has been a tremendous increase in the number and types of instruments to measure language and cognitive skills. The reader is referred to Carroll and Freedle's (1972) text, *Language Comprehension and the Acquisition of*

Knowledge, for an overview of those topics and to Lloyd's (1976) *Communication Assessment and Intervention Strategies* for a review of language assessment procedures and programs.

Summary The usefulness of the BCI with special groups of handicapped children is restricted due to the lack of reliability, validity, and age norms and due to the structure of the items themselves, and the level of interpretation that can be derived from a child's performance on the inventory. As the author indicates, "The various tasks in the Inventory do not measure deficits of equal severity. It is possible for a child to miss 25 tasks on the Inventory and have a deficit far more severe than another child who has the same score" (Manual, p. 17). In addition, the "concepts" measured by the tasks provided are of limited scope in evaluating a child's linguistic or cognitive status.

References

Bereiter, C. and S. Englemann *Teaching Disadvantaged Children in the Preschool.* Englewood Cliffs, N. J.: Prentice-Hall, 1966.

Carroll, J. B. and R. O. Freedle (eds.) *Language Comprehension and the Acquisition of Knowledge.* New York: Halsted Press, 1972.

Englemann, S. *The Basic Concept Inventory Teacher's Manual.* Chicago: Follett Educational Corporation, 1967.

Lloyd, L. L. (ed.) *Communication Assessment and Intervention Strategies.* Baltimore: University Park Press, 1976.

BOEHM TEST OF BASIC CONCEPTS (BTBC)

Ann E. Boehm

The Psychological Corporation, Revised edition, 1971
Two equivalent forms, A and B

Cost $7.75

Manual, 30 pages, $.75; test forms, 8 pages, pack of 30 including 1 copy each of directions, class record form, and key, $7.00; directions, $.25; class record form with key (specify form), $.30; Spanish directions (specify form), $.50.

Time 15–20 minutes per booklet (two for each form), administration; less than 5 minutes, scoring

Elaine P. Hannah *California State University, Northridge*

Purpose The Boehm Test of Basic Concepts (BTBC) is a screening device developed to meet a perceived need for assessment in the cognitive area. The test is composed of 50 items arranged in order of ascending difficulty and is divided into two booklets of 25 items each. The items are said to be suitable for a population of kindergarten to second grade children. Two equivalent forms are available as is a Spanish version of the administration procedure. The test originated with observations by the author that many children arrive at the kindergarten level without an adequate understanding of certain basic concepts which are presumed to be developed by most of the work materials for this level.

Administration, scoring, and interpretation The concepts included in the test are those commonly found in work materials at the preschool and primary grade levels. For each test item or concept, three to six pictures are supplied. The subject is to mark his or her choice with an X after listening to a simple set of verbalized instructions. Usually three or four sets of items appear on each page. Step by step instructions are clear and explicit; the black-and-white pictures are simple and realistic, and distracting clutter is held to a minimum. Three sample questions for initial practice are supplied. The subject receives a point for each correct answer, and the score is compared with normative data that are given in terms of percentages of subjects passing the test at the various age and score levels. Such results may be compared individually, as indicated, or across the total group. Thus one may examine the individual score in terms of age level normative data or relate such a score to the scores achieved by other members of his or her own environmental group. One may thereby identify the individual child who demonstrates a conceptual lag, or identify a lag in the development of specific concepts across a group of children. Deficits can also be identified with the subcategory areas suggested by the author: space, quantity, time, and miscellaneous.

Evaluation of test adequacy Knowledgeable professionals (Proger 1970; Noll 1970; Dahl 1973) generally agree that the reliability data for the BTBC are adequate, Split-half reliability is reported to be within the range of .68 to .90. Split-half equivalence data for each booklet of Form A are listed as approximately .50, with alternate form reliability ranging from .55 to .92.

The validity data are less adequate. Boehm states simply that the concepts chosen are those most frequently found in the academic materials at the early elementary and preschool levels and that they represent abstract ideas or concepts. Recent research by Estes and others (1976), however, indicates that the BTBC scores correlate adequately with appropriate Stanford Achievement Test scores (.39 to .56). This supports Boehm's earlier observation that mastery of the basic concepts is related to academic achievement in the first years of school. Further studies of validity are definitely needed.

Several studies involving the use of the BTBC with differing populations have also been made. The original standardization group was largely eastern and urban. Independent pieces of research indicate that the BTBC is, to a certain extent, culture bound. The study of Mickelson and Galloway (1973) on an American Indian population indicates a significantly different pattern of concept development within this group. This is true, also, of the study by Houck, Biskin, and Regetz (1973) on a rural population. Both substantiate the use of the test as an indicator of directions that might be pursued in terms of classroom training for more adequate use of standardized academic materials. However, normality of development for any one individual must be examined in terms of a comparison with the scores of his or her own culture group.

Other features of the test must also be examined. Although the test items are designed to be within the capabilities of children whose ages range from kindergarten to second grade, the test has, at times, been found to be too easy for groups of higher socioeconomic second and late first grade children. Also some reviewers (e.g., McCandless 1972) feel that the possibility of using it as a group testing measure at the kindergarten level is not realistic without a great deal of assistance. There is also some feeling that an extension into the preschool years, during which much of the preventive type testing is now being done, would be valuable.

Studies still need to be made relating to its use with children who are not developing normally. The test format itself relies totally on the child's ability to attend to a series of pictures on a page. How this would affect the performance of a hyperkinetic child with a visual problem but adequate conceptual development is not certain. Only one study (Ault and others 1977) has investigated the differences between a two-dimensional presentation and a three-dimensional presentation. While final scores did not show a significant difference between the two presentations, it must again be observed that the subject group was a normally developing one.

Boehm also makes some suggestions about the extension of the BTBC into the classroom training situation. This area of application needs a great deal of further investigation. Since most of the concepts being tested are actually representations of a more basic level of cognitive functioning, which may or may not have been achieved, attempts to train specific concepts rather than the total thought processes basic to such concepts may not be the most effective or valid route to take.

Summary   The Boehm Test of Basic Concepts is a screening device with a good potential for indicating the child who is lagging conceptually. Further investigation will usually be needed to indicate whether the deficit is a cultural difference or a true cognitive lag. The test is well structured, is simple in format, and can be given with minimal possibility for administrative error. Therefore, it performs a useful role in the clinical diagnostic area.

References

Ault, R. L., C. C. Cromer, and C. Mitchell   The Boehm Test of Basic Concepts: a three-dimensional version. *J. Educ. Res.* **70**: 186–188, 1977.

Dahl, T. A.   Review of the Boehm Test of Basic Concepts. *Meas. Eval. Guidance* 6: 63–65, 1973.

Estes, G. D., J. Harris, F. Moers, and D. Wodrich   Predictive validity of the Boehm Test of Basic Concepts for achievement in first grade. *Educ. Psych. Meas.* **36**: 1031–1035, 1976.

Houck, C. K., D. S. Biskin, and J. Regetz   A comparison of urban and rural reliability estimates for the Boehm basic concept test. *Psych. Schools* **10**: 430–432, 1973.

McCandless, G.   Review of the Boehm Test of Basic Concepts. In O. K. Buros (ed.), *The Seventh Mental Measurements Yearbook*. Highland Park, N. J.: Gryphon, 1972.

Mickelson, N. I. and C. G. Galloway   Verbal concepts of Indian and non-Indian school beginners. *J. Educ. Res.* **67**: 55–56, 1973.

Noll, V. H.   Review of the Boehm Test of Basic Concepts. *J. Educ. Meas.* **7**: 139–140, 1970.

Proger, B. B.   Test review number 2—The Boehm Test of Basic Concepts. *J. Spec. Ed.* **4**: 249–251, 1970.

DENVER DEVELOPMENTAL SCREENING TEST (DDST)

William K. Frankenburg, Josiah B. Dodds, Alma W. Fandal, Elynor Kazuk, and Marlin Cohrs

LADOCA Project and Publishing Foundation, Revised edition, 1975
Spanish version available

Cost $13.00
Reference manual, 75 pages, $4.00, Spanish version, $4.50; manual workbook, 114 pages, $6.00; test kit (without forms and manual) $7.00; test forms, Engiish or Spanish, 1 page, pack of 100 for $2.00.
Prescreening questionnaire, pads of 100 for $3.00. Separate forms for each of five age groups: 3-5, 9-12, and 16-24 months; 3-4 and 5-6 years

Time 10-20 minutes, administration; 5-10 minutes, scoring

Robert D. Hubbell *California State University, Sacramento*

Purpose The Denver Developmental Screening Test is designed as a screening tool to aid in the early detection of delayed development in young children.

Administration, scoring, and interpretation The test consists of a manual, score sheet, and eight stimulus items, such as wool, raisins, a rattle, and one-inch blocks. After training, an individual can administer the test using the score sheet without reference to the manual. Certain items on the score sheet are footnoted to specific instructions on the reverse side of the sheet. A number of items are marked with an "R," indicating that they can be scored on the basis of a report from the parent, although actual observation of the behavior is recommended.

In terms of content, the test is divided into four sectors: Personal–Social, Fine Motor–Adaptive, Language, and Gross Motor. Examples of the Personal–Social sector are as follows: *smiles spontaneously, works for toy out of reach, removes garments, separates from mother easily.* The Fine Motor–Adaptive sector includes items such as *follows (with gaze) to midline, regards raisin, dumps raisin from bottle, draws man.* The Gross Motor sector samples such items as *rolls over, walks backward, hops on one foot.* The Language sector contains 21 items. Representative items for the first year of life are *laughs, turns to voice, imitates speech sounds,* says *dada or mama (specific).* Comprehension and expression at succeeding ages are assessed with items such as *points to one named body part; uses plurals, gives first and last name, comprehends cold, tired, hungry, and opposite analogies.* The bulk of the items represent semantic knowledge with relatively few items pertaining to syntax or articulation.

The test is administered with the parent present as well as the child. Testing continues until all items at the child's age level have been given, and at least three items passed and three items failed in each of the four sectors. Each item administered is marked in one of four categories: pass, fail, refuse, and no opportunity to perform the item.

The score sheet is constructed so that the normative data for each item are represented in terms of the ages at which 25, 50, 75, and 90 percent of the normative group passed that item. Comparison of a child's performance on individual items with that of the normative sample is easily accomplished through visual inspection. The results of testing may be assigned one of three interpretations: *abnormal,* in which two sectors each have two or more delays, or one sector has two or more delays and one other sector has one delay and in the same sector no item is passed at the child's age level; *questionable,* in which there are two or more delays in one sector, or one or more sectors have one delay and in the same sector(s) no item is passed at the child's age level; and *normal,* in which none of the preceding patterns is found. It is recommended that children whose performance is interpreted as abnormal or questionable be retested in two or three weeks. If the child's performance is found to be at the same level, and the parents indicate that the observed behavior is typical of the child, a referral to a physician should be made.

Evaluation of test adequacy   The DDST was standardized on a sample of 1036 normal children from the Denver area (Frankenburg and Dodds 1967). The subjects were selected to approximate the demographic characteristics of Denver in terms of occupational and ethnic groups according to the 1960 census. The age range was from 16 days to 72 months. Groups of approximately 40 children were tested at each month of age from one to 15 months, at three-month intervals from 15 to 24 months, and at larger intervals from 24 to 72 months. More specific information about the sample is included in the manual so that the individual user can judge the appropriateness of the standardization sample for evaluating specific groups of children the test user may encounter in local clinical applications.

Insufficient data on reliability are included in the manual. In a study reported elsewhere (Frankenburg, Camp, Van Natta, Demersseman, and Voorhees 1971), interexaminer agreement on individual items ranged from 81 to 100 percent ($N = 76$), and test–retest reliability, with a span of one week between administrations, produced Pearson product–moment correlations ranging from .66 to .91. Reliability was poorer with children in their first two years and better with older children. The items with high stability included many that could be passed by parental report, thus making the reliability of the DDST partially dependent on the reliability of parental reporting in general. The reliability of parental reporting was demonstrated empirically by Frankenburg, van Doorninck, Liddell, and Dick (1976). They devised a questionnaire in which DDST items were rewritten so they could be directly administered to mothers. The mothers consistently evaluated their children as being more advanced than did trained aides evaluating the same children with the questionnaire.

A validity study was also published separately from the manual (Frankenburg, Camp, and Van Natta 1971), although some of these data are reported in an appendix to the manual. Scores for 236 children on the DDST were compared with scores on one of the following tests: Stanford–Binet, the Bailey and Cattell scales, and the Revised Yale Developmental Schedule. In comparison with these tests, the DDST classified 81 percent of the children correctly.

In an independent evaluation of the same data, Werner (1972) reports that the DDST may underrefer during the first two years and overrefer during the third year of life. In summary, the reliability and validity of the DDST are not superior but are probably comparable with those of other screening tests.

The authors designed the test so it could be administered by aides. In addition to the Reference Manual (Frankenburg, Dodds, Fandal, Kazuk, and Cohrs 1975), there is a workbook version of the manual for use in training paramedical and nursing personnel (Frankenburg, Dodds, and Fandal 1973). This publication contains the material in the reference manual plus some additional information and some self-quizzes. Training films are also available. The reliability of the instrument when used by aides may be questioned, however. Werner (1972) reports an unpublished study in which mothers trained to give the DDST underreferred by 50 percent, and the correlation between their scores and scores obtained by psychologists was only .30.

Recently, a prescreening questionnaire has been developed, the Denver Prescreening Developmental Questionnaire or PDQ (Frankenburg and others 1976). This questionnaire consists of items revised from the DDST. It is designed to be administered to the parent in a few minutes. Criteria are suggested for selecting children to be evaluated with the full DDST. The questionnaire overrefers at a high rate. It is apparently designed for use in health care settings where large numbers of children are screened. The PDQ will be of little use to speech–language pathologists because it is designed to identify children who need developmental screening. Normally, individuals in the speech and language field will use identification screening devices more specific to their interests.

Summary The DDST is a screening test for developmental delay in young children. It is relatively simple to administer and straightforward in interpretation. The test was standardized on a sample of urban children. The reliability and validity of the test vary somewhat with the age of the child, but are comparable with those of other developmental screening instruments. It is recommended that the DDST be used in conjunction with other assessment procedures, rather than as a sole indicator. Speech–language pathologists will probably find the test most useful in initial evaluations of children between three and six years, particularly children suspected of possible delay in articulation or language development. Interpretation of DDST results should be in relation to general developmental level rather than in terms of specific speech and language parameters.

References

Frankenburg, W. K., B. W. Camp, and P. A. Van Natta Validity of the Denver Developmental Screening Test. *Child Dev.* 42: 475–485, 1971.

——, J. A. Demersseman, and S. F. Voorhees Reliability and stability of the Denver Developmental Screening Test. *Child Dev.* 42: 1315–1325, 1971.

Frankenburg, W. K., J. B. Dodds, and A. W. Fandal *Denver Developmental Screening Test: Manual/Workbook for Nursing and Paramedical Personnel.* Denver: LADOCA Project and Publishing Foundation, 1973.

Frankenburg, W. K. and J. B. Dodds The Denver Developmental Screening Test. *J. Pediat.* 71: 181-191, 1967.

Frankenburg, W. K., W. J. van Doorninck, T. N. Liddell, and N. P. Dick The Denver Prescreening Developmental Questionnaire (PDQ). *Pediatrics* 57: 744-753, 1976.

Werner, E. E. Review of the Denver Developmental Screening Test. In O. K. Buros (ed.), *Seventh Mental Measurements Yearbook,* Highland Park, N. J.: Gryphon, 1972.

IOWA SCALE OF ATTITUDE TOWARD STUTTERING

Robert B. Ammons and Wendell Johnson

Published in W. Johnson, F. L. Darley, and D. C. Spriestersbach, *Diagnostic Methods in Speech Pathology.* New York: Harper & Row, 1963.

Forms The Interstate Printers and Publishers, Inc.

Cost $15.95 for the book; 8¢ each for forms Manual, see book, pages 262–264, 283–287; Forms, 5 pages, 8¢ per form, discount for quantities of 100 or more

Time 20–30 minutes, administration; less than 2 minutes, scoring

Richard F. Curlee *University of Arizona*

Purpose The Iowa Scale of Attitude toward Stuttering attempts to measure the test taker's reaction to stuttering in social speech situations. It was designed to be used with stutterers, members of the family, and other important listeners in their lives.

Administration, scoring, and interpretation The scale presents 45 assertions about stutterers and what they should or should not do or feel in selected speaking situations. The test taker is asked to indicate the extent to which he or she agrees or disagrees with each assertion by circling one of the following responses: strongly agree, moderately agree, undecided, moderately disagree, strongly disagree. Responses are interpreted to reflect one's relative acceptance or nonacceptance of stuttering.

Descriptions of the scale in Johnson, Darley, and Spriestersbach (1963) suggest that persons with junior high school reading ability should be able to grasp the point of each statement and to follow instructions in responding to it. Written instructions accompanying the scale encourage the test taker to answer each item, to respond as rapidly and accurately as possible, and to guess if unsure of attitude. No restrictions on test conditions or supplementary instructions are provided in the directions for administration. Responses are scored as follows: strongly agree = 4, moderately agree = 3, moderately disagree = 2, strongly disagree = 1, undecided = 0. Item scores are summed and divided by the number of items answered minus the number answered "undecided." Lower mean scores are interpreted as indicating better attitudes toward stuttering, with those falling between 1.0 and 1.4 said to reflect very good attitudes and considerable tolerance of stuttering, and those above 2.2, poor attitudes and considerable intolerance of stuttering. Scores between 1.4 and 2.2 are believed to reflect moderate attitudes. It is noted, however, that scores of individuals are of limited value and should be interpreted judiciously. It is also suggested that the scale's major value is in identifying attitudes that should be explored in counseling with stutterers or their families.

Evaluation of test adequacy The development of this scale has been described in detail by Ammons and Johnson (1944). The 45 items were selected from an original 160-item scale administered to 63 stutterers, 61 speech clinicians, 40 university freshmen, and 40 local townspeople. Items that differentiated the upper and lower quartiles of the groups were retained. Internal consistency of the 45-item scale was estimated to be .89 using the Spearman–Brown split-half correlation technique. Test–retest reliability is not known and needed cross-validation studies have not been conducted. Johnson, Darley, and Spriestersbach (1963) reported mean, median, and quartile scores of 162 parents of stutterers and 36 of their children gathered at the University of Iowa Speech Clinic, but these data are not useful in estimating either the reliability or validity of the scale. No basis for interpreting scores as indicative of poor, moderate, or very good attitudes is given. In short, the scale does not meet the standards established for educational and psychological tests and manuals by the American Psychological Association (1966).

The Iowa Scale of Attitude toward Stuttering clearly reflects the theoretical positions of Wendell Johnson and his colleagues about the role of speakers' and listeners' attitudes in the onset and maintenance of stuttering. Agreement with such statements as, "A stutterer should not plan to be a lawyer" is thought to indicate an intolerance of stuttering, and such intolerant attitudes are believed to have causal significance for stuttering. The relationship of attitudes about stuttering is controversial and remains to be clarified by adequately controlled research. As a result, the validity of the construct on which this scale is based is questionable. The original 160-item scale was intended to include a wide range of life situations in which stutterers might find themselves. Nevertheless, the present 45-item scale lacks direct evidence of content validity. Most important, however, neither the criterion-related validity nor test–retest reliability of the scale is known. Essentially, the scale remains in the same state of preliminary development that it occupied when it was first described over 30 years ago by Ammons and Johnson (1944). It must be concluded that the Iowa Scale of Attitude toward Stuttering has little if any clinical value.

Summary The lack of basic reliability and validity information should preclude the use of the scale in clinical practice. Of the scales currently available to assess attitudes about stuttering, the short form of the Erickson Scale of Communication Attitudes (qv)(Erickson 1969; Andrews and Cutler 1974) has undergone the most appropriate development and may be related to treatment outcomes (Guitar 1976). In contrast, no relationship was found between attitude scores of stutterers on the original 160 items of the present scale and their self-ratings of severity of stuttering or the number of years they had received therapy.

References

American Psychological Association *Standards for Educational and Psychological Tests and Manuals.* Washington, D. C.: American Psychological Association, 1966.

Ammons, R. and W. Johnson Studies in the psychology of stuttering: XVIII. The construction and application of a test of attitude toward stuttering. *J. Speech Dis.* 9: 39–49, 1944.

Andrews, G. and J. Cutler Stuttering therapy: the relation between changes in symptom level and attitudes. *J. Speech Hearing Dis.* 39: 312–319, 1974.

Erickson, R. L. Assessing communication attitudes among stutterers. *J. Speech Hearing Res.* 12: 711–724, 1969.

Guitar, B. Pretreatment factors associated with the outcome of stuttering therapy. *J. Speech Hearing Res.* 19: 590–600, 1976.

Johnson, W., F. L. Darley, and D. C. Spriestersbach *Diagnostic Methods in Speech Pathology.* New York: Harper & Row, 1963.

A PROGRAMMED APPROACH TO VOICE THERAPY

Frank B. Wilson and Mabel Rice

Teaching Resources Corporation, 1977

Cost $129.95
Manual, 76 pages, $12.95; unscored voice profiles, 1 page, pad of 50 for $2.50; scored voice profiles, pad of 30 for $1.50; physician referral form, 1 page, pad of 25 for $3.75

Time 5–15 minutes, voice sample; variable time for profiling depending on extent of review of taped voice sample

Susan J. Shanks *California State University, Fresno*

Purpose In the manual the authors state that they developed the Programmed Approach to Voice Therapy to provide the speech–language pathologist with an initial structure for therapy. While this work is addressed primarily to the management of voice disorders, the voice profiling system is of interest here as an assessment procedure.

Administration, scoring, and interpretation The program includes five one-hour audiocassette taped lectures with sequenced slides on voice assessment and management procedures. The listener can rate the deviant voices presented using the scoring profiles. Listener reliability can be determined by comparison of the individual's ratings with the profiles given by the lecturer.

The profiling system is described in detail on Side 1, Reel 1 of the tapes. It involves ratings of laryngeal and resonating cavities, intensity, vocal range, and a judgment of severity. In all of the ratings, 1 represents normal. The laryngeal cavity involves two ratings, one for opening and one for pitch. For laryngeal opening, the scale is from −4 (open) to +3 (closed), and from −3 (low pitch) to +3 (high pitch) for pitch. The resonating cavity scale is from −2 (hyponasal) to +4 (hypernasal). Deviations from normal intensity are either −2 (soft) or +2 (loud), and −2 (monotone) or +2 (variable pitch) for vocal range. The severity judgment is based on a seven-point scale with 1 representing normal and 7 representing severe. The ratings are made on the basis of three trials in sustaining "ah," and a recorded speech sample that includes stating one's name and age, counting to ten, making a few remarks about a favorite pastime, and reading a short passage, if the person is able to read.

Four placement options are described. The options include (1) no further contact, (2) observations, (3) referral, and (4) management. The authors provide criteria for each option.

Evaluation of test adequacy In the Introduction and Developmental History section of the manual, the authors review the initial attempts to standardize the voice profiling system in the St. Louis School District. Fifty speech–language pathologists in the schools were selected for three days of training in distinguishing normal from deviant voices using 30 20-second speech samples. Of these listeners, 41 exceeded 90 percent accuracy; seven of the remaining nine reached or exceeded 83 percent accuracy; and two fell below 75 percent. Listener reliability was "good": the 41 best listeners had a consistency of 97 percent; nine exceeded 85 percent; and one person was below 80 percent.

The authors state that designating the type of deviation and severity was much less accurate and required more extensive training. The training tapes in the program were designed for this purpose. They refer to a recent unpublished study which suggests that the amount of training needed to establish voice profiling reliability has yet to be determined.

The program's slide/tape format is easily adapted to either group or self-paced instruction. The listener can turn off the tape to study a slide or repeat a voice sample to review the profile, symptomatology, and management procedures given. The color coded slides are referred to by number during each lecture, which allows the listener to return to a section for further study. Tape 5, the Dictionary of Voice Disorders, is a clinical supplement to the first four hours. It presents calibration tapes that are recommended for teaching clients self-monitoring behaviors. The demonstration of assessment procedures and pre- and posttherapy samples included in this tape are a strength of the program.

The program lacks directions for coordinating the kit materials and the information in the manual. The manual gives a short description of each tape, assessment procedures, and management sequences, but does not correlate the taped material and the carefully delineated program outlined in Appendix A.

Summary   This voice program is the first commercial product available for improving skills in identification and management of specific vocal disorders. Standardization of the voice profiling system is not currently available. The program has not been reviewed in the literature. Directors of training programs and persons planning in-service training for speech–language pathologists in schools will find it another useful tool for assisting the student and professional in improving listening skills and in understanding voice problems.

Reference

Wilson, F. B. and M. Rice   *A Programmed Approach to Voice Therapy.* Austin: Learning Concepts, Inc., 1977.

SCALE OF COMMUNICATION ATTITUDES (S-SCALE)

Robert L. Erickson

Not available commercially. Published in *J. Speech Hearing Res.* **12**: 711–724, 1969.

Time 2–4 minutes, administration; 1 minute, scoring

Ehud Yairi *University of Illinois at Urbana-Champaign*

Purpose Measuring devices of the reactive aspects of stuttering are potentially useful to a large number of clinicians whose therapeutic regimen includes modifying the stutterer's negative emotions and maladjusted attitudes, as well as to investigators interested in the diagnosis, prognosis, and therapeutic processes of stuttering. Scale of Communication Attitudes (S-Scale) by Robert L. Erickson (1969) represents one of the recent attempts to construct such a device. Its specific goal as set forth by the author is to provide an index of the extent to which an individual stutterer's attitudes toward interpersonal communication deviate from normal attitudes. Published as a part of a scientific article, S-Scale is still unavailable to users on a commercial basis.

Administration, scoring, and interpretation Scale of Communication Attitudes is a 39-item self-administered pencil-and-paper inventory. The items that comprise the scale are short descriptive statements about communication habits, experiences, and emotional reactions associated with speaking and listening. Subjects simply indicate whether or not they agree with each statement. A subject's scale score represents an arithmetic summation of the number of items to which he or she responded in the predicted direction for stutterers. Opposite or omitted responses are weighted as zero. Thus the range of possible scores varies between zero and 39. Instructions for administration are clear and succinct and the inventory takes only several minutes to complete and score. However, there are no guidelines or suggestions for interpretation of scores except for a general notion that higher scores indicate greater discomfort in social situations. Some idea about the standing of individual subjects may be gained by comparing their scores to a table of cumulative relative frequency distribution of S-Scale scores in the stuttering and nonstuttering normative groups used to derive the inventory.

Evaluation of test adequacy Scale of Communication Attitudes serves a useful function by providing clinicians with a means for assessing systematically the impact of the stuttering problem on stutterers' interpersonal attitudes, and the precipitating role of such covert emotional reactions on stutterers' speaking habits. It gives the clinician a quick and more objective view of clients' needs so these can be meaningfully implemented into individualized therapeutic plans. The inventory appears more attractive than other instruments of its kind, such as the Iowa Scale of Attitude toward Stuttering (Ammons and Johnson 1944) (qv) and the Stutterer's Self-Rating of Reactions to Speaking Situations (Shumak 1955), in that it is shorter and less complicated. Because the inventory items are worded so as to avoid any reference to a specific disorder of communication, S-Scale has an additional advantage of usefulness for studying various clinical and normal populations. Unfortunately, in the absence of commercial materials, potential users of this instrument must prepare their own test and key forms adapted from the journal reference.

Scale of Communication Attitudes also appears to be superior to other available scales in the area of stuttering from the standpoint of test construction. Its strength rests on the stringent criteria used in its empirical derivation from an original 1060-item poll. The final items included are those which (1) survived an initial screening for reading difficulty and social desirability, (2) showed the proportion of 50 stutterers responding to them in a given direction exceeding the proportion of 100 nonstutterers responding in the same direction by a margin equal to at least twice the standard error of the difference between the two groups, and (3) indicated a statistically significant ($p \leq .01$) phi correlation with the dichotomy stutterers/nonstutterers (based on responses of a second group of 70 stutterers and 44 nonstutterers).

Concurrent validity was inferred from data showing that high scoring stutterers (the fourth quartile in the entire distribution of 120 stutterers) rated themselves as having significantly more severe stuttering problems, having improved less in therapy, and having experienced greater social discomfort than did low scoring stutterers (the first quartile in the distribution). Qualitative differences between high and low scoring stutterers on an adjective list used to describe themselves provided an additional indicator of validity. Overall correlation coefficient of S-Scale scores with self-rated social discomfort was .66. However, the correlation between scale scores and clinician rating of stuttering severity was only .35; it was .46 with self-rated severity of stuttering. A split-half reliability of .85 and a full-scale reliability estimate of .92 were reported. These values indicate that whatever the inventory is measuring is being measured with a reasonable degree of consistency.

In spite of the commendable efforts that went into the construction of S-Scale there still remain several weaknesses. First, the normative groups of 120 stutterers and 144 nonstutterers were composed exclusively of male college students in the rural midwest United States and cannot be regarded as a representative sample of the general young adult population. This fact must be kept in mind when making interpretations and generalizations. Second, although 95 percent of the stutterers' scores are higher than the median score of nonstutterers, a considerable amount of overlapping is clearly evident in the score distribution of the two groups. Whether or not one accepts the author's contention that the observed overlapping does not exceed tolerable limits, a situation in which 78 percent of nonstutterers' scores falls in the same range that includes 85 percent of stutterers' scores calls for additional item selection processing. Third, as mentioned earlier, not much can be said about the meaning of the range of possible scale scores. In other words, we are not really sure what properties, except for superficial item content, are being measured and their relationships to various facets, types, and severity of stuttering. This conclusion is not surprising in view of the vagueness characterizing some validity measures like self- and clinician-rating of improvement. Undoubtedly, further work on test validity is the most challenging task if the S-Scale is to develop into a serious standardized diagnostic tool.

Summary Scale of Communication Attitudes represents a significant advancement in its area but requires updating and further research and development. Meanwhile, it would seem to merit consideration as an informal accessory clinical tool.

References

Ammons, R. and W. Johnson Studies in the psychology of stuttering: XVIII. The construction and application of a test of attitude toward stuttering. *J. Speech Dis.* **9**: 39–49, 1944.

Erickson, R. L. Assessing communication attitudes among stutterers. *J. Speech Hearing Res.* **12**: 711–724, 1969.

Shumak, I. A speech situation rating sheet for stutterers. In W. Johnson (ed.), *Stuttering in Children and Adults.* Minneapolis: University of Minnesota Press, 1955, Chapter 28.

SYMBOL DIGIT MODALITIES TEST (SDMT)

Aaron Smith

Western Psychological Services, 1973; Adult Norms Supplement, 1976
Two forms, written and oral

Cost $12.50
Manual, 9 pages, $2.50; adult norms supplement, 4 pages, supplied with the manual; scoring key (template), $2.00; test form, 1 page, pad of 100 for $8.50; 2–19 pads for $7.75 each; 20 pads for $7.25 each

Time 5 minutes, administration; 1 minute, scoring

Maryjane Rees *California State University, Sacramento*

Purpose According to the manual (p.1):

> ... the Symbol Digit Modalities Test provides an economic test for early screening of learning and other cerebral disorders in group written administrations for children, as well as providing useful indices of normal capacities in large scale group testing of adults. The SDMT can also be used in diagnostic studies of individual subjects with suspected brain lesions when used in conjunction with standardized intelligence and other tests.

Administration, scoring, and interpretation The test involves coding a set of geometric figures or symbols using numbers as the code. The key, printed at the top of the test form, shows the pairing of the numbers (one to nine) with the symbols. The test form contains eight rows of randomly presented symbols with a box under each symbol for recording the paired digit. Response time is limited to 90 seconds, and responses may be either written or oral. The oral form is used as a retest for children scoring more than one standard deviation below the appropriate age-sex norm on the written test, or it may be used as an initial test for children with motor problems that interfere with writing.

The author recommends group administration of the written form of the test. The manual contains verbatim-type instructions that direct attention to the essential elements of the test and describe how the first three boxes should be filled in. The next seven boxes are completed for practice. If, after checking the practice, the examiner ascertains that anyone does not understand the task, the instructions are repeated and additional examples provided until the task is clearly understood. The children are then instructed to work as quickly as possible and to write the correct response over a mistake rather than erase it. Instructions and practice are the same for the oral test, except that it is necessarily administered individually, and the examiner records the digits spoken by the child. If given shortly after the written test, practice is not repeated. "Shortly" is not defined.

Apparently, the examiner need not have special qualifications. Nonetheless, the instructions seem inadequate for examiners not trained in group administration of timed tests, as they are likely to be unaware of the precautions necessary to ensure that all participants stop immediately when the signal is given, which is a particular problem if groups are large.

The requirement that the examiner repeat instructions and provide additional examples if necessary can cause the amount of time between completing the practice and the signal to begin the test and, therefore, duration of exposure to the key, to vary from group to group. Since the instructions stress speed, control of the time element is critical.

The score is the number of correct responses. It can be determined readily through use of a template placed over the test form.

The norms consist of means and standard deviations for the written and oral forms of the test when given as initial tests. The norms for boys and girls are different and are shown by one-year intervals from eight to 17 years as well as for two-year combinations. The difference between means of the oral retest and initial written test scores is shown for each age group for the sexes combined. Standard deviations for the oral retest are not provided, yet this information is critical to the interpretation of test results as the recommended procedure is to use the oral test as a retest for children who fail to meet the specified criterion. Interpretation of results depends on whether one or both scores are subnormal, which is defined as more than one standard deviation below the age–sex norm.

The author acknowledges that substitution tests are subject to practice effects but found that the interval between the initial test and the oral retest, which was variable for the standardization group, did not significantly affect the amount of gain shown in retest scores. This suggests that the norms for the oral test given as an initial test might be appropriate. Nonetheless, some practice effect is apparent since the mean gain in oral retest scores over initial written test means produces means larger than those for initial oral test scores at each age level tested. For some comparisons, the difference is nearly the size of one standard deviation, which would materially affect the interpretation of individual scores. The failure to provide oral retest norms is particularly perplexing since Smith (1968, p. 85) states:

> The construction of the SDMT was based on the rationale of providing different modality-specific measures of the same mental task and comparing performance as a function of the modalities used in the response.

In interpreting test results, written or oral scores *alone* are not diagnostically definitive. The combination of a subnormal written score and a normal oral score suggests specific writing impairment. Conversely, a normal written score combined with a subnormal oral score suggests impairment in speech performance. Children whose scores are subnormal on both forms of the test should be referred for a visual acuity examination and detailed neuropsychologic studies. If the subnormal scores do not simply reflect performance at the lower end of the scale of a normal distribution, such scores may reflect one or more of the following: (1) impairment of the perceptual processes involved, (2) selective impairment in fine graphomotor movements and difficulties in initiating and quickly shifting spoken responses, (3) minimal brain dysfunction, mental retardation, dyslexia, and/or other learning disorders.

Even though the manual indicates that one of the purposes of the test is that of large-scale screening of adults, it does not contain norms beyond those for 17-year-olds. Norms for adults were not published until three years after the manual appeared. They are contained in the Adult Norms Supplement, which is a four-page leaflet. Means and standard deviations for written and oral retests are shown for groups from 18 to 74 years old by decades, except for the youngest group for which the range is 18 to 24 years. The data are further collapsed into three age groups: 18 to 34, 35 to 54, and 55 to 75. Scores 1 to 1.5 standard deviations below the norm should be considered suggestive of cerebral dysfunction. Neither the manual nor the supplement describes how the test might be used in diagnostic studies of adults with suspected brain lesions.

The norms for adults do not pose the problem of the norms for children in that they do include means and standard deviations for the oral retest. However, norms for the oral test as an initial test are not given; thus the performance of individuals who can respond only to the oral test cannot be evaluated adequately. Further, the norms are for males and females combined, yet mean scores for females were consistently significantly better than for males in the four oldest age groups (14 to 17 years) used to establish children's norms. The manual (p. 8) indicates that sex differences obtain in the scores of adults and cites a number of references to this effect.

Evaluation of test adequacy The test was standardized on 1090 boys and 1011 girls from eight through 17 years old. None had apparent defects that might impair written or oral test performance, and all were attending classes for normal children. Classes were drawn from 15 different public schools in Omaha and were selected to reflect the demographic composition of urban Omaha. Entire classes were tested with the written form. At varying intervals following the written test, the oral test was administered individually to each of the children. A second sample consisting of 784 boys and 795 girls received only the oral form of the test. Though not discussed in the manual, Smith (1967, p. 1081) has pointed out that the demographic character of the midwest differs from that of large coastal cities and concluded, "The extent to which these SDMT findings can be generalized to other more or less similar populations is therefore unknown."

As evidence of validity, the manual cites eight tables containing data from different studies, only three of which pertain to children. One table contains means and standard deviations from the written test for New York City public school children in five age groups that correspond with the age groups for which norms are provided. Group size ranged from seven to 21. Calculated from the data provided, the difference between means of the normative group and the New York sample was significant ($p < .01$) for two comparisons, while the variances differed significantly ($p < .05$) for one comparison.

Another table includes means for several groups of educable retarded and brain-damaged children. Age ranges for the groups differed, and scores for boys and girls are combined. Data for age–sex equated normals are included, but standard deviations are not given, making it impossible to determine the extent to which the groups fall below one standard deviation of the mean for normals.

The other table pertaining to children includes the mean scores of children with "language disorders" displayed in nine categories. Age ranges of the groups are variable, with some extending below and others above the ages for which norms are provided. Considering that the norms are sensitive to both age and sex, data collapsed over both do not provide insight into performance of children with "language disorders."

The five other tables cited as evidence of validity contain data from adults such as speech pathology and liberal arts students, and adults with chronic aphasia, acute cerebrovascular disease, partial commissurotomy, "organics," and "schizophrenics."

The only mention of reliability in the manual is one that refers the reader to Table 10 for reliability data (p. 5). This table contains initial and retest means for treated

($N = 24$) and untreated ($N = 15$) aphasic subjects with a mean interval between tests of about two years. Standard deviations are not shown, nor are correlation coefficents for initial and posttest scores given. Not only are these data irrelevant for the test used with children, they are inadequate to establish reliability of the test for adults.

On the basis of the information contained in the manual, the validity of the test is not adequately established, and its reliability as a test for children is not even addressed. Further, the efficiency of the test in screening has not been established, though from the statement on page 5 of the manual to the effect that the majority of children with subnormal written and oral scores will be essentially normal, the inference that overreferral is high seems warranted, but the extent to which overreferral occurs is not indicated.

Data from a study done in South Africa are cited in the manual in support of the contention that ". . . the SDMT is useful for prediction and early identification of children with potential reading difficulties" (p. 1). In this study, the correlation for SDMT scores of 79 boys and 79 girls after their first two terms of schooling and reading scores obtained one year later was 0.67 ($p < .01$). In the first place, $r = .67$ is not useful for individual prediction. The coefficient of alienation for a correlation coefficient of this magnitude is .74, and its forecasting efficiency is only 26 percent. Second, the lowest age for which norms are available is eight years, which represents age at the end of second grade or the beginning of third grade in schools in this country. By that time, whether a child is having difficulty with reading is already known. Finally, generalizing results from children in South African schools to children in schools in this country is hazardous because the educational systems are different.

The standardization group for adults included 214 women and 206 men from two communities—Florence Township, New Jersey, and Madison Heights, Michigan. None had handicaps or other evidence of neurological involvement.

In addition to the norms, the Adult Norms Supplement includes means and standard deviations for the written and oral retest for 100 adults with chronic cerebral lesions. Additional tables show the number and percentage of normals whose scores on both the written and oral retest would result in negative and false positive classification for different cutoff scores and corresponding positive and false negative identification for those with chronic lesions.

False positive rates for the normal group varied as a function of age and test (written or oral) but were within an acceptable range using −1.5 SD as the cutoff. Rates were somewhat high (9 to 15 percent) with −1 SD as the criterion. False negative rates for those with lesions also varied as a function of age and test and were exceedingly high (61.5 percent written and 38.5 percent oral) for the oldest group, though this rate is probably inflated by the fact that $N = 13$ in this group. False negative rates were between 13 percent and 19 percent for the two younger groups with −1.5 SD as the cutoff. Using −1 SD as the cutoff, the false negative rate remained unacceptably high for the oldest group and was rather high (6.3 percent written and 12.5 percent oral retest) for the youngest group. No false negative identification occurred in the middle group.

The data presented do speak to the validity of the test in that scores of the group with lesions are markedly lower than those of normals, but that does not rule out the possibility that some other groups might also have low scores as will be discussed subsequently. No evidence of the test's stability or temporal reliability is provided.

It is evident from the data that the efficiency of the test in identifying normals and those with cerebral lesions leaves something to be desired, especially because of the false negative rates. What the data do not show is how efficient the test is for screening unselected populations. That it is likely to be quite inefficient can be inferred from studies about the Digit Symbol test included in the Wechsler scales, which involves the same substitution process except that the symbols rather than the digits are written.

The problem is not that coding or substitution tests are insensitive to brain damage, rather such tests are sensitive to a myriad of other conditions as well. With reference to the Digit Symbol test, Zimmerman and Woo-Sam (1973) state, "Low scores have been reported for the brain-damaged, anxious, depressed, dissociated, schizophrenics, and hyperactives unable to attend adequately to the task" (p. 129). According to Wechsler (1958), the inferior performance of neurotics on the Digit Symbol test was noted as long ago as 1923 (p. 81). He further states that the Digit Symbol test is one of the three most sensitive to anxiety states and that mental defectives have consistently low scores on it (p. 170). Rapaport, Gill, and Schafer (1968) say that impaired psychomotor speed as reflected in Digit Symbol scores is ". . . most directly related to the presence of depressive trends or schizophrenic deterioration" (p. 158). Zimmerman and Woo-Sam (1973) have observed that those who are not at ease with tasks requiring speed or who like to work carefully can be seriously penalized by the Digit Symbol test (p. 128), an observation shared by Rapaport, Gill, and Schafer (1968, p. 157).

Additional sources of low scores for reasons other than brain damage or cerebral dysfunction may be inferred from Sattler's (1974, pp. 25–49) review of the extensive literature on testing minority children. It suggests that timed tests tend to penalize minority-group children, including white disadvantaged children, who may have emotional and motivational deficits or whose cultural background stresses passivity and noncompetitiveness. Sattler (p. 187) believes success in this type of test depends partly on the child's skill with pencil and paper. Skill with pencil and paper is usually related to amount of education, an observation that is supported by the evidence that higher scores on the SDMT oral test systematically decreased with age as far as children are concerned. Wechsler (1958) retained the Army Beta form that required writing symbols in order to minimize the advantage that facility with numbers might produce (p. 82). While the effects of socioeconomic background are not discussed in the manual, Smith (1967) indicates that he not only anticipated but found significant differences in children's scores on the SDMT due to socioeconomic status (p. 1081).

In the absence of evidence to the contrary, it seems logical to assume that performance on the SDMT is vulnerable to the same broad spectrum of conditions that affect performance on the Digit Symbol test. This assumption coupled with the false negative and false positive rates reported for preselected groups suggests a very high degree of inefficiency for a screening test.

Some additional considerations deserve mention. The SDMT is a variant of the Digit Symbol test, which is, according to Wechsler (1958, p. 81) ". . . one of the oldest and best established of all psychological tests. It is to be found in a large variety of intelligence scales. . . ." Though the usual form of the test requires writing the symbol, the reverse is not unique, as the revised Army Beta incorporated this feature (Mursell 1949, p. 145). The manual does not discuss such differences as may occur in the underlying processes when numbers rather than symbols must be written, nor does it discuss the choice of symbols. Royer (1971) found that information processing varied as a function of both the type of substitution (digit symbol or symbol digit) and the extent to which the symbols were from different or equivalent sets (different rotations of a single figure). He concluded that the nature of the required task makes differential demands on the psychological processes involved (p. 341).

The use of the SDMT for assessing the effects of various specific therapies for children and adults with speech and language disorders, as suggested in the manual (p. 5), lacks merit. Specific mention is made of its use in this regard for stuttering, voice disorders, cleft palate, and articulation disorders.

To some extent, one would predict improvement in oral SDMT scores following successful stuttering therapy. The test samples the type of speaking situation that the majority of individuals who stutter find exceedingly difficult, demanding as it does an exact response under time pressure. Since stuttering often varies as a function of specific situations, performance on a single task is in no way an adequate measure of the effects of therapy.

Any rationale for using SDMT scores as a measure of effective therapy for hoarseness due to vocal nodules, the most common voice disorder in children, or resonance disorders due to palatal clefts or velar insufficiency is, at best, obscure. Success in eliminating a lateral lisp or a nasal snort has no discernible relation to whatever underlying abilities are measured by the SDMT.

Where language deficits are due to brain damage, one might reasonably expect improvement in these skills to be reflected in better performance on a task requiring oral responses. The critical measurement for evaluating effectiveness of therapy for any disorder is necessarily the amount of change in the specific behaviors to which therapy is addressed.

Summary Coding or substitution tests have long been recognized as intelligence tests; therefore, the use of the SDMT as a screening instrument is questionable in view of present-day controversies and restrictions about the use of intelligence tests, particularly in educational settings. Even so, as a screening device for the purposes described in the manual, the test would be more in the domain of the psychologist than of the speech–language pathologist. The research applications for which it is suggested, such as psychiatric disorders, aging, and sex differences in mental and related physiologic functions, are also more in the psychologist's domain.

The kinds of screening instruments of interest to speech–language pathologists are those that identify or predict communication disorders at an early age, an age long before children can respond to the type of pencil-and-paper test the written form of the SDMT represents or recognize numbers as required by the oral form of the test. As a diagnostic test, it appears to have no application for most speech and language disorders. It may be of interest in research about language disorders in children and adults, as is suggested by Smith's (1971) work with aphasic patients. Its immediate clinical application is not clear, particularly since the author warns that written or oral scores alone are not diagnostically significant and that more detailed neuropsychologic studies should be made in the event of low scores.

Standardization of the SDMT has a number of shortcomings. The standardization group for children's norms was drawn from a single midwestern urban community and from just two communities for the adult norms. Its efficiency in screening unselected populations is not known, and this omission is critical for a test having as its major justification economic screening of large groups. Norms for some of the uses that make the test unique are not provided, specifically, oral retest norms for children and initial oral test norms for adults. The correlation between written and oral test scores is not indicated. Temporal reliability is not reported for either the written or oral test. Finally, the written test has not been validated against similar tests, such as the Digit Symbol and Coding tests of the Wechsler scales.

References

Mursell, J. L. *Psychological Testing* (2nd ed.). New York: Longmans, Green, 1949.

Rapaport, D., M. M. Gill, and R. Schafer *Diagnostic Psychological Testing* (Rev. ed.). New York: International Universities Press, 1968.

Royer, F. L. Information processing of visual figures in the digit symbol substitution task. *J. exp. Psychol.* **87**: 335–342, 1971.

Sattler, J. M. *Assessment of Children's Intelligence.* Philadelphia: W. B. Saunders, 1974.

Smith, A. Consistent sex differences in a specific (decoding) test performance. *Educ. psychol. Measmt.* **27**: 1077–1083, 1967.

—— Objective indices of severity of chronic aphasia in stroke patients. *J. Speech Hearing Dis.* **36**: 167–207, 1971.

—— The symbol-digit modalities test: a neuropsychologic test of learning and other cerebral disorders. In J. Helmuth (ed.), *Learning Disorders.* Seattle, Washington: Special Child Publications, 1968.

Wechsler, D. *The Measurement and Appraisal of Adult Intelligence* (4th ed.). Baltimore: Williams and Wilkins, 1958.

Zimmerman, I. L. and J. M. Woo-Sam *Clinical Interpretation of the Wechsler Adult Intelligence Scale.* New York: Grune and Stratton, 1973.

PUBLISHERS OF TESTS REVIEWED

ACADEMIC TESTS, INC.
P. O. Box 18613
Austin, Tex. 78760

ACADEMIC THERAPY
PUBLICATIONS
1539 Fourth Street
San Rafael, Calif. 94901

ALLINGTON CORPORATION
801 North Pitt Street
Alexandria, Va. 22314

AMERICAN GUIDANCE
SERVICE, INC.
Publishers Building
Circle Pines, Minn. 55014

BOBBS-MERRILL CO., INC.
Test Division
4300 West 62nd Street
Indianapolis, Ind. 46268

CENTRAL INSTITUTE FOR
THE DEAF
818 South Euclid Street
St. Louis, Mo. 63110

CLINICAL PSYCHOLOGY
PUBLISHING CO., INC.
4 Conant Square
Brandon, Vt. 05733

COMMUNICATION RESEARCH
ASSOCIATES, INC.
P. O. Box 11012
Salt Lake City, Utah 84111

COMMUNICATION SKILL
BUILDERS, INC.
817 East Broadway
Tucson, Ariz. 85733

CONSULTING PSYCHOLOGISTS
PRESS
577 College Avenue
Palo Alto, Calif. 94306

EDUCATORS PUBLISHING
SERVICE, INC.
75 Moulton Street
Cambridge, Mass. 02138

FOLLETT EDUCATIONAL
CORPORATION
1000 West Washington Boulevard
Chicago, Ill. 60607

GO-MO PRODUCTS
1906 Main Street
Cedar Falls, Iowa 50613

GRUNE AND STRATTON, INC.
111 Fifth Avenue
New York, N. Y. 10003

HOUGHTON MIFFLIN CO.
110 Tremont Street
Boston, Mass. 02107

THE HOUSTON TEST COMPANY
P. O. Box 35152
Houston, Tex, 77035

INTERSTATE PRINTERS AND
PUBLISHERS
19-27 North Jackson Street
Danville, Ill. 61832

LADOCA PROJECT AND PUBLISHING
FOUNDATION, INC.
East 51st Avenue and Lincoln Street
Denver, Colo. 80216

LANGUAGE RESEARCH
ASSOCIATES, INC.
175 East Delaware Place
Chicago, Ill. 60611

LEA AND FEBIGER
600 Washington Square
Philadelphia, Pa. 19106

LINGUISYSTEMS, INC.
Suite 806
1630 Fifth Avenue
Moline, Ill. 61265

CHARLES E. MERRILL PUBLISHING
COMPANY
1300 Alum Creek Drive
Columbus, Ohio 43216

NATIONAL EDUCATION
LABORATORY PUBLISHERS, INC.
P. O. Box 1003
Austin, Tex. 78767

INSTITUTE OF REHABILITATIVE
MEDICINE
New York University Medical Center
400 East 34th Street
New York, N. Y. 10016

NORTHERN MICHIGAN UNIVERSITY
PRESS
Marquette, Mich. 49855

NORTHWESTERN UNIVERSITY
PRESS
1735 Benson Avenue
Evanston, Ill. 60201

PERCEPTUAL LEARNING SYSTEMS
P. O. Box 864
Dearborn, Mich. 48121

PINNACLE PRESS
P. O. Box 1122
Murfreesboro, Tenn. 37130

THE PSYCHOLOGICAL
CORPORATION
304 East 45th Street
New York, N. Y. 10017

PSYCHOLOGICAL TEST SPECIALISTS
P. O. Box 1441
Missoula, Mont. 59801

SPEECH MATERIALS
P. O. Box 1713
Ann Arbor, Mich. 48106

STANWIX HOUSE, INC.
3020 Chartiers Avenue
Pittsburgh, Pa. 15204

TEACHING RESOURCES
CORPORATION
100 Boylston Street
Boston, Mass. 02116

CHARLES C THOMAS
301–327 East Lawrence Avenue
Springfield, Ill. 62703

THE TREE OF LIFE PRESS
1309 North East Second Street
Gainesville, Fla. 32601

UNIVERSITY OF CHICAGO
INDUSTRIAL RELATIONS CENTER
OR UNIVERSITY OF CHICAGO
EDUCATION INDUSTRY SERVICE
1225 East 60th Street
Chicago, Ill. 60637

UNIVERSITY OF ILLINOIS PRESS
Urbana, Ill. 61801

UNIVERSITY OF IOWA BUREAU OF
EDUCATIONAL RESEARCH AND
SERVICE
Extension Division, C-20 East Hall
Iowa City, Iowa 52242

UNIVERSITY OF MICHIGAN
DEPARTMENT OF COMMUNICATION
DISORDERS
Ann Arbor, Mich. 48104

UNIVERSITY OF MINNESOTA PRESS
2037 University Avenue, S. E.
Minneapolis, Minn. 55455

UNIVERSITY OF VICTORIA
NEUROPSYCHOLOGY LABORATORY
Department of Psychology
Victoria, B. C., Canada

UNIVERSITY OF WASHINGTON
PRESS
Seattle, Wash. 98105

UNIVERSITY PARK PRESS
Chamber of Commerce Building
Baltimore, Md. 21202

WESTERN MICHIGAN UNIVERSITY
CONTINUING EDUCATION OFFICE
Kalamazoo, Mich. 49001

WESTERN PSYCHOLOGICAL
SERVICES
12031 Wilshire Boulevard
Los Angeles, Calif. 90025

WORD MAKING PRODUCTIONS
70 West Louise Avenue
Salt Lake City, Utah 84115